The ABSITE Review

The ABSITE Review

Steven M. Fiser, MD

Resident, Cardiothoracic Surgery
Department of Surgery
Massachusetts General Hospital
Harvard Medical School
Boston, Massachusetts

LIPPINCOTT WILLIAMS & WILKINS
A **Wolters Kluwer** Company
Philadelphia · Baltimore · New York · London
Buenos Aires · Hong Kong · Sydney · Tokyo

Acquisitions Editor: Craig Percy
Developmental/Production Editor: Grace R. Caputo
Manufacturing Manager: Benjamin Rivera
Cover Designer: Brian Crede
Compositor: Dovetail Content Solutions, Maryland Composition
Printer: R.R. Donnelley

© 2004 by LIPPINCOTT WILLIAMS & WILKINS
530 Walnut Street
Philadelphia, PA 19106 USA
LWW.com

All rights reserved. This book is protected by copyright. No part of this book may be reproduced in any form or by any means, including photocopying, or utilized by any information storage and retrieval system without written permission from the copyright owner, except for brief quotations embodied in critical articles and reviews. Materials appearing in this book prepared by individuals as part of their official duties as U.S. government employees are not covered by the above-mentioned copyright.

Printed in the U.S.A.

ABSITE is a trademark of the American Board of Surgery, Inc., which neither sponsors nor endorses this book.

Information contained in this book was obtained from rigorous review of general surgery textbooks and review books, from conferences, and from expert opinions. The ABSITE was not systematically reviewed, nor was it used as an outline for this manual.

All figures are from *Surgery: Scientific Principles and Practice*, eds 2 and 3, edited by Lazar J. Greenfield et al, © 1997 by Lippincott-Raven Publishers and © 2001 by Lippincott Williams & Wilkins.

Library of Congress Cataloging-in-Publication Data
Fiser, Steven M., 1971–
 The ABSITE Review / Steven M. Fiser
  p. ; cm.
 Includes index
 ISBN 13 978-0-7817-5566-5
 ISBN 10 0-7817-5566-2
 1. Surgery—Examinations, questions, etc. 2. Surgery—Handbooks, manuals, etc. 3. Surgery, Operative—Examinations, questions, etc. 4. Surgery, Operative—Handbooks, manuals, etc. I. Title: The American Board of Surgery In-Training Examination review. II. Title.
 [DNLM: 1. Surgical Procedures, Operative—Examination Questions. 2. Clinical Medicine—Examination Questions. WO 18.2 F531a 2004]
 RD28.A1F55 2004
 617'.0076—dc22
                                                            2004044147

Care has been taken to confirm the accuracy of the information presented and to describe generally accepted practices. However, the authors, editors, and publisher are not responsible for errors or omissions or for any consequences from application of the information in this book and make no warranty, expressed or implied, with respect to the currency, completeness, or accuracy of the contents of the publication. Application of this information in a particular situation remains the professional responsibility of the practitioner.

The authors, editors, and publisher have exerted every effort to ensure that drug selection and dosage set forth in this text are in accordance with current recommendations and practice at the time of publication. However, in view of ongoing research, changes in government regulations, and the constant flow of information relating to drug therapy and drug reactions, the reader is urged to check the package insert for each drug for any change in indications and dosage and for added warnings and precautions. This is particularly important when the recommended agent is a new or infrequently employed drug.

Some drugs and medical devices presented in this publication have Food and Drug Administration (FDA) clearance for limited use in restricted research settings. It is the responsibility of the health care provider to ascertain the FDA status of each drug or device planned for use in their clinical practice.

To my family, for their love and support during my residency

CONTENTS

Preface
Acknowledgments

1. Cell Biology	1
2. Hematology	4
3. Blood Products	9
4. Immunology	10
5. Infection	13
6. Antibiotics	17
7. Medicines and Pharmacology	20
8. Anesthesia	22
9. Fluids and Electrolytes	26
10. Nutrition	29
11. Oncology	34
12. Transplantation	37
13. Inflammation and Cytokines	41
14. Wound Healing	46
15. Trauma	49
16. Critical Care	62
17. Burns	68
18. Plastics, Skin, and Soft Tissues	72
19. Head and Neck	77
20. Pituitary	82
21. Adrenal	83
22. Thyroid	87
23. Parathyroid	93
24. Breast	97
25. Thoracic	105
26. Cardiac	111
27. Vascular	116
28. Gastrointestinal Hormones	133
29. Esophagus	135
30. Stomach	142
31. Liver	151
32. Biliary System	159
33. Pancreas	165
34. Spleen	172
35. Small Bowel	175
36. Colorectal	182
37. Anal and Rectal	194
38. Hernias, Abdomen, and Surgical Technology	198
39. Urology	202
40. Gynecology	206
41. Neurosurgery	210
42. Orthopaedics	215
43. Pediatric Surgery	220
44. Statistics	229
Appendix: Abbreviations	*231*
Index	*235*

PREFACE

Each year, thousands of general surgery residents across the country express anxiety over preparation for the American Board of Surgery In-Training Examination (ABSITE), an exam designed to test residents on their knowledge of the many topics related to general surgery.

This exam is important to the future career of general surgery residents for several reasons. Academic centers and private practices searching for new general surgeons use ABSITE scores as part of the evaluation process. Fellowships in fields such as surgical oncology, trauma, and cardiothoracic surgery use these scores when evaluating potential fellows. Residents with high ABSITE results are looked upon favorably by general surgery program directors, as high scorers enhance program reputation, helping garner applications from the very best medical students interested in surgery.

General surgery programs also use the ABSITE scores, with consideration of feedback on clinical performance, when evaluating residents for promotion through residency. Clearly, this examination is important to general surgery residents.

Much of the anxiety over the ABSITE stems from the issue that there are no dedicated outline-format review manuals available to assist in preparation. *The ABSITE Review* was developed to serve as a quick and thorough study guide for the ABSITE, such that it could be used independently of other material and would cover nearly all topics found on the exam. The outline format makes it easy to hit the essential points on each topic quickly and succinctly, without having to wade through the extraneous material found in most textbooks. As opposed to question-and-answer reviews, the format also promotes rapid memorization.

Although specifically designed for general surgery residents taking the ABSITE, the information contained in *The ABSITE Review* is also especially useful for certain other groups:
- General surgery residents preparing for their written American Board of Surgery certification examination
- Surgical residents going into another specialty who want a broad perspective of general surgery and surgical subspecialties (and who may also be required to take the ABSITE)
- Practicing surgeons preparing for their American Board of Surgery recertification examination

The ABSITE Review

CHAPTER 1. CELL BIOLOGY

Cell membrane
Lipid bilayer contains protein channels, enzymes, and receptors.
Cholesterol increases membrane fluidity.
Cells are negative inside compared with outside, based on Na/K ATPase (3 Na^+ out/2 K^+ in).

Electrolyte concentrations of intracellular and extracellular fluid compartments

	Extracellular Fluid (mEq/L)		Intracellular Fluid (mEq/L)
	Plasma	Interstitial Fluid	
CATIONS			
Na^+	140	146	12
K^+	4	4	150
Ca^+	5	3	10^{-7}
Mg^+	2	1	7
ANIONS			
Cl^-	103	114	3
HCO_3^-	24	27	10
SO_4^{2-}	1	1	—
HPO_4^{3-}	2	2	116
Protein	16	5	40
Organic anions	5	5	—

(Wait RB et al. Fluids and electrolytes and acid–base balance. In: Greenfield LJ et al, eds. Surgery: scientific principles and practice. Ed 3. Philadelphia: Lippincott Williams & Wilkins, 2001:245)

Desmosomes/hemidesmosomes – adhesion molecules, cell–cell and cell–extracellular matrix, anchor cells
Tight junctions – cell–cell occluding junctions, impermeable barrier (i.e., epithelium)
Gap junctions – allow communication between cells

G proteins – intramembrane protein, transduce signal from receptor to response enzyme
Tyrosine kinase receptors – receptor and response enzyme are a single transmembrane protein

ABO blood type antigens – glycolipids on cell membrane
HLA type antigens – glycoproteins (Gp) on cell membrane

Cell cycle
G1, S (protein synthesis, chromosomal duplication), G2, M (mitosis, nucleus divides)
G1 most variable, determines cell cycle length
Growth factors affect cell during G1
Cells can also go to G0 (quiescent) from G1

Mitosis
Prophase – centromere attachment, spindle formation, nucleus disappears
Metaphase – chromosome alignment
Anaphase – chromosomes pulled apart
Telophase – separate nucleus re-forms around each set of chromosomes

Nucleus, transcription, and translation
Nucleus – double membrane, outer membrane continuous with rough endoplasmic reticulum
Nucleolus – inside the nucleus, no membrane, ribosomes are made here

Transcription – DNA strand used as a template by **RNA polymerase** for synthesis of mRNA strand
Transcription factors – bind DNA and help initiate transcription of genes
  Steroid hormones – binds receptor in cytoplasm, then enters nucleus and acts as transcription factor
  Thyroid hormone – binds receptor in nucleus, then acts as a transcription factor

The ABSITE Review

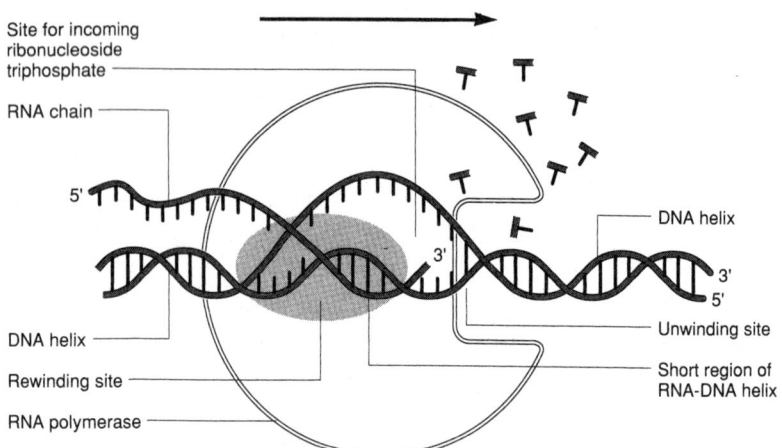

Transcription of DNA. RNA polymerase acts to unwind the DNA helix, catalyzes the formation of a transient RNA–DNA helix, and then releases the RNA as a single-strand copy while the DNA rewinds. In the process, the polymerase moves along the DNA from a start sequence to a stop sequence.

DNA polymerase chain reaction – uses oligonucleotides to amplify specific DNA sequences

Purines – guanine, adenine
Pyrimidines – cytosine, thymidine (only in DNA), uracil (only in RNA)

Translation – mRNA used as a template by **ribosomes** for synthesis of protein
Ribosomes – have small and large subunits that read mRNA, then bind appropriate tRNAs that have amino acids, and eventually make proteins

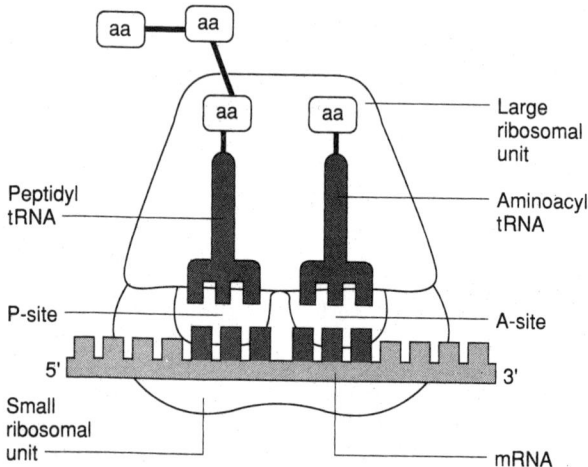

Schematic view of the elongation phase of protein synthesis on a ribosome. As the ribosome moves along the mRNA, incoming aminoacyl–tRNA complexes bind to the A-site on the ribosome, after which a new peptide bond is formed with the nascent polypeptide chain previously attached to the peptide tRNA. The ribosome then moves, ejecting the now-empty tRNA and opening the A-site for the next aminoacyl–tRNA complex.

Chapter 1. Cell Biology

Cellular metabolism

Glycolysis – 1 glucose molecule generates 2-ATP and 2 lactic acid molecules
- **Lactic acid** – can be converted to pyruvate by pyruvate kinase; can then enter Krebs cycle

Mitochondria – 2 membranes, Krebs cycle on inner matrix, NADH/FADH$_2$ created
- **Krebs cycle** – the 2 pyruvate molecules (from the breakdown of one glucose) create NADH and FADH$_2$
- NADH and FADH$_2$ enter the electron transport chain to create ATP.
- Overall, 1 molecule of glucose produces 36-ATP.

Gluconeogenesis – **lactic acid** (Cori cycle) and **amino acids** are converted to glucose
- Used in times of starvation or stress (basically the glycolysis pathway goes in reverse)
- **Fat and lipids** are not available for gluconeogenesis because acetyl CoA (breakdown product of fat metabolism) cannot be converted back to pyruvate

Other cell organelles, enzymes, and structural components

Rough endoplasmic reticulum – synthesizes proteins that are exported (increased in pancreatic acinar cells)
Smooth endoplasmic reticulum – lipid/steroid synthesis, detoxifies drugs (increased in liver and adrenal cortex)

Golgi apparatus – modifies proteins with carbohydrates
Phagosome – engulfed particle

Protein kinase C – activated by **c**alcium and diacylglycerol (DAG)
- Phosphorylates other enzymes and proteins

Protein kinase A – activated by c**A**MP
- Phosphorylates other enzymes and proteins

Myosin – thick filaments, uses ATP to slide along actin to cause muscle contraction
Actin – thin filaments
Intermediate filaments – keratin (hair/nails), desmin (muscle), vimentin (fibroblasts)

CHAPTER 2. HEMATOLOGY

Normal Coagulation

Three initial responses to vascular injury: vascular vasoconstriction, platelet adhesion, thrombin generation

Intrinsic pathway: exposed collagen + prekallikrein + HMW kininogen + factor XII
↓
activate XI
↓
activates IX + VIII
↓
activate X + V
↓
convert **prothrombin (factor II) to thrombin**
↓
thrombin then converts **fibrinogen to fibrin**

Extrinsic pathway: tissue factor (injured cells) + factor VII
↓
activate X + V
↓
convert **prothrombin to thrombin**
↓
thrombin then converts **fibrinogen to fibrin**

Prothrombin complex (for intrinsic and extrinsic pathways)
  X, V, Ca, platelet factor 3, and prothrombin
  Forms on platelets
  Catalyzes the formation of <u>thrombin</u>

Factor X is convergence point and common for both paths.
Tissue factor pathway inhibitor – inhibits factor X

Fibrin – combines with platelets to form <u>platelet plug</u> → hemostasis
XIII – helps crosslink fibrin

Thrombin
  Key to coagulation
  Converts **fibrinogen to fibrin and fibrin split products**
  Activates **factors V and VIII**
  Activates **platelets**

Factor VII – shortest half-life
Factors V and VIII – labile factors, activity lost in stored blood, <u>activity not lost in FFP</u>
Factor VIII – only factor not synthesized in liver (synthesized in endothelium)

Vitamin K–dependent factors – II, VII, IX, and X; proteins C and S

Vitamin K – takes <u>6 hours</u> to take effect
FFP – effect is <u>immediate</u> and lasts 6 hours

Factor II – prothrombin
Normal half-life – RBCs: 120 days; platelets: 7 days; PMNs: 1–2 days

Chapter 2. Hematology

Normal Anticoagulation

Antithrombin III
   Key to anticoagulation
   Binds and inhibits **thrombin**
   Inhibits **factors IX, X, XI**
   Heparin binds AT-III

Protein C – vitamin K–dependent; degrades factors V and VIII; degrades fibrinogen
Protein S – vitamin K–dependent, protein C cofactor

Fibrinolysis
   Tissue plasminogen activator – released from endothelium and converts plasminogen to plasmin
   Plasmin – degrades factors V and VIII, fibrinogen, and fibrin → lose platelet plug
   Alpha-2 antiplasmin – natural inhibitor of plasmin, released from endothelium

---

Prostacyclin (PGI$_2$)
   From endothelium
   Decreases platelet aggregation and promotes vasodilation (antagonistic to TXA$_2$)

Thromboxane (TXA$_2$)
   From platelets
   Increases platelet aggregation and promotes vasoconstriction
   Triggers release of **calcium** in platelets → exposes **GpIIb/IIIa receptor** and causes platelet-to-platelet binding, platelet-to-collagen binding
   Activates **PIP system** to further increase calcium

Coagulation factors
   Cryoprecipitate – contains highest concentration of vWF VIII; used in von Willebrand's disease and hemophilia A (factor VIII deficiency), also contains fibrinogen
   FFP – has high levels of all factors (including labile factors V and VIII), protein C, protein S, and AT-III
   DDAVP and conjugated estrogens – cause release of VIII and vWF from endothelium

Coagulation measurements
   PT – measures II, V, VII, and X; fibrinogen; best for **liver synthetic function**
   PTT – measures most factors **except VII and XIII (thus does not pick up factor VII deficiency)**; also measures fibrinogen
   Want **PTT 60–90** for anticoagulation

   ACT = activated clotting time
   Want **ACT 150–200** for routine anticoagulation, **350–400** for cardiopulmonary bypass

   INR >1.5 – relative contraindication to performing surgical procedures
   INR >1.3 – relative contraindication to central line placement, percutaneous needle biopsies, and eye surgery

Conditions causing abnormal bleeding
   Incomplete hemostasis – most common cause of surgical bleeding

   Von Willebrand's disease
      Most common congenital bleeding disorder
      Types I and II are autosomal dominant; type III is autosomal recessive.
      vWF links **GpIb receptor on platelets to collagen**.
      PT normal; PTT can be normal or abnormal
      Have long **bleeding time** (ristocetin test)
      Type I is most common (70% of cases) and often has only mild symptoms.
      Type III causes the most severe bleeding.

Type I and III – reduced quantity of circulating vWF
  Tx: cryoprecipitate, DDAVP, conjugated estrogens
Type II – defect in vWF molecule itself, have enough vWF but doesn't work well.
  Tx: cryoprecipitate

Hemophilia A (VIII deficiency)
Sex-linked recessive
Need levels 100% preoperatively; keep 30% after surgery
Prolonged PTT and normal PT
Factor VIII crosses placenta → newborns may not bleed at **circumcision**
Hemophiliac joint – no aspiration
  Tx: ice, keep joint mobile with range of motion exercises, factor VIII concentrate
Epistaxis, intracerebral hemorrhage, and hematuria may occur.
  Tx: factor VIII concentrate or cryoprecipitate

Hemophilia B (IX deficiency) – Christmas disease
Sex-linked recessive
Need level 50% preoperatively
Prolonged PTT and normal PT
Tx: factor IX concentrate or FFP

Factor VII deficiency – prolonged PT and normal PTT, bleeding tendency. Tx: FFP

Platelet disorders – cause bruising, epistaxis, mucosal bleeding, petechiae, purpura
  Acquired thrombocytopenia – can be caused by H_2 blockers, heparin
  Glanzmann's thrombocytopenia – GpIIb/IIIa receptor deficiency on platelets (can't bind to each other)
    Fibrin links the GpIIb/IIIa receptors together. Tx: platelets
  Bernard Soulier – GpIb receptor deficiency on platelets (can't bind to collagen)
    vWF links GpIb to collagen. Tx: platelets
  Uremia – inhibits GpIb, GpIIb/IIIa, vWF. Tx: hemodialysis (1st), DDAVP, conjugated estrogens, cryoprecipitate, platelets

  Ticlopidine – decreases ADP in platelets, prevents exposure of GpIIb/IIIa. Tx: platelets
  Dipyridamole – inhibits cAMP phosphodiesterase, increases cAMP, decreases ADP-induced platelet aggregation. Tx: platelets
  Pentoxifylline – inhibits platelet aggregation. Tx: platelets
  Clopidogrel (Plavix) – ADP receptor antagonist. Tx: platelets
  PCN/cephalosporins – bind platelets, can **increase bleeding time**

Heparin-induced thrombocytopenia (HIT)
Thrombocytopenia due to antiplatelet antibodies (IgG) results in platelet destruction.
Can also cause platelet aggregation and thrombosis (HITT; **T** = thrombosis)
Forms a **white clot**
Can occur with low doses of heparin
Low-molecular-weight heparin may have a decreased risk of causing HIT.
Tx: stop heparin; hirudin, ancrod, or dextran to anticoagulate

Disseminated intravascular coagulation (DIC)
Decreased platelets, prolonged PT, prolonged PTT
Low fibrinogen, high fibrin split products, high D-dimer
Often initiated by tissue factor
Need to treat underlying cause

ASA – stop 7 days before surgery; patients will have **prolonged bleeding time**
  Inhibits cyclooxygenase in platelets, ↓ TXA_2
Coumadin – stop 7 days before surgery
Platelets – keep >50,000 before surgery, >20,000 after surgery

Prostate surgery – can release urokinase, activates plasminogen → thrombolysis
  Tx: Amicar (aminocaproic acid)
H and P – best way to predict bleeding risk
Normal circumcision – does not rule out bleeding disorders; can still have clotting factors from mother

Chapter 2. Hematology

Abnormal bleeding with tooth extraction or tonsillectomy – picks up 99% patients with bleeding disorder
Epistaxis – common with vWF deficiency and platelet disorders
Menorrhagia – common with bleeding disorders

Conditions causing abnormal hypercoagulability
Leiden factor – 30% spontaneous venous thromboses
    Most common congenital hypercoagulability disorder
    Resistance to activated protein C, **defect on factor V**
    Tx: heparin, warfarin

Protein C or S deficiency – 5% spontaneous venous thromboses. Tx: heparin, warfarin

Anti-thrombin III deficiency – 2%–3% spontaneous venous thromboses
    Heparin doesn't work in these patients.
    Can develop after previous heparin exposure
    Tx: AT-III concentrate or FFP (highest concentration of AT-III) followed by heparin or hirudin or ancrod; warfarin

Polycythemia vera – defect in platelet function; usually have thrombosis, can have bleeding
    Keep Hct <48 and platelets <400 before surgery.
    Tx: ASA

Lupus anticoagulant – antiphospholipid antibodies
    Not all of these patients have SLE.
    Procoagulant (get prolonged PTT but are hypercoagulable)
    Dx: prolonged PTT (not corrected with FFP), positive Russell viper venom time, false-positive RPR test for syphilis
    Tx: heparin, warfarin

Acquired hypercoagulability – tobacco (most common factor causing acquired hypercoagulability), malignancy, inflammatory states, inflammatory bowel disease, infections, oral contraceptives, pregnancy, rheumatoid arthritis, postop patients, myeloproliferative disorders

Cardiopulmonary bypass – factor XII (Hageman factor) activated; results in hypercoagulable state
    Tx: heparin

Warfarin-induced skin necrosis
    Occurs when placed on coumadin without being heparinized first
    Due to short half-life of proteins C and S, which are first to decrease in levels compared with the procoagulation factors; results in relative hyperthrombotic state
    Patients with relative protein C deficiency are especially susceptible.
    Tx: heparin if it occurs; prevent by placing patient on heparin before starting warfarin

Deep venous thrombosis (DVT)
Stasis, venous injury, and hypercoagulability risk factors
Treatment
    1st – warfarin for 6 months
    2nd – warfarin for 1 year
    3rd or significant PE – warfarin for lifetime
Greenfield filters – for patients with contraindications to anticoagulation; with documented PE while on anticoagulation; with free-floating iliofemoral, IVC, or femoral DVT; or who have undergone pulmonary embolectomy

Pulmonary embolism
If patient has coded, go to OR; otherwise give heparin (thrombolytics have not shown an improvement in survival) or suction catheter-based intervention
⅓ of positive V/Q scans have negative duplexes.
Most common from the **iliofemoral region**

Hematologic drugs
Anticoagulation agents
Warfarin – prevents vitamin K–dependent decarboxylation of glutamic residues on vitamin K–dependent factors
Dextran – inhibits platelets and coagulation factors
Sequential compression devices – improve venous return but also induce fibrinolysis with compression (release of tPA)

Heparin
Activates antithrombin III
Reversed with **protamine** (1–1.5 protamine/100 U heparin (or 1 mg heparin) follow PTT
Half-life of heparin is 60–90 minutes; **cleared by reticuloendothelial system**
Long-term heparin – osteoporosis, alopecia; does not cross placental barrier → warfarin does
Protamine – cross-reacts with NPH insulin or previous protamine exposure; 4%–5% of all patients (regardless of previous exposure) get protamine reaction – hypotension, bradycardia, and decreased heart function

Hirudin (Hirulog) – leeches, thrombin inhibitor; want PTT 60–90
Ancrod – Malayan pit viper venom; stimulates tPA release

Procoagulant agents (antifibrinolytics)
ε-Aminocaproic acid (Amicar)
Inhibits fibrinolysis by inhibiting **plasmin**
Used in DIC, persistent bleeding following cardiopulmonary bypass, thrombolytic overdoses
Aprotinin (Trasylol) – inhibits fibrinolysis by inhibiting **plasminogen activation**

Thrombolytics
Streptokinase – has high antigenicity; **urokinase, tPA (tissue plasminogen activator)**
For thrombolytics to work, a **guidewire** must get past the obstruction.
Need to follow fibrinogen levels – fibrinogen <100 associated with increased risk and severity of bleeding

Contraindications to thrombolytic use (urokinase, streptokinase, TPA)
Degree	Contraindications
Absolute	Active internal bleeding; recent CVA (<2 months); intracranial pathology
Major	Recent (<10 days) surgery, organ biopsy, or obstetric delivery; left heart thrombus; active peptic ulcer or gastrointestinal abnormality; recent major trauma; uncontrolled hypertension
Minor	Minor surgery; recent CPR; atrial fibrillation with mitral valve disease; bacterial endocarditis; hemostatic defects (i.e., renal or liver disease); diabetic hemorrhagic retinopathy; pregnancy

(Data from NIH Consensus Development Conference. Thrombolytic therapy in treatment. Ann Intern Med 1980;93:141.)

CHAPTER 3. BLOOD PRODUCTS

All blood products carry risk of HIV and hepatitis, except **albumin and serum globulins** (these are heat treated).

CMV-negative blood – use in low-birthweight infants, bone marrow transplant patients, other transplant patients

Clerical error leading to ABO incompatibility is #1 cause of death from transfusion reaction.

Stored blood is low in 2,3-DPG → causes left shift (increased affinity for oxygen)

Hemolysis reactions
Acute hemolysis – ABO incompatibility; antibody mediated
  Back pain, chills, tachycardia, fever, hemoglobinuria
  Can lead to ATN, DIC, shock
  Haptoglobin <50 (binds Hgb, then gets degraded), free hemoglobin >5, increase in unconjugated bilirubin
  Tx: fluids, diuretics, HCO_3^-, pressors
  In anesthetized patients, transfusion reactions may present as **diffuse bleeding**.
Delayed hemolysis – antibody-mediated against minor antigens
  Tx: observe if stable
Nonimmune hemolysis – from squeezed blood
  Tx: fluids and diuretics

Other reactions
Febrile nonhemolytic transfusion reaction – <u>most common transfusion reaction</u>
  Usually recipient antibody reaction against **WBCs** in donor blood
  Tx: discontinue transfusion if patient had previous transfusions or if it occurs soon after transfusion has begun
  Use WBC filters for subsequent transfusions.
Anaphylaxis – bronchospasm, hypotension, urticaria
  Usually IgG against IgA in IgA-deficient recipient
  Tx: fluids, Lasix, pressors, steroids, epinephrine
Urticaria – usually nonhemolytic
  Usual reaction against plasma proteins or IgA
  Tx: Benadryl, supportive
Transfusion-related acute lung injury (TRALI) – rare
  Caused by antibodies to recipient's WBCs, clot in pulmonary capillaries

Other transfusion problems
Poor clotting – caused by cold products or cold body temp
Dilutional thrombocytopenia – occurs after 10 units PRBCs
Hypocalcemia – occurs with massive transfusion
Antiplatelet antibodies – develop in 20% of patients after 10–20 platelet transfusions
Hetastarch (Hespan) – can use up to 1 L without risk of bleeding complications

Most common bacterial contaminate – **GNRs (usually *E. coli*)**
Most common blood product source of contamination – **platelets (not refrigerated)**
Chagas' disease – can be transmitted with blood transfusion

Risk of transfer of infectious diseases

Disease	Approximate Risk per Unit of Blood
HIV	1 : 1,000,000–2,000,000
Hepatitis B or C	1 : 250,000–500,000

CHAPTER 4. IMMUNOLOGY

T cells (thymus) – cell-mediated immunity
    Helper T cells (CD4)
        Release **IL-4**, which causes **B cell** maturation into **plasma cells**
        Release **IL-2**, which causes maturation of **cytotoxic T cells**
        Involved in **delayed-type hypersensitivity** (brings in inflammatory cells by chemokine secretion)

        Th1 helper T cells
            Predominant release of proinflammatory cytokines (IL-2, INF-gamma)
            Involved in cell-mediated responses
        Th2 helper T cells
            Predominant release of anti-inflammatory cytokines (IL-4 → inhibits macrophages)
            Involved in atopy and allergic responses

    Suppressor T cells (CD8) – regulate CD4 and CD8 cells
    Cytotoxic T cells (CD8) recognizes and attacks non–self-antigens attached to <u>MHC class I receptors</u>

    Intradermal skin test (i.e., TB skin test) – used to test cell-mediated immunity
    Infections associated with defects in cell mediated immunity – intracellular pathogens (TB, viruses)
    Nucleotides – can ↑ T-cell–mediated immunity

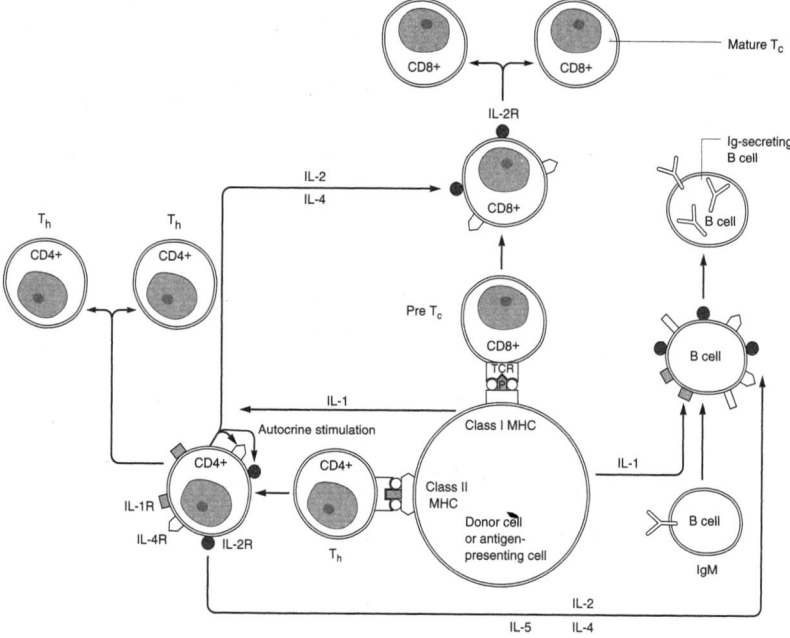

T- and B-cell activation. Two signals are required. First, alloantigen binds to antigen-specific receptors—the TCR (T cells) or surface IgM (B cells). The second, or costimulatory, signal is provided by IL-1 released by the antigen-presenting cell. CD4+ helper T cells (T_h) release IL-2, IL-4, and IL-5, which provide help for CD8+ T cells (T_c) and for B-cell activation.

B cells (bone) – antibody-mediated (humoral) immunity
    IL-4 from helper T cells stimulates B cells to become plasma cells (antibody secreting).

MHC classes
MHC class I (A, B, and C)
- CD8 cell activation
- Present on all nucleated cells
- Single chain with 5 domains
- Target for cytotoxic T cells

MHC class II (DR, DP, and DQ)
- CD4 cell activation
- Present on B cells, dendrites, monocytes, and antigen-presenting cells
- 2 chains with 4 domains each
- Activator for helper T cells
- Stimulate antibody formation

Viral infection – endogenous viral proteins produced, are bound to class I MHC, go to cell surface, and are recognized by CD8 cytotoxic T cells

Bacterial infection – endocytosis, proteins get bound to class II MHC molecules, go to cell surface, recognized by CD4 helper T cells and B cells → B cells then produce antibody to that antigen and are transformed to plasma cells and memory B cells

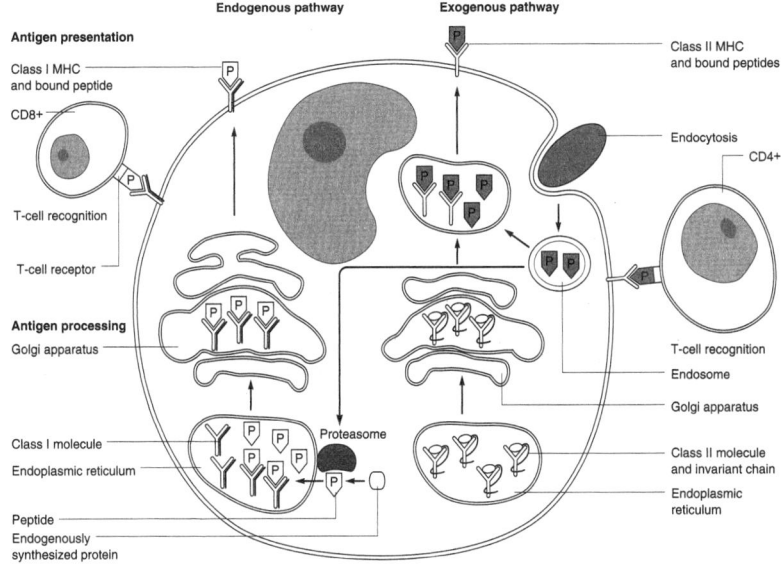

Antigen processing and presentation. Endogenously synthesized or intracellular proteins are degraded into peptides that are transported to the ER. These peptides bind to class I MHC molecules and are transported to the surface of the antigen-presenting cell. CD8+ cells recognize the foreign peptide bound to class I MHC by way of the TCR complex. Exogenous antigen is endocytosed and broken down into peptide fragments in endosomes. Class II molecules are transported to the endosome in association with the invariant chain, bind the peptide, and are delivered to the surface of the antigen-presenting cell, where they are recognized by CD4+ cells.

Activation sequence

Macrophage (antigen-presenting cell) → helper T cell → killer T cell, natural killer cell, memory T cell, cytotoxic T cell
↓
B cell → forms plasma cells (release antibody) and memory B cells

Natural killer cells
Not restricted by MHC, do not require previous exposure, do not require antigen presentation
Not considered T or B cells
Recognize cells that **lack self-MHC**
Part of the body's natural immunosurveillance for cancer

Antibodies
IgM – initial antibody made after exposure to antigen. Is the largest antibody, having 5 domains (10 binding sites)
IgG – most abundant antibody in body. Responsible for secondary immune response. Can cross the placenta and provides protection in newborn period
IgA – found in secretions, in Peyer's patches in gut, and in breast milk (additional source of immunity in newborn); helps prevent microbial adherence and invasion in gut
IgD – membrane-bound receptor on B cells (serves as an antigen receptor)
IgE – allergic reactions, parasite infections (see table on hypersensitivity reactions, below)

IgM and IgG are opsonins.
IgM and IgG fix complement (requires 2 IgGs or 1 IgM)
Variable region – antigen recognition
Constant region – recognized by PMNs and macrophages
  Fc fragment does not carry variable region.
Polyclonal antibodies have multiple binding sites to the antigen at multiple epitopes.
Monoclonal antibodies have only one binding site to one epitope.

Hypersensitivity reactions

Type	Description	Examples
I	Immediate hypersensitivity reaction (allergic reaction) IgE mediated: mast and basophils release histamine, serotonin, and bradykinin in response to release of major basic protein from eosinophils, which have IgE receptors for the antigen.	Bee stings, peanuts, hay fever
II	IgG or IgM reacts with cell-bound antigen	ABO blood type incompatibility, Rh incompatibility, Graves' disease, myasthenia gravis, ITP
III	Immune complex deposition	Serum sickness, rheumatoid arthritis, SLE
IV	Delayed-type hypersensitivity Antigen stimulation of previously sensitized T cells	TB skin test, contact dermatitis

Basophils – major source of histamine in blood
Mast cells – major source of histamine in tissue (other than stomach)
Primary lymphoid organs – liver, bone, thymus
Secondary lymphoid organs – spleen and lymph nodes
Immunologic chimera – 2 different cell lines in one individual (bone marrow transplant patients)

IL-2
Converts lymphocytes to lymphokine-activated killer (LAK) cells by enhancing their immune response to tumor
Also converts lymphocytes into tumor-infiltrating cells
Has been shown to be successful for melanoma

Tetanus
Non–tetanus-prone wounds – give tetanus toxoid only if patient has received <3 doses or tetanus status unknown
Tetanus-prone wounds (>6 hours old; obvious contamination and devitalized tissue; crush, burn, frostbite, or missile injuries) – always give tetanus toxoid unless patient has had ≥3 doses and it has been <5 years since last booster
Tetanus immune globulin – give only to patient with tetanus-prone wounds who have not been immunized or if immunization status unknown

CHAPTER 5. INFECTION

Malnutrition – most common immune deficiency

Microflora
Stomach – virtually sterile; some GPCs, some yeast
Proximal small bowel – 10^5 bacteria, mostly GPCs
Distal small bowel – 10^7 bacteria, GPCs, GPRs, GNRs
Colon – 10^{11} bacteria, almost all anaerobes, some GNRs, GPCs

Anaerobes
Most common organism in the GI tract
More common than bacteria in colon (1000:1)
Bacteroides fragilis – most common anaerobe in the colon
E. coli – most common aerobic bacteria in the colon

Gram-negative sepsis
E. coli most common
Endotoxin (lipopolysaccharide lipid A) is released.
Triggers release of TNF-alpha (from macrophages), activates complement and coagulation cascade.
Early gram-negative sepsis – ↓ insulin, ↑ glucose (impaired utilization)
Late gram-negative sepsis – ↑ insulin, ↑ glucose secondary to insulin resistance
Hyperglycemia – often occurs just before patient becomes clinically septic
Optimal glucose level in a septic patient – 100–120

Clostridium difficile **colitis**
Dx: fecal leukocytes in stool, *C. difficile* toxin
Tx: oral – vancomycin or Flagyl; IV – Flagyl; lactobacillus can also help
Stop other antibiotics or change them.

Abscesses
90% of abdominal abscesses have anaerobes.
80% of abdominal abscesses have both anaerobic and aerobic bacteria.
Abscesses are treated by **drainage**.
Usually occur 7–10 days after operation

Wound infection
Clean (hernia): 2%
Clean contaminated (elective colon resection with prepped bowel): 3%–5%
Contaminated (gunshot wound to colon with repair): 5%–10%
Gross contamination (abscess): 30%

Staphylococcus aureus – coagulase-positive
Most common organism overall in surgical wound infections
Staphylococcus epidermidis – coagulase-negative
Exoslime released by staph species is an **exopolysaccharide matrix**.

E. coli – most common GNR in surgical wound infections
Bacteroides fragilis – **most common anaerobe in surgical wound infections**
Recovery from tissue indicates necrosis (only grows in low redox state)
Also implies translocation from the gut

$\geq 10^5$ bacteria needed for wound infection; less bacteria needed if foreign body present
Risk factors for wound infection: long operations, hematoma or seroma formation, advanced age, chronic disease (COPD, renal failure, liver failure, diabetes mellitus), malnutrition, immunosuppressive drugs

Surgical infections within 48 hours of procedure
  Injury to bowel with leak
  Invasive soft tissue infection – *Clostridium perfringens* and beta-hemolytic strep can present within hours postoperatively (produce exotoxins)

Most common nonsurgical infection – **urinary tract infection (most commonly *E. coli*)**
  Biggest risk factor – urinary catheters

Leading cause of infectious death after surgery – **nosocomial pneumonia**
  Related to length of ventilation; aspiration from duodenum thought to have a role
  Most common organisms in ICU pneumonia – **#1 *S. aureus***, #2 *Pseudomonas*
  GNRs #1 class of organisms in ICU pneumonia

Line infections
  #1 *S. epidermidis*, #2 *S. aureus*, #3 yeast
  Femoral lines at higher risk for infection compared with subclavian and intrajugular lines
  50% line salvage rate with antibiotics; much less likely with yeast line infections
  Central line cultures – >15 colony forming units = line infection → need new site
  Site shows signs of infection → move to new site
  If worried about line infection, best to pull out the central line and place peripheral IVs if central line not needed

Necrotizing soft tissue infections
  Beta-hemolytic *Streptococcus* (group A), *Clostridium perfringens*, and mixed organism
  Usually occur in patients who are immunocompromised (diabetes mellitus) or who have poor blood supply
  Can present very quickly after surgical procedures (within hours)

  Necrotizing fasciitis – beta-hemolytic group A strep; can be polyorganismal
    Overlying skin may be pale red and progress to purple with blister or bullae development.
    Overlying skin can look normal in the early stages.
    Thin, gray, foul-smelling drainage; crepitus
    Tx: early debridement, high-dose penicillin; may want broad spectrum if thought to be polyorganismal

  ***Clostridium perfringens* infections**
    Necrotic tissue decreases oxidation-redux potential, setting up environment for *Clostridium perfringens*.
    Clostridium perfringens has alpha toxin.
    Pain out of proportion to exam
    May not show skin signs with deep infection
    Gram stain shows GPRs without WBCs.
    Myonecrosis and gas gangrene – common presentations
    Can occur with farming injuries
    Tx: early debridement, high-dose penicillin

  Fournier's gangrene
    Severe infection in perineal and scrotal region
    Risk factors – diabetes mellitus and immunocompromised state
    Caused by mixed organisms (GPCs, GNRs, anaerobes)
    Tx: early debridement; try to preserve testicles if possible; antibiotics

  Mixed organism infection can also cause necrotizing soft tissue infections.

Fungal infection
  Need fungal coverage for positive blood culture, 2 sites other than blood, 1 site with severe symptoms, endophthalmitis, patients on prolonged bacterial antibiotics with failure to improve

  Actinomyces **(not a true fungus)** – pulmonary symptoms most common; can cause tortuous abscesses in cervical, thoracic, and abdominal areas. Tx: drainage and penicillin G

Chapter 5. Infection

Nocardia (not a true fungus) – pulmonary and CNS symptoms most common
    Tx: drainage and sulfonamides (Bactrim)
Histoplasmosis – pulmonary symptoms most common; Mississippi and Ohio River valleys
    Tx: amphotericin for severe infections
Cryptococcus – CNS symptoms most common
    Tx: amphotericin for severe infections
Coccioidomycosis – pulmonary symptoms; Southwest
    Tx: amphotericin for severe infections
Candida – common inhabitant of the respiratory tract
    Tx: fluconazole (some *Candida* resistant), amphotericin for severe infections

Spontaneous (primary) bacterial peritonitis
Protein <1 g/dl in peritoneal fluid – risk factor
Monobacterial (50% *E. coli*, 30% *Streptococcus*, 10% *Klebsiella*)
Secondary to decreased host defenses (intrahepatic shunting, impaired bactericidal activity in ascites); not due to transmucosal migration
Fluid cultures negative in many cases
PMNs >500 cells/cc diagnostic
Tx: ceftriaxone or other 3rd generation cephalosporin
Need to rule out intra-abdominal source (diverticular abscess, perforation) if not getting better on antibiotics or if cultures are polymicrobial
Liver transplantation not an option with active infection
Fluoroquinolones good for short-term prophylaxis

Secondary bacterial peritonitis
Intra-abdominal source (transmucosal migration, perforated viscus)
Polymicrobial – *Bacteroides fragilis, E. coli, Enterococcus* most common organisms
Tx: need laparotomy to find source

HIV
Exposure risk – HIV blood transfusion 70%, infant from positive mother 30%, needle stick from positive patient 0.3%, mucous membrane exposure (1%)[1]
Seroconversion occurs in 6–12 weeks
AZT and lamivudine can help ↓ seroconversion after exposure
Should be given within 1–2 hours of exposure

Opportunistic infections – most common cause for laparotomy in HIV patients (CMV infection most common)
Neoplastic disease – 2nd most common reason for laparotomy
CMV colitis – most common intestinal manifestation of AIDS (can present with pain, bleeding, or perforation)
Lymphoma in HIV patients – stomach most common followed by rectum; mostly non-Hodgkin's, 70% B cell
Tx: chemotherapy
Lower GI bleeds more common than upper GI bleeds in HIV patients
    Upper GI bleeds – Kaposi's sarcoma, lymphoma
    Lower GI bleeds – CMV, bacterial, HSV

CD4 counts: 800–1200 normal; 300–400 symptomatic disease; <200 opportunistic infections

Hepatitis C
Now rarely transmitted with blood transfusion (0.0001%/unit)
1%–2% of population infected
Fulminant hepatic failure rare
Chronic infection occurs in 80%; fulminant hepatic failure rare; cirrhosis in 15% over 20 years; hepatocellular carcinoma in 1%–5%
Interferon may help prevent development of cirrhosis.

---

[1] Deziel DJ et al. Rush University review of surgery. Ed 3. Philadelphia: WB Saunders, 2000:149.

Other infections
Brown recluse spider bites – Tx: dapsone initially; may need resection of area and skin graft for large ulcers later
Acute septic arthritis – *Gonococcus*, staph, *H. influenzae*, strep
   Tx: drainage, 3rd generation cephalosporin and vancomycin until cultures show organism
Diabetic foot infections – mixed staph, strep, GNRs, and anaerobes
   Tx: broad-spectrum antibiotics (Unasyn, Zosyn)
Cat/dog/human bites – polymicrobial
   Eikinella found only in human bites; can cause permanent joint injury
   Pasteurella multocida found in cat and dog bites
   Tx: broad-spectrum antibiotics (Augmentin)

Impetigo, erysipelas, cellulitis, and folliculitis – staph and strep most common organisms
Furuncle – boil; usually *S. epidermidis* or *S. aureus*. Tx: drainage +/– antibiotics
Carbuncle – a multiloculated furuncle

Peritoneal dialysis catheter infections
S. aureus and *S. epidermidis* most common
Fungal infections hard to treat
Tx: intraperitoneal vancomycin and gentamicin; intraperitoneal amphotercin for fungus; increased dwell time and intraperitoneal heparin may help
Removal of catheter for peritonitis that lasts for 4–5 days
Fecal peritonitis requires laparotomy to find perforation
Some say need removal of peritoneal dialysis catheter for all fungal, tuberculous, and *Pseudomonas* infections

Sinusitis
Risk factors – nasoenteric tubes, intubation, patients with severe facial fractures
Usually polymicrobial
CT head shows air-fluid levels in the sinus
Tx: broad-spectrum antibiotics; rare to have to tap sinus percutaneously for systemic illness

Use **clippers** preoperatively instead of razors to decrease chance of wound infection.

CHAPTER 6. ANTIBIOTICS

Antiseptic – kills and inhibits organisms on body
Disinfectant – kills and inhibits organisms on inanimate objects
Sterilization – all organisms killed
Common antiseptics in surgery
    Iodophors (Betadine) – good for GPCs, GNRs, poor fungi
    Chlorhexidine gluconate (Hibiclens) – good for GPCs, GNRs, and fungi

Mechanism of action
    Inhibitors of cell wall synthesis – penicillins, cephalosporins, carbapenems, monobactams, vancomycin
    Inhibitors of the 30s ribosome and protein synthesis – tetracycline, aminoglycosides (tobramycin, gentamicin), linezolid
    Inhibitors of the 50s ribosome and protein synthesis – erythromycin, clindamycin, chloramphenicol, Synercid
    Inhibitor of DNA helicase (DNA gyrase) – quinolones (BID dosing)
    Inhibitor of RNA polymerase – rifampin
    Produces oxygen radicals that breakup DNA – metronidazole (Flagyl)

    Sulfonamides – PABA analogue, inhibit purine synthesis
    Trimethoprim – inhibits dihydrofolate reductase, inhibits purine synthesis
    Bacteriostatic antibiotics – chloramphenicol, tetracycline, clindamycin, erythromycin (all have reversible ribosomal binding), Bactrim
    Aminoglycosides – have irreversible binding to ribosome and are considered **bactericidal**

Mechanism of antibiotic resistance
    PCN resistance – plasmids for beta-lactamase
    Transfer of plasmids – most common method of antibiotic resistance
    Methicillin-resistant *S. aureus* (MRSA) – resistance to methicillin caused by **mutation of cell wall–binding protein**
    Vancomycin-resistant *Enterococcus* – resistance develops from **mutation in cell wall binding protein**
    Gentamicin resistance – resistance due to modifying enzymes leading to decrease active transport

Appropriate drug levels
    Vancomycin – peak 20–40; trough 5–10
    Gentamicin – peak 6–10; trough <1
    Peak too high → decrease amount of each dose
    Trough too high → decrease frequency of doses (increase time interval between doses)

Specific antibiotics
Penicillin
    GPCs – streptococci, syphilis, *Neisseria meningitides* (GPR), *Clostridium perfringens* (GPR), beta-hemolytic *Streptococcus*, anthrax
    Not effective against *Staphylococcus* or *Enterococcus*

Oxacillin/nafcillin
    Anti-staph penicillins (staph only)

Ampicillin/amoxicillin
    Same as penicillin but also picks up <u>enterococci</u>

Unasyn (ampicillin/sulbactam) and Augmentin (amoxicillin/clavulanic acid)
    Broad spectrum – pick up GPCs (staph and strep), GNRs, +/– anaerobic coverage
    Effective for enterococci; <u>not</u> effective for *Pseudomonas*, *Acinetobacter*, or *Serratia*
    Sulbactam and clavulanic acid are beta-lactamase inhibitors.

Ticarcillin/piperacillin (antipseudomonal penicillins)
    GNRs – enterics, *Pseudomonas, Acinetobacter*, and *Serratia*
    Side effects: inhibits platelets; high salt load

Timentin (ticarcillin/clavulanic acid) and Zosyn (piperacillin/sulbactam)
  Broad spectrum – pick up **GPCs** (staph and strep), **GNRs, anaerobes**
  Effective for enterococci; effective for *Pseudomonas, Acinetobacter,* and *Serratia*
  Side effects: inhibits platelets; high salt load

First-generation cephalosporins (cefazolin, cephalexin)
  GPCs – staph and strep
  Not effective for *Enterococcus*; does not penetrate CNS
  Ancef (cefazolin) has the longest half-life → best for prophylaxis
  Side effects: can produce positive Coombs test

Second-generation cephalosporins (cefoxitin, cefotetan, cefuroxime)
  GPCs, GNRs, +/– anaerobic coverage; lose some staph activity
  Not effective for *Enterococcus, Pseudomonas, Acinetobacter,* or *Serratia*
  Effective only for community-acquired GNRs
  Cefotetan has longest half-life → best for prophylaxis
  Side effects: prolonged PT

Third-generation cephalosporins (ceftriaxone, ceftazidime, cefepime, cefotaxime)
  GNRs mostly, +/– anaerobic coverage
  Not effective for *Enterococcus*; effective for *Pseudomonas, Acinetobacter,* and *Serratia*
  Side effects: cholestatic jaundice (ceftriaxone), sludging in gallbladder (ceftriaxone)

Monobactam (aztreonam)
  GNRs; picks up *Pseudomonas, Acinetobacter,* and *Serratia*

Carbapenems (meropenem/imipenem)
  Broad spectrum – GPCs, GNRs, and anaerobes
  Not effective for **MEPP**: MRSA, *Enterococcus, Proteus,* and *Pseudomonas* (which can develop resistance)
  Cilastatin – prevents renal hydrolysis of the drug and increases half-life
  Side effects: carbapenems can cause seizures

Bactrim
  GNRs, +/– GPCs
  Not effective for *Enterococcus, Pseudomonas, Acinetobacter,* and *Serratia*
  Side effects (numerous): teratogenic, allergic reactions, renal damage, Stevens-Johnson syndrome (erythema multiforme), hemolysis in G6PD-deficient patients

Quinolones
  GPCs, mostly GNRs
  Not effective for *Enterococcus*; picks up *Pseudomonas, Acinetobacter,* and *Serratia*
  40% of MRSA sensitive; same efficacy PO and IV

Aminoglycosides (gentamicin, tobramycin)
  GNRs
  Disrupt calcium homeostasis; need oxygen to work
  Good for *Pseudomonas, Acinetobacter,* and *Serratia*; not effective for anaerobes (need O_2)
  Resistance due to modifying enzymes leading to decreased active transport
  Synergistic with ampicillin for *Enterococcus* – beta-lactams (ampicillin/amoxicillin) facilitate aminoglycoside penetration
  Side effects: reversible nephrotoxicity, irreversible ototoxicity

Erythromycin (macrolides)
  GPCs; best for community-acquired pneumonia and atypical pneumonias
  Side effects: nausea (PO), cholestasis (IV)
  Also binds motilin receptor and is prokinetic for bowel

Vancomycin (glycopeptides)
  GPCs, *Enterococcus, Clostridium difficile* (with PO intake), MRSA
  Binds cell wall proteins
  Resistance develops from change in cell wall binding sites.
  Side effects: HTN, Redman syndrome (histamine release), nephrotoxicity, ototoxicity

Chapter 6. Antibiotics

Synercid (streptogramin – quinupristin-dalfopristin)
GPCs; includes MRSA, VRE

Linezolid (oxazolidinones)
GPCs; includes MRSA, VRE

Tetracycline
GPCs, GNRs, syphilis
Side effects: tooth discoloration in children

Chloramphenicol
Anaerobes
Side effects: gray baby syndrome, decreased bone marrow, aplastic anemia

Clindamycin
Anaerobes, some GPCs
Good for aspiration pneumonia
Can be used to treat *Clostridium perfringens*
Side effects: pseudomembranous colitis

Metronidazole
Anaerobes
Side effects: disulfiram-like reaction, peripheral neuropathy

Carbenicillin and ticarcillin can interfere with aminoglycosides.
Tetracyclines can interfere with beta-lactams.
Broad-spectrum antibiotics can lead to **superinfection**.

Antifungal drugs
   Amphotericin – binds sterols in wall and alters membrane permeability
      Side effects: nephrotoxic, fever, decreased potassium, hypotension, anemia
   Fluconazole – not all *Candida* spp. are sensitive
   Ketoconazole – not all *Candida* spp. are sensitive
   Prolonged broad-spectrum antibiotics +/– fever → **fluconazole**
   Possible fungal sepsis → **amphotericin**

Antituberculosis drugs
   Isoniazid – inhibits mycolic acids
      Side effects: hepatotoxicity, B_6 deficiency
   Rifampin – inhibits RNA polymerase
      Side effects: hepatotoxicity; GI symptoms; high rate of resistance
   Pyrazinamide
      Side effect: hepatotoxicity
   Ethambutol
      Side effect: retrobulbar neuritis

Antiviral drugs
   Acyclovir – inhibits DNA polymerase, usually used for HSV infections; can be used for EBV
   Ganciclovir – used for CMV infections
      Side effects: decreased bone marrow, CNS toxicity

Effective for *Enterococcus* – vancomycin, Timentin/Zosyn, ampicillin/amoxicillin, gentamicin with ampicillin

Effective for *Pseudomonas*, *Acinetobacter*, and *Serratia* – ticarcillin/piperacillin, Timentin/Zosyn, 3rd generation cephalosporins, aminoglycosides (gentamicin and tobramycin), meropenem/imipenem (resistance can develop in *Pseudomonas*), fluoroquinolones
Double cover *Pseudomonas*.

Perioperative antibiotics
Used to prevent incisional wound infections
Need to be given within 2 hours before incision

CHAPTER 7. MEDICINES AND PHARMACOLOGY

Sublingual and rectal drugs – do not pass through the liver first
Skin absorption – based on lipid solubility through the epidermis
CSF absorption – restricted to nonionized, lipid-soluble drugs

Albumin – largely responsible for binding drugs (PCNs and warfarin 90% bound)
Sulfonamides – will displace unconjugated bilirubin in newborns
Tetracycline and heavy metals – stored in bone

0 order kinetics – constant amount of drug is eliminated regardless of dose
1st order kinetics – drug eliminated proportional to dose
Takes 5 half-lives for a drug to reach steady-state
Volume of distribution = amount of drug in the body divided by amount of drug in plasma or blood
    Drugs with a high volume of distribution have higher concentrations in the **extravascular compartment** (e.g., fat tissue) compared with **intravascular concentrations**.
Bioavailability – fraction of unchanged drug reaching the systemic circulation
    Assumed to be 100% for intravenous drugs, less for other routes (i.e., oral)

ED_{50} – drug level at which <u>desired effect</u> occurs in 50% of patients
LD_{50} – drug level at which <u>death</u> occurs in 50% of patients

Hyperactive – effect at an unusually low dose
Tachyphylaxis – tolerance after only a few doses
Potency – dose required for effect
Efficacy – ability to achieve result without untoward effect

Microsomal drug metabolism (hepatic cell endoplasmic reticulum, P-450 system)
    Phase I – demethylation, oxidation, reduction, hydrolysis reactions (mixed function oxidases, requires NADPH/oxygen)
    Phase II – glucuronic acid (**#1**) and sulfates attached (forms **water-soluble metabolite**); often inactive and ready for excretion. Biliary excreted drugs may become deconjugated in intestines with reabsorption, some in active form

    Inhibitors of P-450 – cimetidine, isoniazid, ketoconazole, erythromycin, Cipro, Flagyl, allopurinol, verapamil, amiodarone, MAOIs, disulfiram
    Inducers of P-450 – cruciform vegetables, ETOH, insecticides, cigarette smoke, phenobarbital (barbiturates), dilantin, theophylline, warfarin

    P-450 system transforms aromatic hydrocarbons into carcinogens

Kidney – most important organ for eliminating drugs (glomerular filtration and tubular secretion)

Polar drugs (ionized) – more <u>water soluble</u> and more likely to be eliminated in unaltered form
Nonpolar drugs (nonionized) – more <u>fat soluble</u> and more likely to be metabolized before excretion

Gadolinium – side effect: nausea

Gout – caused by uric acid buildup; end product of purine metabolism
    Colchicine – anti-inflammatory; binds tubulin and inhibits migration
    Indomethacin – anti-inflammatory
    Allopurinol – xanthine oxidase inhibitor, blocks uric acid formation from xanthine; used in chronic setting for <u>overproducers</u>
        Probenecid – ↑ renal secretion of uric acid; used for <u>undersecreters</u>

Cholestyramine – can bind vitamin K and cause bleeding tendency
HMG-CoA reductase inhibitors (-statin drugs) – can cause liver dysfunction, rhabdomyolysis
Niacin (inhibits cholesterol synthesis) – can cause flushing. Tx: ASA
Promethazine (Phenergan, antiemetic) – causes tardive dyskinesia (inhibits dopamine receptors)
    Tx: diphenhydramine (Benadryl)

Chapter 7. Medicines and Pharmacology

Metoclopramide (Reglan, prokinetic) – dopamine receptor blocker that can be used to increase gastric motility and gut motility in general
Ondansetron (Zofran) – serotonin receptor inhibitor; antiemetic
Omeprazole – proton pump inhibitor; blocks H/K ATPase in stomach
Cimetidine/ranitidine – histamine H_2 receptor blockers; decrease acid in stomach
Octreotide – somatostatin analog that is longer acting

Digoxin
 Inhibits Na/K ATPase and increases myocardial calcium
 ↑ atrial contraction rate but **slows AV conduction**
 Also acts as an **inotrope**
 ↓ **blood flow** to intestines – has been implicated in causing **mesenteric ischemia**
 Hypokalemia – ↑ sensitivity of heart to digitalis; can precipitate arrhythmias or AV block
 Is not cleared with dialysis
 Other side effects: visual changes (yellow hue), fatigue, arrhythmias

Procainamide – can cause lupus-like syndrome, pulmonary fibrosis, and torsades
  Magnesium – used to treat torsades
 Follow drug levels and QT intervals: >400 msec is concerning
 Normal procainamide level: 4–12
 Normal NAPA level: <30

Adenosine – causes transient interruption of AV node

ACE (angiotensin-converting enzyme) inhibitors (captopril)
 Best single agent shown to reduce mortality in patients with CHF
 Can prevent CHF post-MI
 Can prevent progression of renal dysfunction in patients with hypertension and DM
 Can precipitate renal failure in patients with renal artery stenosis

Beta-blockers – may prolong life in patients with severe LV failure
 Reduce risk of MI and atrial fibrillation postoperatively

Atropine – acetylcholine antagonist; increases heart rate

Metyrapone and aminoglutethimide – inhibit adrenal steroid synthesis
 Used in patients with adrenocortical CA

Leuprolide – analog of GnRH and LHRH; inhibits release of LH and FSH from pituitary when given continuously (paradoxic effect)

Vasopressin (ADH) – acts on V-1 receptors found on vascular smooth muscle (constriction)
 Can be used in patients with <u>gastrointestinal bleeding</u> by reducing intestinal blood flow

Indomethacin – inhibits prostaglandin production
 Used to close patent ductus arteriosus (PDA) in children and used in patients with gout

Misoprostol – PGE_1 derivative; a protective prostaglandin used to prevent peptic ulcer disease
 Consider use in patients on chronic NSAIDs

NSAIDs – inhibit prostaglandin synthesis and lead to ↓ mucus and HCO_3^- secretion and ↑ acid production

Haldol – can cause extrapyramidal manifestations; inhibits dopamine receptors

ASA poisoning – tinnitus, headaches, nausea and vomiting
 1st – respiratory alkalosis
 2nd – metabolic acidosis

Tylenol overdose – Tx: N-acetylcysteine

Activated protein C (Xigris) – used for sepsis
 Mechanism is **fibrinolysis**.
 Drug inactivates the inhibitor of protein C, creating activated protein C.

CHAPTER 8. ANESTHESIA

Inhalational agents
MAC – minimum alveolar concentration = smallest concentration of inhalational agent at which 50% of patients will not move with incision
Small MAC → more lipid soluble = more potent
Speed of induction is inversely proportional to solubility.
Nitrous is fastest but has high MAC (low potency).

Inhalational agents cause unconsciousness, amnesia, and some degree of analgesia.
Blunt hypoxic drive
Most are associated with some degree of **myocardial depression**, ↑ **cerebral blood flow**, and ↓ **renal blood flow**.

NO_2 **(nitrous oxide)** – fast, minimal myocardial depression
Halothane – slow, highest degree of cardiac depression and arrhythmias; least pungent, which is good for children
  Halothane hepatitis – fever, eosinophilia, jaundice, ↑ LFTs
Enflurane – can cause seizures
Isoflurane – good for neurosurgery; higher cost
Sevoflurane – less myocardial depression, fast onset/offset, less laryngospasm; higher cost

Induction agents
Sodium thiopental (barbiturate) – fast acting
  Side effects: ↓ cerebral blood flow and metabolic rate, ↓ blood pressure

Propofol – very rapid distribution and on/off; amnesia; sedative
  Side effects: hypotension, respiratory depression
  Not an analgesic
  Do not use in patients with egg allergy.
  Metabolized in liver and by plasma cholinesterases

Ketamine – dissociation of thalamic/limbic systems; places patient in a cataleptic state (amnesia, analgesia)
  No respiratory depression
  Side effects: hallucinations, catecholamine release (↑ carbon monoxide, tachycardia), ↑ airway secretions, and ↑ cerebral blood flow
  Contraindicated in patients with head injury
  Good for **children**

Etomidate – fewer hemodynamic changes; fast acting
Continuous infusions can lead to adrenocortical suppression.

Rapid sequence intubation – can be indicated for recent oral intake, GERD, delayed gastric emptying, pregnancy, bowel obstruction

Muscle relaxants (paralytics)
Diaphragm – last muscle to go down and 1st muscle to recover from paralytics
Neck muscles and face – 1st to go down and last to recover from paralytics

Depolarizing agent – the only one is succinylcholine
Succinylcholine – fast, short-acting; causes fasciculations at first, ↑ ICP; many side effects
  Malignant hyperthermia
    Defect in calcium metabolism
    Calcium released from sarcoplasmic reticulum causes muscle excitation–contraction syndrome.
    Side effects: 1st sign is ↑ **end-tidal CO_2**, then fever, tachycardia, rigidity, acidosis, hyperkalemia
    Tx: **dantrolene** (10 mg/kg) inhibits Ca release and decouples excitation complex), cooling blankets, HCO_3, glucose, supportive care

Chapter 8. Anesthesia

Hyperkalemia – depolarization releases K (see also Chap. 9, Fluids and Electrolytes)
Don't use in burn patients, neurologic injury, neuromuscular disorders, spinal cord injury, massive trauma, acute renal failure.
Open-angle glaucoma can become closed-angle glaucoma.
Atypical pseudocholinesterases – causes prolonged paralysis (Asians)

Nondepolarizing agents
Inhibit neuromuscular junction by competing with acetylcholine
Can get prolongation of these agents with hypothermia, hypercarbia, certain antibiotics, electrolyte abnormalities, myasthenia gravis

Cis-atracurium – undergoes Hoffman degradation
  Can be used in liver and renal failure
Mivacurium – fast, short acting; degradation by **plasma cholinesterases**
  Histamine release
Rocuronium – fast, intermediate duration; hepatic metabolism
Pancuronium – slow acting, long-lasting; renal metabolism
  Most common side effect – **tachycardia**

Reversing drugs for nondepolarizing agents
Neostigmine – counters nondepolarizing agents, blocks **acetylcholinesterase**, increasing acetylcholine
Edrophonium – counters nondepolarizing agents, blocks **acetylcholinesterase**, increasing acetylcholine
Atropine or glycopyrrolate should be given with neostigmine or edrophonium to counteract effects of generalized acetylcholine overdose

Local anesthetics
Work by increasing action potential threshold, preventing Na influx
Can use 0.5 cc/kg of 1% lidocaine
Infected tissues hard to anesthetize secondary to **acidosis**
Length of action – bupivacaine > lidocaine > procaine
Epinephrine allows higher doses to be used, stays locally.
  Side effects: tremors, seizures, tinnitus, arrhythmias (CNS symptoms occur before cardiac)
  No epinephrine with arrhythmias, unstable angina, uncontrolled hypertension, poor collaterals (penis and ear), uteroplacental insufficiency

Amides (all have an "i" in first part of name) – lidocaine, bupivacaine, mepivacaine; rarely allergic reactions
Esters – tetracaine, procaine, cocaine; ↑ allergic reactions secondary to PABA analogue

Narcotics (opioids)
Morphine, fentanyl, Demerol, codeine
Act on mu receptors
Profound analgesia, respiratory depression (↓ CO_2 drive), no cardiac effects, blunt sympathetic response
Metabolized by the liver and excreted via kidney
Overdose of narcotic drugs – Tx: **Narcan**
Avoid use of narcotics in patients on **MAOIs** → can cause **hyperpyrexic coma**

Morphine – analgesia, euphoria, respiratory depression, miosis, ↓ cough, constipation, histamine release
  Active metabolites can build up in patients with renal failure.
Demerol – analgesia, euphoria, respiratory depression, miosis, tremors, fasciculations, convulsions
  No histamine release
  Avoid in patients with renal failure → can get buildup of **normeperidine analogue and result in seizures** (also need to be careful with the amount given)
Methadone – simulates morphine, less euphoria
Fentanyl – 80x strength of morphine (does not cross react in patients with morphine allergy)
  No histamine release
Sufentanil, alfentanil, remifentanil – very fast-acting narcotics with short half-lives

Benzodiazepines
Hepatically metabolized; anticonvulsant, amnesic, anxiolytic, respiratory depression; not analgesic
Versed (midazolam) – short acting; contraindicated in pregnancy, crosses placenta
Ativan (lorazepam) – long acting
Valium (diazepam) – long acting
Overdose of these drugs – Tx: flumazenil (competitive inhibitor; may cause seizures and arrhythmias; contraindicated in patients with elevated ICP or status epilepticus)

Epidural and spinal anesthesia
Epidural – causes sympathetic denervation, vasodilation
 Morphine in epidural can cause **respiratory depression**.
 Lidocaine in epidural can cause **decreased heart rate and blood pressure**.
 Dilute concentrations allow sparing of motor function.
 Tx for acute hypotension and bradycardia: turn epidural down; fluids, phenylephrine, atropine
 T-5 epidural can affect cardiac accelerator nerves
 Epidural contraindicated with hypertrophic cardiomyopathy, cyanotic heart disease → can get inadvertent spinal anesthesia
Spinal anesthesia – injection into subarachnoid space, spread determined by baricity and patient position
 Neurologic blockade is above motor blockade.
 Spinal contraindicated with hypertrophic cardiomyopathy, cyanotic heart disease
Caudal block – through sacrum, good for pediatric hernias and perianal surgery

Epidural and spinal complications – hypotension, headache, urinary retention, abscess/hematoma formation, neurologic impairment
High spinal – respiratory depression
Spinal headaches – Tx: rest, increased fluids, caffeine, analgesics; blood patch to site if persists >24 hours. Headache gets worse sitting up.

Perioperative complications
CHF and renal failure – associated with most postoperative hospital mortality
Postop MI – may have no pain or EKG changes; can have hypotension, arrhythmias, ↑ filling pressures, oliguria, bradycardia

Patients that need cardiology workup – angina, previous MI, shortness of breath, CHF, walks <2 blocks due to shortness of breath or chest pain, FEV_1 <70%, aortic stenosis murmur, PVCs >5/min, age >70, patients undergoing major vascular surgery

ASA classes

Class	Description
I	Healthy
II	Mild disease without limitation (controlled hypertension, obesity, diabetes mellitus, significant smoking history, older age)
III	Severe disease (angina, previous MI, poorly controlled hypertension, diabetes mellitus with complications, moderate COPD)
IV	Severe constant threat to life (unstable angina, CHF, renal failure, liver failure, severe COPD)
V	Moribund (ruptured AAA, saddle pulmonary embolus, ascending aortic dissection resulting in heart failure)
VI	Donor
E	Emergency

Most **vascular procedures** are considered moderate- to high-risk surgery.
Biggest risk factors for postop MI: age >70, DM, previous MI, CHF, and unstable angina

Best determinant of esophageal vs tracheal intubation – **end-tidal CO_2**

Intubated patient undergoing surgery with sudden transient rise in ETCO$_2$
  Dx: most likely alveolar hypoventilation
  Tx: ↑ tidal volume (most likely do to atelectasis) or ↑ respiratory rate

Intubated patient with sudden drop in ETCO$_2$ – likely became disconnected from the vent; could also be due to pulmonary embolism or significant hypotension

CHAPTER 9. FLUIDS AND ELECTROLYTES

Total body water
 Roughly ⅔ of total body weight is water (men); **infants** have a little more body water, **women** have a little less.
 ⅔ of water weight is intracellular (mostly muscle).
 ⅓ of water weight is extracellular.
  ⅔ of extracellular water is interstitial.
  ⅓ of extracellular water is in plasma.

 Proteins – determine plasma/interstitial compartment osmotic pressures
 Na – determines intracellular/extracellular osmotic pressure

 Volume overload – most common cause is iatrogenic; first sign is **weight gain**
 Cellular catabolism – can release a significant amount of H_2O

 0.9% normal saline: Na 154 and Cl 154
 Lactated Ringer's solution (LR; ionic composition of plasma): Na 130, K 4, Ca 2.7, Cl 109, bicarb 28

 Plasma osmolarity: $(2 \times Na) + (glucose/18) + (BUN/2.8)$
  Normal: 280–295

Estimates of volume replacement
 4 cc/kg/day for 1st 10 kg
 2 cc/kg/day for 2nd 10 kg
 1 cc/kg/day for each kg after that
 Best indicator of adequate volume replacement is **urine output**.

 During open abdominal operations, fluid loss is **0.5–1.0 L/hr** unless there are measurable blood losses.
 Usually don't have to replace blood lost unless it's **>500 cc.**
 Insensible fluid losses – 10 cc/kg/day, 75% skin, 25% respiratory, pure water

 IV replacement after major adult gastrointestinal surgery
  During operation and 1st 24 hours, use **LR**.
  After 24 hours, switch to **D5 ½ NS with 20 mEq K⁺**.
   5% dextrose will stimulate **insulin release**, resulting in amino acid uptake and protein synthesis.

GI fluid secretion
Stomach	1–2 L/day
Biliary system	500–1000 ml/day
Pancreas	500–1000 ml/day
Duodenum	500–1000 ml/day

 Normal K⁺ requirement: 0.5–1.0 mEq/kg/day
 Normal Na⁺ requirement: 1–2 mEq/kg/day

GI electrolyte losses
 Sweat – hypotonic
 Saliva – K⁺ (highest concentration of K⁺ in body)
 Stomach – H⁺ and Cl⁻
 Pancreas – HCO_3^-
 Bile – HCO_3^-
 Small intestine – HCO_3^-, K⁺
 Large intestine – K⁺

 Gastric losses – replacement is D5 ½ NS with 20 mg K⁺
 Pancreatic/biliary/small intestine losses – replacement is LR with HCO_3^-
 Large intestine (diarrhea) losses – replacement is LR with K⁺

Chapter 9. Fluids and Electrolytes

GI losses – should generally be replaced cc/cc
Urine output – should be kept at least 0.5 cc/kg/hr; should not be replaced, usually a sign of normal postoperative diuresis

Potassium (normal 3.5–5.0)
Hyperkalemia – peaked T waves initial finding on EKG
  Calcium gluconate (membrane stabilizer for heart)
  Sodium bicarbonate (causes alkalosis, K enters cell in exchange for H)
  10 U insulin and 1 ampule of 50% dextrose (K driven into cells along with glucose)
  Kayexalate
  Dialysis if refractory
Hypokalemia – T waves disappear

Sodium (normal 135–145)
Hypernatremia – correct with ½ NS slowly to avoid brain swelling
Hyponatremia – Na deficit = 0.6 x (weight in kg) x (140 – Na)
  Water restriction is the first treatment for hyponatremia, then **diuresis,** then NaCl replacement.
  Correct Na slowly to avoid **central pontine myelinosis**.
  Hyperglycemia can cause pseudohyponatremia – for each 100 increment of glucose over normal, add 2 points to the Na value.

Calcium (normal 8.5–10.0; normal ionized Ca 4.4–5.5)
Hypercalcemia (Ca usually >13 or ionized >6–7) – causes lethargic state
  Breast cancer most common malignant cause
  Tx: NS at 200–300 cc/hr, Lasix
  For **malignant disease** → mithramycin, calcitonin, aldaronic acid
Hypocalcemia (Ca usually <8 or ionized Ca <4) – hyperreflexia, Chvostek's sign (tapping on face produces twitching), perioral tingling and numbness, Trousseau's sign (carpopedal spasm), prolonged QT interval.
  May need to **correct Mg** before being able to correct Ca
  Protein adjustment for calcium – for every 1 g decrease in protein, add 0.8 to Ca

Magnesium (normal 2.0–2.7)
Hypermagnesemia – causes lethargic state; burn, trauma and renal dialysis patients
  Tx: calcium
Hypomagnesemia – signs similar to hypocalcemia

Metabolic acidosis
Anion gap = Na – (HCO_3 + Cl)
  Normal: <10–15
Anion gap acidosis – "MUDPILES" = **m**ethanol, **u**remia, **d**iabetic ketoacidosis, **p**araldehydes, **i**soniazid, **l**actic acidosis, **e**thylene glycol, **s**alicylates

Normal gap acidosis usually due to loss of Na/HCO_3^- (ileostomies, small bowel fistulas)

Tx: underlying cause; keep pH >7.20 with bicarbonate; severely ↓ pH can affect myocardial contractility

Metabolic alkalosis
Usually a contraction alkalosis
Nasogastric suction – results in **hypochloremic, hypokalemic, metabolic alkalosis,** and paradoxical **aciduria**
Loss of Cl⁻ and H ion from stomach secondary to nasogastric tube (hypochloremia and alkalosis)
Loss of water causes kidney to reabsorb Na in exchange for K^+ (Na/K ATPase), thus losing K^+ (hypokalemia)
Na^+/H^+ exchanger activated in an effort to reabsorb water along with K^+/H^+ exchanger in an effort to reabsorb K^+ → results in paradoxical aciduria

Acid–base balance

Condition	pH	CO_2	HCO_3
Respiratory acidosis	↓	↑	↑
Respiratory alkalosis	↑	↓	↓
Metabolic acidosis	↓	↓	↓
Metabolic alkalosis	↑	↑	↑

Henderson-Hesselbach equation
$pH = pK + \log [HCO_3^-] / [CO_2]$
Ratio of base to acid (HCO_3^- to CO_2) of 20:1 = pH of 7.4

Acute renal failure
FeNa = (urine Na/Cr) / (plasma Na/Cr) – <u>best test for azotemia</u>

Prerenal – FeNa <1%, urine Na <20, BUN/Cr ratio >20, urine osmolality >500 mOsm
70% of renal mass must be damaged before ↑ Cr and BUN

Contrast dyes – <u>volume expansion</u> best prevents renal damage
Myoglobin – converted to <u>ferrihemate</u> in acidic environment, which is toxic to renal cells
  Tx: <u>alkalinize urine</u>

Tumor lysis syndrome
Release of purines and pyrimidines leads to ↑ **PO_4 and uric acid**, ↓ Ca
Can result in ↑ BUN and Cr, EKG changes
Tx: hydration, allopurinol (↓ uric acid production), diuretics, alkalinization of urine

Vitamin D (cholecalciferol)
Made in skin (UV sunlight) from 7-dehydrocholesterol
Goes to liver for (25-OH), then **kidney for (1-OH)**. This creates the active form of vitamin D.
Active form of vitamin D – ↑ **calcium-binding protein**, leading to ↑ intestinal Ca absorption

Chronic renal failure
↓ **active vitamin D** (↓ 1-OH hydroxylation) → ↓ Ca reabsorption from gut (↓ Ca binding protein)
Anemia – from low erythropoietin

Transferrin – transporter of iron
Ferritin – storage form of iron

CHAPTER 10. NUTRITION

Caloric need
  Approximately 25 kcal/kg/day
  Fat   9 kcal/g
  Protein   4 kcal/g
  Oral carbohydrates 4 kcal/g
  Dextrose   3.4 kcal/g

10% lipid solution contains 1.1 kcal/cc; 20% lipid solution contains 2 kcal/cc.
1 g protein/kg/day is needed, of which 20% should be essential amino acids.
30% fat calories – important for essential fatty acids
Rest of calories should be as **carbohydrates**.

Trauma or sepsis stress can increase kcal requirement 20%–40%.
Pregnancy increases kcal requirement 300 kcal/day.
Lactation increases kcal requirement 500 kcal/day.
Protein requirement also increases with these.

Burns
  Calories: 25 kcal/kg/day + (30 kcal/day x % burn)
  Protein: 1–1.5 g/kg/day + (3 g x % burn)

Much of the energy expenditure is used for **heat production**.
Basal metabolic rate **increases 10%** for each degree above 38.0°C.

If overweight, use equation: weight = [(actual weight – ideal body weight) x 0.25] + IBW
Harris-Benedict equation calculates basal energy expenditure based on **weight, height, age, and gender**

Central line TPN – glucose based; **maximum glucose administration** – 3 g/kg/hr
Peripheral line parenteral nutrition (PPN) – fat based

Short-chain fatty acids – fuel for **colonocytes**
Glutamine – fuel for **small bowel enterocytes**
  Most common amino acid in **bloodstream and tissue**
  Releases NH_4 in kidney, thus helping with **nitrogen excretion**
  Can be used for gluconeogenesis

Primary fuel for neoplastic cell – glutamine

Preoperative nutritional assessment
  Approximate half-lives
    Albumin – 20 days
    Transferrin – 10 days
    Prealbumin – 2 days

  Normal **protein** level: 6.0–8.5
  Normal **albumin** level: 3.5–5.5

  Ideal body weight (IBW)
    Men = 106 lb + 6 lb for each inch over 5 feet
    Women = 100 lb + 5 lb for each inch over 5 feet

  Preoperative signs of poor nutritional status
    Acute weight loss >10% in 6 months
    Weight <85% of IBW
    Albumin <3.0
    Low albumin (<3.0) – **strong risk factor for morbidity and mortality after surgery**

Respiratory quotient (RQ)
Ratio of CO_2 produced to O_2 consumed – measurement of energy expenditure

RQ >1 = lipogenesis (overfeeding)
  Tx: ↓ carbohydrates and caloric intake
  High carbohydrate intake can lead to CO_2 buildup and ventilator problems.
RQ <0.7 = ketosis and fat oxidation (starving)
  Tx: ↑ carbohydrates and caloric intake

Pure fat metabolism – RQ = 0.7
Pure protein metabolism – RQ = 0.8
Pure carbohydrate metabolism – RQ = 1.0

Postoperative phases
Diuresis phase – postoperative days 2–5
Catabolic phase – postoperative days 0–3 (negative nitrogen balance)
Anabolic phase – postoperative days 3–6 (positive nitrogen balance)

Starvation or major stress (surgery, trauma, systemic illness)
Glycogen stores
Depleted after 24–36 hours of starvation (⅔ in skeletal muscle, ⅓ in liver) → **body then switches to fat**
Skeletal muscle lacks **glucose-6-phosphatase** (found only in **liver**).
Glucose-6-phosphate stays in muscle after breakdown from glycogen and is utilized.

Gluconeogenesis precursors – amino acids (especially alanine), lactate, pyruvate, glycerol
  Alanine is the simplest amino acid precursor for gluconeogenesis.
    Primary substrate for gluconeogenesis
  Alanine and phenylalanine – only amino acids to increase during times of stress
  Late starvation – gluconeogenesis occurs in <u>kidney</u>

Starvation
Protein-conserving mechanisms **do not occur after trauma** (or surgery) secondary to catecholamines and cortisol.
Protein-conserving mechanisms do occur with **starvation**.
Fat (ketones) is the main source of energy in trauma and starvation.

Most patients can tolerate a 15% weight loss without major complications.
Patients can tolerate about **7 days** without eating; if longer than that, place a **Dobbhoff tube or start TPN**.
Try to feed gut to avoid **bacterial translocation** (bacterial overgrowth, increased permeability due to starved enterocytes).
Elemental formula – all protein given in the form of amino acids (given IV, expensive)
PEG – consider when regular feeding not possible (e.g., CVA) or predicted to not occur for >4 weeks

Brain – utilizes <u>ketones</u> with progressive starvation (normally uses glucose)
Peripheral nerves, adrenal medulla, red blood cells, and white blood cells – obligate glucose users

Refeeding syndrome
Occurs when feeding after prolonged starvation/malnutrition
Results in ↓ K, Mg, and PO_4; causes cardiac dysfunction and fluid shifts
Prevent this by starting at a **low rate** (10–15 kcal/kg/day).

Cachexia – anorexia, weight loss, wasting
  Thought to be mediated by TNF-alpha
  Glycogen breakdown, lipolysis, protein catabolism

Kwashiorkor – protein deficiency

Marasmus – starvation

Metabolic differences in bodily response to starvation and injury

Parameter	Simple Starvation	Severe Injury
Basal metabolic rate	–	++
Presence of mediators	–	+++
Major fuel oxidized	Fat	Mixed
Ketone body production	+++	±
Hepatic ureagenesis	+	+++
Negative nitrogen balance	+	+++
Gluconeogenesis	+	+++
Muscle proteolysis	+	+++
Hepatic protein synthesis	+	+++

(Smith JS Jr et al. Nutrition and metabolism. In: Greenfield LJ et al, eds. Surgery: scientific principles and practice. Ed 3. Philadelphia: Lippincott Williams & Wilkins, 2001:50.)

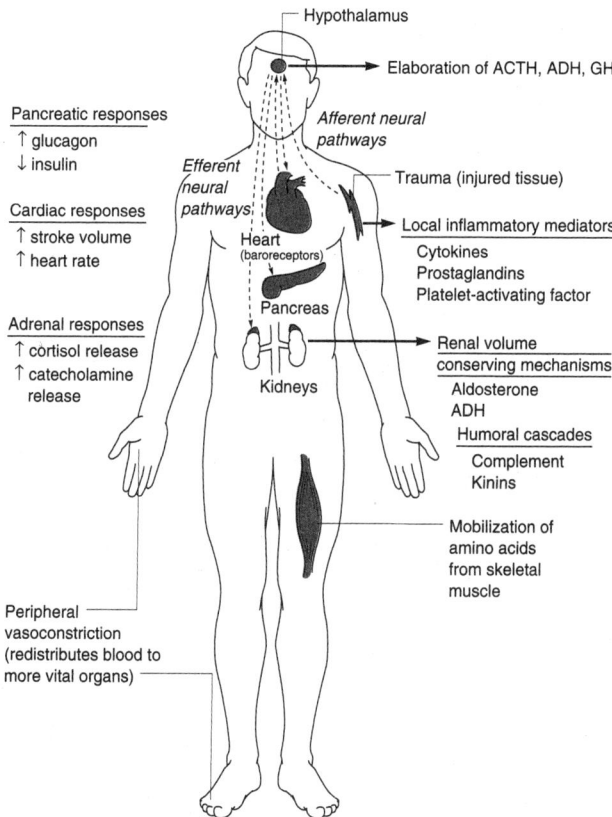

Homeostatic adjustments initiated after injury.

Nitrogen balance
6.25 g of protein contains 1 g of nitrogen.
N balance = (N in – N out) = ([protein/6.25] – [24 hr urine N + 4 g])
  Positive N balance – more protein ingested than excreted (anabolism)
  Negative N balance – more protein excreted than taken in (catabolism)
Total protein synthesis for a healthy, normal 70-kg male is **250 g/day**.

Liver
Responsible for amino acid production and breakdown
Urea production to get rid of ammonia from amino acid breakdown
Majority of protein breakdown from skeletal muscle is **glutamine and alanine**.

Fat digestion
Triacylglycerides (TAGs), cholesterol, and lipids
Broken down by pancreatic lipase, cholesterol esterase, and phospholipase to micelles and free fatty acids
Micelles – aggregates of bile salts, long-chain free fatty acids, and monoacylglycerides
Enter enterocyte by fusing with membrane
Bile salts – increase absorption area for fats, helping form **micelles**
Cholesterol – used to synthesize bile salts
Fat-soluble vitamins (A, D, E, K) – absorbed in micelles
Medium- and short-chain fatty acids – enter enterocyte by simple diffusion

Micelles and other fatty acids enter enterocytes → chylomicrons are formed, which enter **lymphatics** (thoracic duct)
Chylomicrons – 90% TAGs, 10% phospholipids/proteins/cholesterol
Medium- and short-chain fatty acids – enter **portal system** (same as amino acids and carbohydrates).
Long-chain fatty acids – enter **lymphatics** along with chylomicrons

Lipoprotein lipase – on liver endothelium; clears chylomicrons and TAGs from the blood, breaking them down to fatty acids and glycerol, which are then taken up by hepatocyte
Free fatty acid–binding protein – on liver endothelium; binds short- and medium-chain fatty acids

VLDL – most important route of entry for dietary cholesterol; synthesized in the liver

Saturated fatty acids – used for fuel by cardiac and skeletal muscles
Fatty acids (ketones – acetoacetate, beta-hydroxybutyrate) – preferred source of energy for the liver, heart, and skeletal muscle
Unsaturated fatty acids – used as structural components for cells

Hormone-sensitive lipase – in fat cells; breaks down **TAGs** (storage form of fats) **to fatty acids and glycerol**; released into blood (sensitive to growth hormone, catecholamines, glucocorticoids)

Essential fatty acids – linolenic, linoleic
Needed for prostaglandin synthesis (long-chain fatty acids)
Important for immune cells

Omega-3 fatty acids – PGI_3, TXA_3, LTB_5 (all odd) – thought to have antioxidant properties
Omega-6 fatty acids – PGE_2, TXA_2, LTB_4 (all even)

Carbohydrate digestion
Begins with **salivary amylase**, then pancreatic amylase and disaccharidases
Glucose and galactose – absorbed by secondary active transport; released into portal vein
Fructose – facilitated diffusion; released into portal vein
Sucrose = fructose + glucose
Lactose = galactose + glucose
Maltose = glucose + glucose

Protein digestion
Begins with **stomach pepsin**, then trypsin, chymotrypsin, and carboxypeptidase
Trypsinogen released from pancreas and activated by enterokinase released from duodenum
Other pancreatic protein enzymes are then activated by trypsin.
Trypsin can then also autoactivate other trypsinogen molecules.
Protein broken down to amino acids, dipeptides, and tripeptides by proteases
Absorbed by secondary active transport; released as free amino acids into portal vein
May want to limit protein intake in patients with **liver failure and renal failure to avoid ammonia buildup** and possible worsening encephalopathy

Chapter 10. Nutrition

Nonessential <u>amino acids</u> – those that begin with **A or G, plus proline and serine**

Branched-chain <u>amino acids</u> – **leucine, isoleucine, valine** ("LIV")
　Metabolized in **muscle**
　Possibly important in patients with liver failure
　Are **essential amino acids**

Deficiencies

Deficiency	Effect
Chromium	Hyperglycemia, encephalopathy, neuropathy
Selenium	Cardiomyopathy, weakness, hair loss
Copper	Pancytopenia
Zinc	Hair loss, poor healing, rash
Trace elements	Poor wound healing
Phosphate	Weakness (failure to wean of ventilator), encephalopathy, decreased phagocytosis
Thiamine (B_1)	Wernicke's encephalopathy, cardiomyopathy, peripheral neuropathy
Pyridoxine (B_6)	Sideroblastic anemia, glossitis, peripheral neuropathy
Cobalamin (B_{12})	Megaloblastic anemia, peripheral neuropathy, beefy tongue
Folate	Megaloblastic anemia, glossitis
Niacin	Pellagra (diarrhea, dermatitis, dementia)
Essential fatty acids	Dermatitis, hair loss, thrombocytopenia
Vitamin A	Night blindness
Vitamin K	Coagulopathy
Vitamin D	Rickets, osteomalacia
Vitamin E	Neuropathy

Cori cycle
　Glucose is utilized and converted to **lactate** in muscle.
　Lactate then goes to the liver and is converted back to **pyruvate** and eventually **glucose** via gluconeogenesis.
　Glucose is then transported back to muscle.

CHAPTER 11. ONCOLOGY

Cancer #2 cause of death in the US

PET (positron emission tomography) **scan** – used to identify metastases → **detects fluorodeoxyglucose molecules**

T cells need MHC complex to attack tumor.
Natural killer cells can independently attack tumor cells.
Tumor antigens are random unless viral-induced tumor.

Hyperplasia – increased number of cells
Metaplasia – replacement of one tissue with another (GERD squamous epithelium in esophagus changed to columnar gastric tissue)
Dysplasia – altered size, shape, and organization (Barrett's esophagus)

Tumor markers
  CEA – colon CA
  AFP – liver CA
  CA 19-9 – pancreatic CA
  CA 125 – ovarian CA
  Beta-HCG – testicular CA, choriocarcinoma
  PSA – prostate CA (thought to be the tumor marker with the **highest sensitivity**)
  NSE – small cell lung CA, neuroblastoma
  BRCA I and II – breast CA
  Half-lives – CEA: 18 days; PSA: 18 days; AFP: 5 days

Oncogenesis
  Cancer transformation
    Heritable alteration in genome
    Loss of growth regulation
  Latency period – time between exposure and formation of clinically detectable tumor
  Initiation – carcinogen acts with DNA
  Promotion of cancer cells
  Progression of cancer cells to clinically detectable tumor

  Neoplasms can arise from **carcinogenesis** (smoking), **viruses** (EBV), or **immunodeficiency** (HIV).
  Retroviruses contain oncogenes
    Epstein-Barr virus – associated with Burkitt's lymphoma (8:14 translocation) and nasopharyngeal CA (c-myc)
  Proto-oncogenes are human genes with malignant potential.

Radiation therapy (XRT)
  M phase – most vulnerable stage of cell cycle for XRT
  Most damage done by formation of **oxygen radicals** → maximal effect with **high oxygen levels**
  Main target is **DNA** – oxygen radicals cause damage of DNA and other molecules
  XRT itself can also cause some damage by causing small breaks in DNA

  Higher-energy radiation has skin-preserving effect (maximal ionizing potential not reached until deeper structures).
  Fractionate doses
    Allows **repair** of normal cells
    Allows **reoxygenation** of tumor
    Allows **redistribution** of tumor cells in cell cycle

  Very radiosensitive tumors – **seminomas, lymphomas**
  Very radioresistant tumors – **epithelial, sarcomas**
  Kidneys, lungs, liver, and lymphocytes have increased sensitivity to XRT.

Large tumors – less responsive to XRT due to lack of oxygen in the tumor
Brachytherapy – source of radiation in or next to tumor (Au-198, I-128); delivers high, concentrated doses of radiation

Chemotherapy agents
Cell cycle–specific agents (5FU, methotrexate) – exhibit plateau in cell-killing ability
Cell cycle–nonspecific agents – linear response to cell killing

Tamoxifen (blocks estrogen receptor) – decreases short-term risk of breast CA by 45%
   1% risk of blood clots
   1% risk of endometrial CA
Taxol promotes microtubule formation and stabilization that cannot be broken down; cells are ruptured
Bleomycin and busulfan – can cause pulmonary fibrosis

Cisplatin (platinum alkylating agent) – nephrotoxic, neurotoxic, ototoxic
Carboplatin (platinum alkylating agent) – **bone** (myelo) suppression

Vincristine (microtubule inhibitor) – peripheral neuropathy, neurotoxic
Vinblastine (microtubule inhibitor) – **bone** (myelo) suppression

Alkylating agents – transfer alkyl groups; form covalent bond
   Cyclophosphamide – acrolein is the active metabolite
      Side effects: gonadal dysfunction, SIADH, hemorrhagic cystitis
      Mesna can help with hemorrhagic cystitis.
   Isofosfamide
Levamisole – **anthelminthic drug** thought to stimulate immune system against cancer
Methotrexate – inhibits dihydrofolate reductase (DHFR), which inhibits purine and DNA synthesis
   Side effects: renal toxicity, radiation recall
   Leucovorin rescue – ↓ folate (tetrahydrofolic acid); reverses effects of methotrexate
5-Fluorouracil (5FU) – inhibits thymidalate synthesis, which inhibits purine and DNA synthesis
   Leucovorin – ↑ toxicity of 5FU
Doxorubicin – DNA intercalator, O_2 radical formation
   Heart toxicity secondary to O_2 radicals at >500 mg/m^2
Etoposide (VP-16) – inhibits topoisomerase (which normally unwinds DNA)

Least myelosuppression – bleomycin, vincristine, busulfan, cisplatin
GCSF (granulocyte colony-stimulating factor) – used for neutrophil recovery after chemo
   Side effects: Sweet's syndrome (acute febrile neutropenic dermatitis)

Resection of a normal organ to prevent cancer
   Colon – FAP
   Breast – BRCA I or II with strong family history
   Thyroid – RET proto-oncogene or MENIN gene with family history of MEN or thyroid CA

Tumor suppressor genes
   Retinoblastoma (Rb1) – chromosome 13; involved in **cell cycle**
   p53 – chromosome 17; involved in **cell cycle** (normal gene induces cell cycle arrest and apoptosis; abnormal gene allows unrestrained cell growth)
   APC – chromosome 5; involved with **cell adhesion and cytoskeleton function**
   DCC – chromosome 18; involved in **cell adhesion**
   bcl – involved in **apoptosis** (programmed cell death)
   BRCA

Proto-oncogenes
   ras proto-oncogene – G protein defect
   src proto-oncogene – tyrosine kinase defect
   sis proto-oncogene – platelet-derived growth factor receptor defect
   erb B proto-oncogene – epidermal growth factor receptor defect
   myc (c-myc, n-myc, l-myc) proto-oncogenes – nuclear factors

LiFraumeni syndrome – defect in p53 gene → patients get childhood sarcomas, breast CA, brain tumors, leukemia, adrenal CA
Medullary CA of the thyroid (see also Chap. 22, Thyroid)
    Associated with Ret proto-oncogene (chromosome 10)
    Patients with Ret gene defect plus family history → 90% get medullary CA of thyroid; need prophylactic total thyroidectomy
    MENIN gene also associated with thyroid medullary CA

Colon CA
Genes involved in development include **APC, p53, DCC, and K-ras**.
APC involved in cell adhesion and cytoskeleton function – thought to be the initial mutation in the development of colon CA
Colon CA does not go to bone.

Carcinogens
Coal tar – larynx, skin, bronchial CA
Beta-naphthylamine – urinary tract CA (bladder CA)
Benzene – leukemia
Asbestos – mesothelioma

Cancer spread
Suspicious supraclavicular nodes – breast, lung, stomach (Virchow's node), pancreas
Suspicious axillary node – lymphoma (#1), breast, melanoma
Suspicious periumbilical node – pancreas (Sister Mary Joseph's node)
Ovarian metastases – stomach (Krukenberg tumor), colon
Bone metastases – breast (#1), prostate
Skin metastases – breast, melanoma
Small bowel metastases – melanoma (#1)

Clinical trials
Phase I – is it safe and at what dose?
Phase II – is it effective?
Phase III – is it better than existing therapy?
Phase IV – implementation and marketing

Types of therapy
Induction – sole treatment; often used for advanced disease or when no other treatment exists
Primary (neoadjuvant) – chemotherapy given 1st, followed by another (secondary) therapy
Adjuvant – combined with another modality; given after other therapy is used
Salvage – for tumors that fail to respond to initial chemotherapy

Lymph nodes have poor barrier function → better to view them as signs of **probable metastasis**

En bloc multiorgan resection can be attempted for some tumors (colon into uterus, adrenal into liver, gastric into diaphragm).
Aggressive local invasiveness is different from metastatic disease.

Palliative surgery – tumors of hollow viscus causing obstruction or bleeding (colon CA), pancreatic CA with biliary obstruction, breast CA with skin or chest wall involvement
Sentinel lymph node biopsy – no role in patients with clinically palpable nodes; you need to go after and sample these nodes

Colon metastases to the liver – 25% 5-year survival rate if successfully resected

Most successfully cured metastases with surgery – colon CA in liver, sarcoma to the lung, melanoma to lung; <u>but</u> survival still low overall for these
Ovarian CA – one of the few tumors for which **surgical debulking** improves chemotherapy (not seen in other tumors)
Curable solid tumors with chemotherapy only – Hodgkin's disease, non-Hodgkin's lymphoma
Most lymphomas are **B cell**.
T-cell lymphomas – HTLV-1 (skin lesions), mycosis fungoides (Sezary cells)
HIV-related malignancies – Kaposi's sarcoma, non-Hodgkin's lymphoma

CHAPTER 12. TRANSPLANTATION

Transplant immunology
  HLA-A, -B, and -DR – most important in recipient/donor matching
  HLA-DR – most important overall
  ABO blood compatibility – required for all transplants (except liver)

  Crossmatch
    Detects preformed recipient antibodies by mixing recipient serum with donor lymphocytes → would cause **hyperacute rejection**
    Required for all transplants

  Panel reactive antibody (PRA)
    Techniques identical to crossmatch; detects preformed recipient antibodies using a panel of typing cells
    Get a percentage of cells that the serum reacts with
    Transfusions, pregnancy, previous transplant, and autoimmune diseases can all increase PRA.

  Mild rejection – pulse steroids
  Severe or secondary rejection – OKT3 or other drugs

  Skin cancer – #1 malignancy following any transplant (squamous cell CA #1)

  Posttransplant lymphoproliferative disorder (PTLD) – next most common malignancy following transplant – **Epstein-Barr virus related**
    Tx: withdrawal of immunosuppression; may need chemotherapy and XRT for aggressive tumor

Drugs
  Azathioprine (Imuran)
    Inhibits de novo purine synthesis, which inhibits T cells
    6-mercaptopurine is the active metabolite (formed in the liver).
    Side effects: myelosuppression
    Keep WBCs >3

  Mycophenalate – similar action to azathioprine

  Steroids – inhibit genes for cytokine synthesis (IL-1, IL-6) and macrophages

  Cyclosporin (CSA)
    Binds **cyclophilin protein** and inhibits genes for cytokine synthesis (IL-2, IL-3, IL-4, INF-gamma)
    Side effects: nephrotoxicity, hepatotoxicity, HUS, tremors, seizures
    Keep trough 200–300
    Undergoes **hepatic metabolism and biliary excretion**

  FK-506 (Prograf)
    Binds **FK binding protein**; actions similar to CSA but 10–100x more potent
    Side effects: nephrotoxicity, mood changes; more GI and neurologic changes than CSA
    Keep trough 10–15

  ATGAM
    Equine polyclonal antibodies directed against antigens on T cells (CD2, CD3, CD4, CD8, CD11/18)
    Used for induction therapy
    Complement dependent
    Keep peripheral T cell count >3

  Thymoglobulin
    Rabbit polyclonal antibodies
    Similar action as ATGAM

OKT3
Monoclonal antibodies that block antigen recognition function of T cells by binding CD3, inhibiting T cell receptor complex
Interferes with both class I and II MHC
Cause CD3 opsonization that is complement dependent
Used for severe rejection
Follow peripheral CD3 cells
Side effects: fever, chills, pulmonary edema, shock

Zenepax – human monoclonal antibody against IL-2 receptors
Used with induction and to treat rejection

Types of rejection
Hyperacute rejection (occurs within minutes to hours)
Caused by preformed antibodies that should have been picked up by the crossmatch
Activates the complement cascade and thrombosis of vessels occurs
Tx: emergent retransplant
Accelerated rejection (occurs <1 week)
Caused by sensitized T cells to donor antigens
Produces a secondary immune response
Tx: ↑ immunosuppression, pulse steroids, and possibly OKT3
Acute rejection (occurs 1 week to 1 month)
Caused by T cells (cytotoxic and helper T cells)
Tx: ↑ immunosuppression, pulse steroids, and possibly OKT3
Chronic rejection (months to years)
Partially a type IV hypersensitivity reaction (sensitized T cells)
Antibody formation also plays a role; leads to graft fibrosis and vascular damage
Monocytes and cytotoxic T cells have a role
Tx: ↑ immunosuppression or OKT3 – no really effective treatment

Kidney transplantation
Can store kidney for 48 hours
Need ABO type and crossmatch
UTI – can still use kidney
Acute ↑ in creatinine (1.0–3.0) – can still use kidney
Mortality primarily from **stroke and MI**
Attach to **iliac vessels**

Complications
Urine leaks (#1) – Tx: drainage and stenting usually first; may need reoperation
Renal artery stenosis – diagnose with ultrasound
  Tx: PTA with stent
Lymphocoele – most common cause of external compression
  Tx: 1st **percutaneous drainage**; if that fails then need **intraperitoneal marsupialization** (90% successful)
Postop oliguria – usually due to ATN (pathology shows hydrophobic changes)
Postop diuresis – usually due to urea and glucose
New proteinuria – suggestive of renal vein thrombosis
Postop diabetes – side effect of CSA, FK, steroids
Viral infections – **CMV** – Tx: gangciclovir; **HSV** – Tx: acyclovir

Acute rejection – usually occurs in 1st 6 months; pathology shows tubulitis or vasculitis with more severe form
Kidney rejection workup – usually for ↑ in Cr
  Ultrasound with duplex (to rule out vascular problem and ureteral obstruction) and biopsy; empiric ↓ in CSA or FK (these can be nephrotoxic); pulse steroids
Chronic rejection – usually don't see until after 1 year; no good treatment
5-year graft survival overall – 70% (cadaveric 65%, living donors 75%)

Living kidney donors
Most common complication – wound infection (1%)
Most common cause of death – fatal PE
The remaining kidney hypertrophies.

Liver transplantation
Can store for 24 hours
Need crossmatch only
Contraindications to liver TXP – **current ETOH abuse, acute ulcerative colitis**
Chronic hepatitis – most common reason for liver TXP in adults
Criteria for emergent TXP – **stage III (stupor), stage IV (coma)**
Patients with hepatitis B antigenemia can be treated with **HBIG (hepatitis B immunoglobulin) and lamivudine (protease inhibitor)** postoperatively
Hepatocellular CA – if single tumor <5 cm or up to 3 tumors each <3 cm, can still consider TXP
Portal vein thrombosis – not a contraindication to TXP
APACHE score – best predictor of 1-year survival

Hepatitis C – disease most likely to recur in the new liver allograft; reinfects essentially all grafts
Hepatitis B – reinfection rate has been reduced to 20% with use of HBIG

ETOH – 20% will start drinking again (recidivism)
Macrosteatosis – extracellular fat globules in the liver allograft
    #1 predictor of primary nonfunction
    If 50% of cross section is macrosteatatic in potential donor live, there's a 50% chance of primary nonfunction.

Duct-to-duct anastamosis is performed.
Hepaticojejunostomy in kids
Right subhepatic, right and left subdiaphragmatic drains
Biliary system (ducts, etc) depends on **hepatic artery** blood supply.
Most common arterial anomaly – **right hepatic coming off SMA**

Complications
Bile leak (#1) – Tx: PTC tube and stent
Primary nonfunction
    1st 24 hours – total bilirubin >10, bile output <20 cc/12 hr, PT and PTT 1.5x normal
    After 96 hours – hyperkalemia, mental status changes, ↑ LFTs, renal failure, respiratory failure
    Usually requires retransplantation
Hepatic artery thrombosis – Tx: angio (potentially treated with angiography and balloon dilatation +/− stent), surgery
    Hepatic vein thrombosis rare
Abscesses – most common from hepatic artery thrombosis
IVC stenosis – edema, ascities, renal insufficiency
Cholangitis – get PMNs around portal triad, <u>not</u> mixed infiltrate

Acute rejection – T cell mediated against blood vessels
    Clinical – fever, jaundice, ↓ bile output, change in bile consistency
    Labs – leukocytosis, eosinophilia, ↑ LFTs, total bilirubin, and PT
    Pathology – shows **portal lymphocytosis, endothelitis (mixed infiltrate), and bile duct injury**
    Usually occurs in 1st 2 months
Chronic rejection – disappearing bile ducts (antibody and cellular attack on bile ducts); gradually get bile duct obstruction with ↑ in alkaline phosphatase, portal fibrosis
Acute rejection most common predictor

Retransplantation rate – 20%
5-year survival rate – 70%

Pancreas transplantation
Need **donor celiac and SMA** for arterial supply
Need **donor portal vein** for venous drainage
Attach to iliac vessels
Most use **enteric drainage** for pancreatic duct. Take second portion of duodenum from donor along with ampulla of Vater and pancreas, then perform anastomosis of donor duodenum to recipient bowel.

Successful pancreas/kidney TXP results in stabilization of retinopathy, ↓ neuropathy, ↑ nerve conduction velocity, ↓ autonomic dysfunction (gastroparesis), ↓ orthostatic hypotension
No reversal of vascular disease

Complications
  Thrombosis (#1) – hard to treat
  Rejection – hard to diagnose if patient does not also have a kidney transplant
    Can see ↑ glucose, amylase, or trypsinogen; fever, leukocytosis

Heart transplantation
Can store for 6 hours
Need ABO compatibility and crossmatch
For patients with life expectancy <1 year
Persistent pulmonary hypertension after heart transplantation
  Tx: Flolan (PGI$_2$); ECMO if severe
  Associated with ↑ morbidity and mortality after heart TXP
Acute rejection – shows perivascular infiltrate with ↑ grades of myocyte inflammation and necrosis
Chronic rejection – progressive diffuse coronary **atherosclerosis**

Lung transplantation
Can store 6 hours
Need ABO compatibility and crossmatch
For patients with life expectancy <1 year
#1 cause of early mortality – **reperfusion injury**
Indication for double-lung TXP – **cystic fibrosis**
Exclusion criteria for using lungs – aspiration, moderate to large contusion, infiltrate, purulent sputum, PO$_2$ < 350 on 100% FiO$_2$ and PEEP 5
Acute rejection – perivascular lympocytosis
Chronic rejection – **bronchiolitis obliterans**

Opportunistic infection
Viral – CMV, HSV, VZV
Protozoan – *Pneumocystis jeroveci* (*P. carinii*) pneumonia (reason for Bactrim prophylaxis)
Fungal – *Aspergillus, Candida, Cryptococcus*

CHAPTER 13. INFLAMMATION AND CYTOKINES

Inflammation phases
    Injury – leads to exposed <u>collagen</u>, <u>platelet activating factor</u> release, <u>tissue factor</u> release from endothelium
    Platelets bind – release important growth factors, including <u>TGF-beta and PDGF</u>; leads to PMN, macrophage recruitment
    Macrophages – dominant role in wound healing, release important growth factors (TGF-beta and PDGF) and cytokines (IL-1 and TNF-alpha)

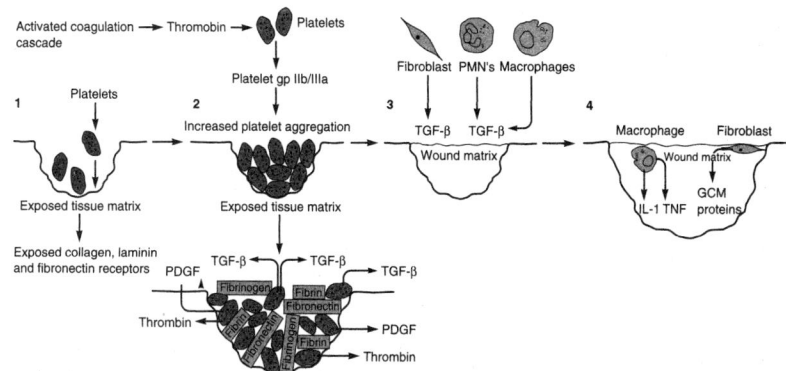

Establishment of a provisional wound matrix. (1) Platelets bind to exposed wound matrix through interaction of beta-1 and beta-3 integrins and collagen, laminin, and fibrinonectin receptors. (2) After wounding, the coagulation cascade is activated, generating thrombin, which activates platelet glycoprotein (gp) IIb/IIIa and increases platelet aggregation. A provisional wound matrix is formed, made up of platelets, fibrin, fibrinogen, and fibronectin. The activated platelets in the wound generate transforming growth factor-beta (TGF-β), platelet-derived growth factor (PDGF), and thrombin. (3) TGF-beta is strongly chemotactic for neutrophils, macrophages, and fibroblasts, recruiting these cells into the provisional wound matrix, where they are also subsequently activated by TGF-beta. (4) Increasing concentrations of TGF-beta result in macrophage activation, producing increased amounts of tumor necrosis factor-alpha (TGF-α) and interleukin-1 (IL-1). TGF-beta also stimulates fibroblast production of extracellular matrix proteins. These reactions further enhance migration of macrophages and fibroblasts into the wound, facilitating repair.

Growth and activating factors
    TGF-beta (transforming growth factor-beta) – <u>key component of tissue repair</u>
        First released by platelets but eventually released by many types of cells
        Chemotactic and activates inflammatory cells (PMNs and macrophages)
        Chemotactic and activates fibroblasts → collagen and extracellular matrix (ECM) proteins
        Angiogenesis
        Epithelialization
        Overproduction can result in fibrosis

    PDGF (platelet-derived growth factor) – similar effect as TGF-beta
        Chemotactic and activates inflammatory cells (PMNs and macrophages)
        Chemotactic and activates fibroblasts → collagen and ECM proteins
        Angiogenesis
        Epithelialization
        Chemotactic for smooth muscle cells
        Has been shown to accelerate wound healing

    EGF (epidermal growth factor) – acts on similar receptors as TGF-beta; less potent
        Chemotactic and activates fibroblasts → collagen and ECM proteins
        Angiogenesis – V-EGF stimulates angiogenesis and is involved in tumor metastasis
        Epithelialization

FGF (fibroblastic growth factor)
    Chemotactic and activates fibroblasts → collagen and ECM proteins
    Angiogenesis
    Epithelialization

PAF (platelet-activating factor) – not stored, generated by **phospholipase** in endothelium and other cells
    Stimulates many types of inflammatory cells; chemotactic; ↑ adhesion molecules

Chemotactic factors
    For inflammatory cells – TGF-beta, PDGF, IL-8, LTB-4, C5a and C3a, PAF
    For fibroblasts – TGF-beta, PDGF, EGF, FGF
Angiogenesis factors – TGF-beta, EGF, FGF, TGF-alpha, IL-8, hypoxia
Epithelialization factors – TGF-beta, PDGF, EGF, FGF, TGF-alpha

PMNs – last 1–2 days in tissues
Platelets – last 7–10 days
Lymphocytes – involved in chronic inflammation (T cells), and antibody production (B cells)

TXA_2 and PGI_2 – see Chap. 2, Hematology

Cell types in type I hypersensitivity reactions
Eosinophils – primary effectors in **type I hypersensitivity reactions** (allergic reactions)
    Have IgE receptors that bind to allergen
    Release major basic protein, which stimulates basophils and mast cells to release histamine
    Eosinophils increased in parasitic infections
Basophils – have IgE receptors
    Main source of histamine in **blood**; not found in tissue
Mast cells – primary cell in **type I hypersensitivity reactions**
    Main source of histamine in **tissues** other than stomach

Histamine – vasodilation, tissue edema, postcapillary leakage
Bradykinin – vasodilation, increased permeability, pain, contraction of pulmonary arterioles
    Angiotensin-converting enzyme (ACE) – inactivates bradykinin

Nitric oxide (NO)
Has arginine precursor
Activates guanylate cyclase and increases cGMP, resulting in vascular smooth muscle dilation
Is also called endothelium-derived relaxing factor (EDRF)
Endothelin – vascular smooth muscle constriction

Important cytokines
Main initial cytokine response to injury and infection is release of **TNF-alpha and IL-1**.
Tumor necrosis factor-alpha (TNF-alpha)
    Macrophages – largest producers of TNF
    Increases adhesion molecules
    Overall, a procoagulant
    Causes cachexia in patients with cancer
    Activates neutrophils and macrophages → more cytokine production, cell recruitment
        Can also cause myocardial depression
    Fever, hypothermia, tachycardia, ↑ cardiac output, ↓ SVRI → high concentrations can cause circulatory collapse and multisystem organ failure
IL-1
    Main source also macrophages; effects similar to TNF and synergizes TNF
    Responsible for **fever** (PGE_2 mediated in hypothalamus)
        Raises thermal setpoint, causing fever
        NSAIDs ↓ fever, reducing PGE_2 synthesis.
    Alveolar macrophages – cause fever with atelectasis by **releasing IL-1**
    IL-1 also increases IL-6 production

IL-6
    ↑ **hepatic acute phase proteins** (C-reactive protein, amyloid A)
    Lymphocyte activation

Interferons
    Released by **lymphocytes** in response to viral infection or other stimulates
    Activate macrophages, natural killer cells, and cytotoxic T cells
    Inhibit viral replication

Hepatic acute phase response proteins
    IL-6 – most potent stimulus
    Increased – C-reactive protein (an opsonin, activates complement), amyloid A and P, fibrinogen, haptoglobin, ceruloplasmin, alpha-1 antitrypsin, alpha-1 antichymotrypsin and C3 (complement)
    Decreased – albumin and transferrin

Cell adhesion molecules
    Selectins – L-selectins, located on leukocytes, bind to E- (endothelial) and P- (platelets) selectins; rolling adhesion
    Beta-2 integrins (CD 11/18 molecules) – on leukocytes; bind ICAMs, etc, anchoring adhesion
    ICAM, VCAM, PECAM, ELAM – on endothelial cells, bind beta-2 integrin molecules located on leukocytes and platelets

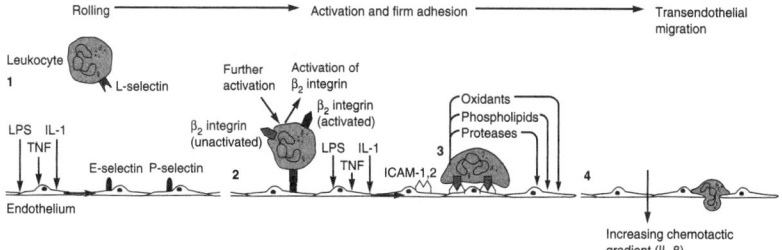

Neutrophil recruitment and activation into areas of inflammation. (1) Selectins mediate early loose adhesion or "rolling." This is a low-affinity adherence between constituitively expressed L-selectin on the neutrophil and E-selectin or P-selectin on the activated vascular endothelium. (2) This rolling slows the neutrophil enough to allow it to be activated, with expression and activation of beta-2 integrins on the cell surface. Further activation of the endothelium by TNF, IL-1, or LPS leads to increased expression of ICAM-1 and ICAM-2, with subsequent firm adherence of the neutrophil to the endothelium. This is mediated through ICAM–beta-2 integrin interaction. (3) The activated adherent neutrophil can then release proteases, oxidants, and phospholipids, resulting in endothelial cell injury and increased microvascular permeability. (4) Neutrophils then diapedese into the extra-vascular space via established chemotactic gradients. PECAM-1 may be important in transendothelial migration.

Complement
    Classic pathway (IgG or IgM) – antigen–antibody complex activates
        Factors C1, C2, and C4 – found only in the classic pathway
    Alternative pathway – endotoxin, bacteria, other stimuli activate
        Factors B, D, and P (properdin) – found only in the alternate pathway
    C3 – common to and is the convergence point for both pathways
    Mg – required for both pathways
    Anaphylatoxins – C3a, C4a, C5a; ↑ vascular permeability, smooth muscle contraction (bronchi); activate mast cells and basophils
    Membrane attack complex – C5b–9b
    Opsonization – C3b
    Chemotaxis – C3a and C5a

Prostaglandins
PGI$_2$ and PGE$_2$ – vasodilation, bronchodilation, ↑ permeability; inhibit platelets
PGD$_2$ – vasodilation, bronchoconstriction, ↑ permeability

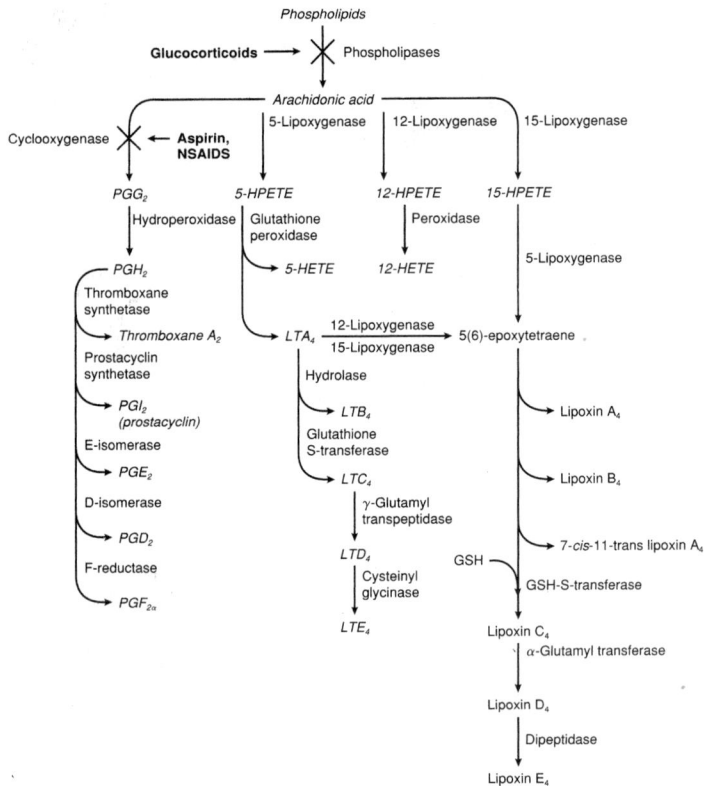

Pathways of eicosanoid production. Inflammatory mediators derived from arachidonic acid. NSAIDs, nonsteroidal anti-inflammatory drugs (e.g., ibuprofen).

NSAIDs – inhibit cyclooxygenase (reversible)
Aspirin – inhibits cyclooxygenase (irreversible), inhibits platelet adhesion by decreasing TXA$_2$
Steroids – inhibit phospholipase, which converts phospholipids to arachadonic acid → inhibits inflammation

Leukotrienes
LTC$_4$, LTD$_4$, LTE$_4$ – <u>slow-reacting substances of anaphylaxis</u>; bronchoconstriction, vasoconstriction followed by increased permeability (wheal and flare)
LTB$_4$ – chemotactic

Catecholamines
Peak 24–48 hours after injury
Norepinephrine released from sympathetic postganglionic neurons and epinephrine released from adrenal medulla (neural response to injury)

Chapter 13. Inflammation and Cytokines

Neuroendocrine response to injury – afferent nerves from site of injury stimulate CRF, ACTH, ADH, growth hormone, epinephrine, and norepinephrine release
Thyroid hormone – does not play a major role in injury

CXC chemokines – chemotaxis, angiogenesis, wound healing
 IL-8 and platelet factor 4 are CXC chemokines.
 C = cysteine X → another amino acid

Oxidants generated in inflammation

$O_2 + 1e^- \xrightarrow[\text{oxidase}]{\text{NADPH}} O_2^{\bullet-}$ Superoxide anion

$2H^+ + O_2^{\bullet-} + O_2^{\bullet-} \xrightarrow[\text{or superoxide dismutase}]{\text{spontaneous}} O_2 + H_2O_2$ Hydrogen peroxide

$H_2O_2 + +Fe^{2+} \rightarrow Fe^{3+} + OH^- + OH\bullet$ Hydroxyl radical

$H_2O_2 + Cl^- + H^+ \xrightarrow{\text{myeloperoxidase}} H_2O + HOCl$ Hypochlorous acid

$R'RNH + HOCl \rightarrow H_2O + R'RNCl$ Chloramines

Cellular defenses against antioxidants

$H_2O_2 + 2\,GSH \xrightarrow{\pm \text{GSH peroxidase}} 2H_2O_2 + GSSG$

$ROOH + 2\,GSH \xrightarrow{\text{GSH peroxidase}} ROH + GSSG + H_2O$

$GSSG \xrightarrow[\text{GSH reductase}]{\text{NADPH}} 2GSH$

$O_2^{\bullet-} + O_2^{\bullet-} + 2H^+ \xrightarrow[\text{dismutase}]{\text{superoxide}} O_2 + H_2O_2$

Red blood cells – have some antioxidant properties (superoxide dismutase and catalase)
Reperfusion injury – **PMNs** are the primary mediator
Chronic granulomatous disease – NADPH-oxidase system enzyme defect in PMNs
 Results in ↓ superoxide radical (O_2^-) formation

CHAPTER 14. WOUND HEALING

Wound healing phases
    Inflammation (days 1–10) – PMNs, macrophages; epithelialization 1–2 mm/day
    Proliferation (5 days to 3 weeks) – fibroblasts, neovascularization, production of collagen, granulation tissue
    Remodeling (3 weeks to 1 year) – type III collagen replaced with type I; decreased vascularity
        Net amount of collagen does not change, although significant production and degradation occurs
        Collagen cross-linking occurs
    Peripheral nerves regenerate at **1 mm/day**.

Order of cell arrival in wound
    Platelets
    PMNs
    Macrophages
    Fibroblasts
    Lymphocytes

Macrophages are essential for wound healing (release of growth factors, cytokines, etc).
Fibroblasts – replace fibronectin-fibrin with **collagen**
Fibronectin – chemotactic for macrophages; anchors fibroblasts
Thrombin and fibrin – also act as growth factors for endothelial cells and fibroblasts
Predominant cell type by day
    Days 0–2 – PMNs
    Days 3–4 – macrophages
    Days 5 and on – fibroblasts
Platelet plug – platelets and fibrin
Provisional matrix – platelets, fibrin, and fibronectin
Accelerated wound healing – reopening a wound results in quicker healing the 2nd time (healing cells there already)

Platelet granules
    Alpha granules
        Platelet factor 4 – aggregation
        Beta-thrombomodulin – binds thrombin
        PDGF – chemoattractant
        TGF-beta – key component of tissue repair
    Dense granules – adenosine, serotonin, and calcium
    Platelet aggregation factors – **TXA$_2$, thrombin, platelet factor 4**
    Other factor released from platelets
        Platelet-activating factor
        Transforming growth factor-alpha
        Fibroblast growth factor
        Beta lysin (antimicrobial)
        PGE$_2$ and PGI$_2$ (vasodilators)
        PGF$_2$ (vasoconstriction)

Epithelial integrity – most important factor in healing **open wounds (secondary intention)**
    <u>Migration</u> from wound edges, sweat glands, and hair follicles
    Dependent on granulation tissue
    Unepithelialized wounds leak serum and protein, promote bacteria

Tensile strength – most important factor in healing **closed incisions (primary intention)**
    Depends on collagen deposition and cross-linking of collagen
    Submucosa – strength layer of bowel
    Weakest time point for small bowel anastamosis – 3–5 days

Myofibroblasts (smooth muscle cell–fibroblast, communicate by gap junctions) – involved in wound contraction and **healing by secondary intention**
    Perineum has better wound contraction than leg.

Chapter 14. Wound Healing

Collagen

Type	Description
I	Most common type of collagen: skin, bone, and tendons Primary collagen in a healed wound
II	Cartilage
III	Increased in healing wound, also in blood vessels and skin
IV	Basement membranes
V	Widespread, particularly found in the cornea

Alpha-ketoglutarate, vitamin C, oxygen, and iron are required for <u>hydroxylation of proline</u> (prolyl hydroxylase) and subsequent <u>cross-linking of proline residues</u>.
Hydroxylysine also undergoes cross-linking.
Collagen – has **proline every 3rd amino acid**; also has abundant **lysine**
Scurvy – vitamin C deficiency

Tensile strength never equal to prewound (80%)
    Type III collagen – predominant collagen type synthesized for days 1–2
    Type I collagen – predominant collagen type synthesized by day 3–4
    Type III replaced by type I collagen by 3 weeks
        At 6 weeks, wound is 80% of its final strength and 60% of its original strength.
        At 8 weeks, wound reaches maximum tensile strength, which is 80% of its original strength.
        Maximum collagen accumulation at 2–3 weeks after that → the amount of collagen stays the same but continued cross-linking improves strength
        d-Penicillamine – inhibits collagen cross-linking

Essentials for wound healing
    Moist environment (avoid desiccation)
    Oxygen delivery – optimal fluids, no smoking, pain control, arterial reconstruction, supplemental oxygen
        Want transcutaneous oxygen measurement (TCOM) >25 mmHg
    Avoid edema – leg elevation, compression
    Remove necrotic tissue

Impediments to wound healing
    Bacteria >10^5/cm^2 – ↓ oxygen content, collagen lysis, prolonged inflammation
    Devitalized tissue and foreign bodies – retards granulation tissue formation and wound healing
    Cytotoxic drugs – 5FU, methotrexate, cyclosporine, FK-506, etc, can impair wound healing
    Diabetes – can contribute to poor wound healing by impeding the early-phase response
    Albumin <3.0 – risk factor for poor wound healing
    Steroids – prevent wound healing by inhibiting macrophages, PMNs, and collagen synthesis by fibroblasts; ↓ wound tensile strength as well
        Vitamin A (25,000 IU qd) – counteracts effects of steroids on wound healing

Diseases associated with abnormal wound healing
    Osteogensis imperfecta – type I collage defect
    Ehlers-Danlos syndrome – 10 types identified, all collagen disorders
    Marfan's syndrome – fibrillin (collagen) defect
    Epidermolysis bullosa – excessive fibroblasts. Tx: phenytoin
    Scurvy
    Pyoderma gangrenosum

Diabetic foot ulcers – Charcot's joint (2nd MTP joint); secondary to neuropathy
    Pressure leads to ischemia
Leg ulcers – 90% of leg ulcers due to venous insufficiency. Tx: Unna boot, elastic wrap
Pressure sores – see Chap. 18, Plastics, Skin, and Soft Tissues
Scars – contain a lot of proteoglycans, hyaluronic acid, and water
    Scar revisions – wait for 1 year to allow maturation; may improve with age
        Infants heal with little or no scarring.
Cartilage – contains no blood vessels
Denervation – has no effect on wound healing

Chemotherapy – has no effect on wound healing after 14 days
Keloids – autosomal dominant; dark skinned
    Collagen goes beyond original scar.
    Tx: XRT, steroids, silicone, pressure garments
Hypertrophic scar tissue – dark skinned; flexor surfaces of upper torso
    Collagen stays within confines of scar.
    Often occurs in burns or wounds that take a long time to heal
    Tx: steroids, silicone, pressure garments

CHAPTER 15. TRAUMA

1st peak for trauma deaths (0 to 30 minutes) – deaths due to lacerations of heart, aorta, brain, brain stem, spinal cord. Can't really save these patients, death is too quick
2nd peak for trauma deaths (30 minutes to 4 hours) – deaths due to head injury (#1) and hemorrhage (#2). These are the patients you can save with rapid assessment (golden hour).
3rd peak for trauma deaths (days to weeks) – deaths due to multisystem organ failure and sepsis

Blunt injury – 80% of all trauma; liver most commonly injured
　Kinetic energy = $\frac{1}{2} MV^2$, where M = mass, V = velocity
　Falls – age and body orientation biggest predictors of survival. LD_{50} is 4 stories.
Penetrating injury – small bowel most commonly injured
Hemorrhage – most common cause of death in 1st hour
　Blood pressure is usually OK until 30% of total blood volume is lost.
Head injury – most common cause of death after reaching the ER alive
Infection – most common cause of death in the long term
Tongue – most common cause of upper airway obstruction → perform jaw thrust
Seat belts – small bowel perforations, lumbar spine fractures, sternal fractures
Saphenous vein at ankle – best site for cutdown for access

Diagnostic peritoneal lavage (DPL)
　Used in hypotensive patients with blunt trauma
　Positive if >10 cc blood, >100,000 RBCs/cc, food particles, bile, bacteria, >500 WBC/cc
　Need laparotomy if DPL is positive
　DPL needs to be supraumbilical if pelvic fracture present.
　DPL misses – retroperitoneal bleeds, contained hematomas

FAST scan (focused abdominal sonography for trauma)
　Ultrasound scan used in lieu of DPL
　Checks for blood in perihepatic fossa, perisplenic fossa, pelvis, and pericardium
　Examiner dependent
　Obesity can obstruct view.
　May not detect free fluid <50–80 ml
　Need laparotomy if FAST scan is positive
　FAST scan misses – retroperitoneal bleeding, hollow viscous injury

Need a CT scan following blunt trauma in patients with abdominal pain, need for general anesthesia, closed head injury, intoxicants on board, paraplegia, distracting injury, hematuria.
　Patients requiring DPL that turned out negative will need an abdominal CT scan.
　CT scan misses – hollow viscous injury, diaphragm injury

Need laparotomy with peritonitis, evisceration, positive DPL, clinical deterioration, uncontrolled hemorrhage, free air, diaphragm injury, intraperitoneal bladder injury, positive contrast studies, specific renal, pancreas, and biliary tract injuries

Possible penetrating abdominal injuries – local exploration and observation if fascia not violated
　Can also go with diagnostic laparoscopy to see if fascia was violated

Abdominal compartment syndrome
　Occurs after massive fluid resuscitation, trauma, or abdominal surgery
　Bladder pressure >25–30
　IVC compression is final common pathway for ↓ cardiac output.
　Gut malperfusion
　Renal vein compression leading to ↓ urine output
　Upward displacement of diaphragm affecting ventilation
　Tx: decompressive laparotomy

Pneumatic antishock garment – controversial; use in patients with SBP <50 and no thoracic injury.
　Release compartments one at a time after reaching ER.

ER thoracotomy
　Blunt trauma – use only if pressure/pulse lost **in ER**
　Penetrating trauma – use only if pressure/pulse lost **on way to ER or in ER**

Catecholamines – peak 24–48 hours after injury
ADH, ACTH, and glucagon – also ↑ after trauma (fight or flight response)

Head injury (see also Chap. 41, Neurosurgery)
Glasgow Coma Scale (GCS)
Motor
  6 – follows commands
  5 – localizes pain
  4 – withdraws from pain
  3 – flexion with pain (decorticate)
  2 – extension with pain (decerebrate)
  1 – no response
Verbal
  5 – oriented
  4 – confused
  3 – inappropriate words
  2 – incomprehensible sounds
  1 – no response
Eye opening
  4 – spontaneous opening
  3 – opens to command
  2 – opens to pain
  1 – no response

GCS score – ≤14: head CT; ≤10: intubation; ≤8: ICP monitor

Epidural hematoma – arterial bleeding from the **middle meningeal artery**
  Head CT – shows lenticular (lens-shaped) deformity
  Patients initially have loss of consciousness (LOC) → then lucid interval → then sudden deterioration (vomiting, restlessness, LOC)
  Operate for significant neurologic degeneration or significant mass effect (shift >5 mm)

Subdural hematoma – most common; tearing of **venous plexus (bridging veins)** between dura and arachnoid
  Head CT – shows crescent-shaped deformity
  Operate for significant mass effect
  Chronic subdural hematomas – usually in elderly after minor fall
    Need drainage if >1 cm or causing significant symptoms

Intracerebral hematoma – usually frontal or temporal
  Can cause significant mass effect requiring operation
Cerebral contusions – can be coup or contracoup
Traumatic intraventricular hemorrhage – need ventriculostomy if causing hydrocephalus
Diffuse axonal injury – shows up better on MRI than CT scan
  Tx: supportive; may need craniectomy if ICP elevated
  Very poor prognosis

Cerebral perfusion pressure (CPP)
CPP = mean arterial pressure (MAP) *minus* intracranial pressure (ICP)
Signs of elevated ICP – ↓ ventricular size, loss of sulci, loss of cisterns
ICP monitors – indicated for GCS ≤8, suspected ↑ ICP, or patient with moderate to severe head injury and inability to follow clinical exam (e.g., is intubated)

Supportive treatment for elevated ICP
Normal ICP is 10; >20 needs treatment
Want cerebral perfusion pressure >60
  Sedation and paralysis
  Raise head of bed
  Relative hyperventilation for modest cerebral vasoconstriction (CO_2 30–35); don't want to overhyperventilate and cause cerebral ischemia from too much vasoconstriction
  Keep Na 140–150, serum Osm 295–310 – may need to use normal saline at times (draws fluid out of brain)

Chapter 15. Trauma

Mannitol – load 1 g/kg, give 0.25 mg/kg q4h after that (draws fluid from brain)
Barbituate coma – consider if above not working
Craniotomy decompression – if not able to get ICP down medically

Phenytoin – given prophylactically to prevent seizures to most patients with traumatic brain injury
Peak intracranial pressure – occurs <u>48–72 hours after injury</u>
Dilated pupil – uncal herniation on same side (CN III compression)

Basal skull fractures
Racoon eyes – anterior fossa fracture
Battle's sign – middle fossa fracture → can injure facial nerve
 If acute, need exploration
 If delayed, likely secondary to edema and exploration not needed
Can also have hemotympanum, CSF rhinorrhea/otorrhea, or injury to CN I, VII, and VIII
Temporal skull fractures – can injure CN VII and VIII
 Most common site of facial nerve injury – geniculate ganglion
 Temporal skull fractures most commonly associated with lateral skull or orbital blows
Most skull fractures do <u>not</u> require surgical treatment
 Operate if significantly depressed (8–10 mm), contaminated, or persistent CSF leak not responding to conservative therapy
CSF leaks – treat expectantly

Spine trauma (see also Chap. 41, Neurosurgery)
Cervical spine
C-1 burst (Jefferson fracture) – caused by axial loading
 Tx: rigid collar
C-2 hangman's fracture – caused by distraction and extension
 Tx: traction and halo
C-2 odontoid fracture
 Type I – above base, stable
 Type II – at base, unstable (will need fusion or halo)
 Type III – extends into vertebral body (will need fusion or halo)
Facet fractures or dislocations – can cause cord injury; usually associated with hyperextension and rotation and with ligamentous disruption

Thoracolumbar spine
3 columns of the thoracolumbar spine
 Anterior – anterior longitudinal ligament and anterior ½ of the vertebral body
 Middle – posterior ½ of the vertebral body and posterior longitudinal ligament
 Posterior – facet joints, lamina, spinous processes, interspinous ligament

If more than 1 column is disrupted, the spine is considered unstable.
 Compression (wedge) fractures usually involve the anterior column only and are considered stable.
 Burst fractures are considered unstable (>1 column) and require spinal fusion.

MRI for neurologic deficits without bony injury to check for ligamentous injury

Indications for emergent surgical spine decompression
Fracture or dislocation not reducible with distraction
Acute anterior spinal syndrome
Open fractures
Soft tissue or bony compression of the cord
Progressive neurologic dysfunction

Maxillofacial trauma
Facial nerve injuries need repair.
Fracture of temporal bone is most common cause of <u>facial nerve injury</u>.
Try to preserve skin and not trim edges with facial lacerations.

Le Fort classification of facial fractures

Type	Description	Treatment
I	Maxillary fracture straight across (–)	Reduction, stabilization, intramaxillary fixation (IMF) +/– circumzygomatic and orbital rim suspension wires
II	Lateral to nasal bone, underneath eyes, diagonal toward maxilla (/ \)	Same as Le Fort I
III	Lateral orbital walls (- -)	Suspension wiring to stable frontal bone; may need external fixation

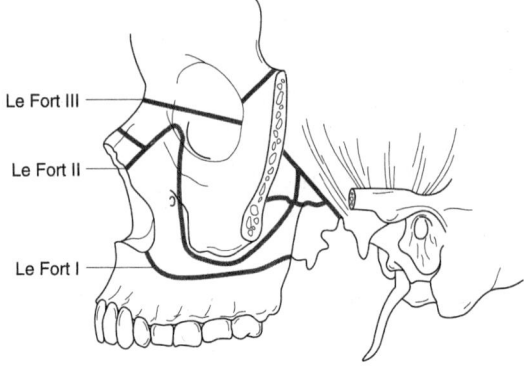

Le Fort classification system of maxillofacial fractures.

Nasoethmoidal orbital fractures – 70% have a CSF leak
  Conservative therapy for 2 weeks
  Can try epidural catheter to ↓ CSF pressure and help it close
  May need surgical closure
Nosebleeds
  Anterior – packing
  Posterior – can be hard to deal with; try balloon tamponade 1st
    May need angioembolization of internal maxillary artery or ethmoidal artery
Orbital blowout fractures – patients with impaired upward gaze or diplopia with upward vision need repair, with restoration of orbital floor with bone fragments or bone graft
Mandibular injury – malocclusion #1 indicator of injury
  Panorex film is often used to assess injury along with fine-cut facial CT scans with reconstruction.
  Most repaired with IMF (metal arch bars to upper and lower dental arches, 6–8 weeks) or open reduction and internal fixation [ORIF])
Tripod fracture (zygomatic bone) – ORIF for cosmesis

Neck trauma
Asymptomatic blunt – neck CT scan
Asymptomatic penetrating – controversial; most common method below

Zone	Method
I	Clavicle to cricoid cartilage; need angiography, bronchoscopy, rigid esophagoscopy, barium swallow. May need sternotomy to reach these lesions
II	Cricoid to angle of mandible. Exploration in OR
III	Angle of mandible to base of skull. Need angio, laryngoscopy. May need jaw subluxation/digastric and sternocleidomastoid muscle release/mastoid sinus resection to reach vascular injuries in this location

Chapter 15. Trauma

Symptomatic blunt or penetrating neck trauma – shock, bleeding, expanding hematoma, losing or lost airway, subcutaneous air, stridor, dysphagia, hemoptysis, neurologic deficit
Need neck exploration.

Esophageal injury
   Hardest neck injury to find
   Rigid esophagoscopy and esophagogram – best combined modality (find essentially 95% of injuries when using both methods)
   Contained injuries – can be observed
   Noncontained injuries – if small injury, <24 hours, without significant contamination, and patient is stable → primary closure; otherwise make spit fistula and drain leak with chest tube
   Always drain esophageal and hypopharyngeal repairs – 20% leak rate
   Approach to esophageal injuries
      Neck – **left side**
      Upper ⅔ of thoracic esophagus – **right thoracotomy**
      Lower ⅓ of the thoracic esophagus – **left thoracotomy**

Laryngeal fracture and tracheal injuries
   These are airway emergencies.
   Symptoms: crepitus, stridor, respiratory compromise
   Need to secure airway emergently in ER
   Tx: primary repair, can use strap muscle for airway support; tracheostomy necessary for most to allow edema to subside and to check for stricture

Thyroid gland injuries – control bleeding and drain
Recurrent laryngeal nerve injury – can try to repair or can reimplant in cricoarytenoid muscle (hoarseness)
Shotgun injures to neck – need angiogram and neck CT
Vertebral artery bleeds – can ligate or embolize without sequela
Common carotid bleeds – ligation will cause stroke in 20%

Chest trauma
Chest tube
   >1500 cc after initial insertion, >250 cc/hr for 3 hours, 2500 cc/24 hr, or bleeding with instability – all relative indications for thoracotomy in OR
   Need to drain all of the blood (in <48 hours) to prevent fibrothorax, pulmonary entrapment, infected hemothorax
   Unresolved hemothorax after 2 well-placed chest tubes → thoracoscopic or open drainage

Sucking chest wound
   Needs to be at least ⅔ the diameter of the trachea to be significant
   Cover wound with dressing that has tape on three sides → prevents development of tension pneumothorax while allowing lung to expand with inspiration

Tracheobronchial injury
   Patient has worse oxygenation after chest tube placement.
   One of the very few indications in which clamping the chest tube may be indicated
   Bronchial injuries are more common on **right**.
   May need to mainstem intubate patient on unaffected side
   Dx: bronchoscopy
   Tx: repair if large air leak and respiratory compromise or after 2 weeks of persistent air leak
   Right thoracotomy for right mainstem, trachea, and proximal left mainstem injuries
   Left thoracotomy for distal left mainstem injuries

Esophageal injury – see section on neck trauma, above

Diaphragm
   Injuries are more likely to be found on **left** and to result from **blunt trauma**.
   CXR – see **air-fluid level** in chest from stomach herniation through hole (diagnosis can be made essentially with CXR)

Transabdominal approach if <1 week
Chest approach if >1 week
May need mesh

Aortic transection
  Signs – widened mediastinum, 1st rib fractures, apical capping, loss of aortopulmonary window, loss of aortic contour, left hemothorax, trachea deviation to right
  Tear is usually at the **ligamentum arteriosum** (just distal to subclavian takeoff). Other areas include near the aortic valve and where the aorta traverses the diaphragm.
  CXR normal in 5% of patients with aortic tears – need aortic evaluation in patients with significant mechanism (head on car crash >45 mph, fall >15 feet)
  Dx: aortogram or CT angiogram of chest
  Tx: need to **control blood pressure** with nipride and esmolol
  Operative approach – left thoracotomy with partial left heart bypass
  Important to treat other life-threatening injuries 1st → patient with positive DPL or other life-threatening injury needs to have that addressed before the aortic transection

Approach for specific injuries
  Median sternotomy – for injuries to ascending aorta, innominate artery, proximal right subclavian artery, innominate vein, proximal left common carotid
  Left thoracotomy – for injuries to left subclavian artery, descending aorta
  Distal right subclavian artery – midclavicular incision +/– resection of medial clavicle

Myocardial contusion – V-tach and V-fib most common causes of death
  Risk highest in 1st 24 hours
  SVT – most common arrhythmia overall in these patients
  Need monitoring

Flail chest – ≥2 consecutive ribs broken at ≥2 sites → results in paradoxical motion
  Underlying pulmonary contusion – biggest pulmonary impairment

Aspiration – may not produce CXR findings immediately

Penetrating chest injury
  Penetrating "box" injuries – borders are clavicles, xyphoid process, nipples
    Need pericardial window, bronchoscopy, esophagoscopy (some say this must be a rigid scope), barium swallow
  Penetrating chest wound outside "box" without pneumothorax or hemothorax
    Need chest tube if patient required intubation
    Otherwise follow patient's CXRs
  Pericardial window – if you find blood, need sternotomy to fix possible injury to heart; place pericardial drain
  Penetrating injuries anterior-medial to midaxillary line and below nipples
    Need laparotomy or laparoscopy
    May also need evaluation for penetrating "box" injury depending on exact location

Traumatic causes of cardiogenic shock – cardiac tamponade (see Chap. 16, Critical Care), cardiac contusion, tension pneumothorax

Tension pneumothorax
  Hypotension, ↑ airway pressures, ↓ breath sounds, bulging neck veins, tracheal shift
  Can see bulging diaphragm during laparotomy
  Cardiac compromise secondary to ↓ venous return
  Tx: chest tube

Pelvic trauma
  Pelvic fractures can be a major source of blood loss.
  If hemodynamically unstable with pelvic fracture and negative DPL, negative CXR, and no other signs of blood loss or reasons for shock → stabilize pelvis (C-clamp, external fixator, or sheet) and go to angio for embolization.
  Patients at high risk for **GU and abdominal injuries**

Chapter 15. Trauma 55

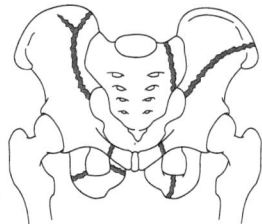

Type I: Unstable (crush)
Mortality: 20%–30%
Blood loss: >10 units
Complications: 60%–75%

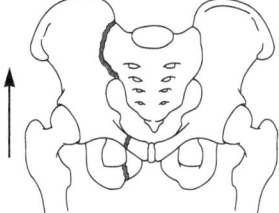

Type II: Unstable
Mortality: 8%–12%
Blood loss: 2–10 units
Complications: 30%–50%

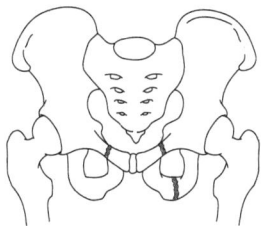

Type III: Stable.
Mortality: <5%
Blood loss: 1–4 units
Complications: 10%–20%

Classification of pelvic fractures with relative stability, mortality rates, and blood loss indicated.

Anterior pelvic fractures – more likely to have venous bleeding
Posterior pelvic fractures – more likely to have arterial bleeding
May need colostomy for open pelvic fractures with rectal tears and perineal lacerations
Pelvic fracture repair itself may need to be delayed until other associated injuries are repaired.
Penetrating injury pelvic hematomas – open
Blunt injury pelvic hematomas – leave unless expanding and patient unstable
    If unstable, stabilize pelvic fracture, pack pelvis if in OR, and get patient to angiography embolization.

Duodenal trauma
Usually blunt from crush or deceleration injury
2nd portion of the duodenum (descending portion, near ampulla of Vater) – most common area of injury
Can also get tears near ligament of Treitz
70%–80% of injuries requiring surgery can be treated with **debridement and primary closure**.
Segmental resection with primary end-to-end closure possible with all **segments except second portion of the duodenum**
25% mortality in these patients because of associated **shock**
Fistulas are the major source of morbidity.

Paraduodenal hematomas (usually in third portion of duodenum overlying spine in blunt injury) – for blunt and penetrating injuries need to open these up if in the OR

Missed hematomas can present with high SBO 12–72 hours after injury.
  UGI study will show "stacked coins" or "coiled spring" appearance.
  Conservative treatment (TPN and NGT) cures 90% of these over 2–3 weeks.

If at laparotomy and injury suspected, perform **Kocher maneuver and open lesser sac**, check for hematoma, bile, petechiae, sucus, and fat necrosis. If found, need formal inspection of the entire duodenum.

Diagnosing suspected duodenal injury – abdominal CT with contrast initially. UGI contrast study best. CT scan may show bowel wall thickening, hematoma, air, contrast leak, retroperitoneal fluid/air.
  If CT scan is worrisome for injury but nondiagnostic, can repeat the CT in 8–12 hours to see if the finding is getting worse.

Tx: Try to get **primary repair**; may need to divert with pyloric exclusion and gastrojejunostomy to allow healing. Place a distal feeding jejunostomy and possibly a proximal draining jejunostomy tube that threads back to duodenal injury site. **Place drains.**

  If not enough duodenum is present for repair or is in 2nd portion of duodenum, need pyloric exclusion and gastrojejunostomy.
    Can then place jejunal patch over hole; may need Whipple procedure in future.
    Consider feeding and draining jejunostomies.

  Trauma Whipple – rarely if ever indicated
  Drains – remove when patient tolerating diet without an increase in drainage
  Fistulas – often close with time
    Tx: bowel rest, TPN, decompression, octreotide, fistulogram to rule out abscess, conservative management for 4–6 weeks. Consider distal obstruction.

Small bowel trauma
Most common organ injured with penetrating injury
These injuries can be hard to diagnose early if associated with blunt trauma.
Occult small bowel injuries
  Abdominal CT scan showing **intra-abdominal fluid not associated with a solid organ injury, bowel wall thickening, or a mesenteric hematoma** is suggestive of injury.
  Need close observation and possibly repeat abdominal CT after 8–12 hours or so to make sure finding is not getting worse
  Need to make sure patients with these nonconclusive findings can **tolerate a diet before discharge**
Repair lacerations **transversely → avoids stricture**
Large lacerations >50% of the circumference or results in lumen diameter <⅓ normal – perform resection and reanastamosis
Multiple close lacerations – just resect that segment
Mesenteric hematomas – open if expanding or large (>2 cm)

Colon trauma
Most associated with penetrating injury
Right and transverse colon – can perform primary reanastamosis
Left colon – colostomy and Hartman's pouch or mucous fistula the safest procedure
Paracolonic hematomas – both blunt and penetrating need to be opened
10% abscess rate after colon injury; 2% fistula rate, higher with primary repair

Rectal trauma
Most associated with penetrating injury
High rectal
  Extraperitoneal – generally not repaired because of inaccessibility
    Tx: presacral drainage and fecal diversion with colostomy
  Intraperitoneal – Tx: repair defect, presacral drainage, fecal diversion with colostomy
Low rectal (<5 cm) – can probably be repaired transanally

Liver trauma

Lobectomy rarely necessary
Common hepatic artery – can be ligated with collaterals through gastroduodenal artery
Hepatic lobar arteries can be ligated without complication unless the patient is hypotensive, which could lead to liver ischemia.
Pringle maneuver (clamping portal triad) does not stop bleeding from **hepatic veins**.

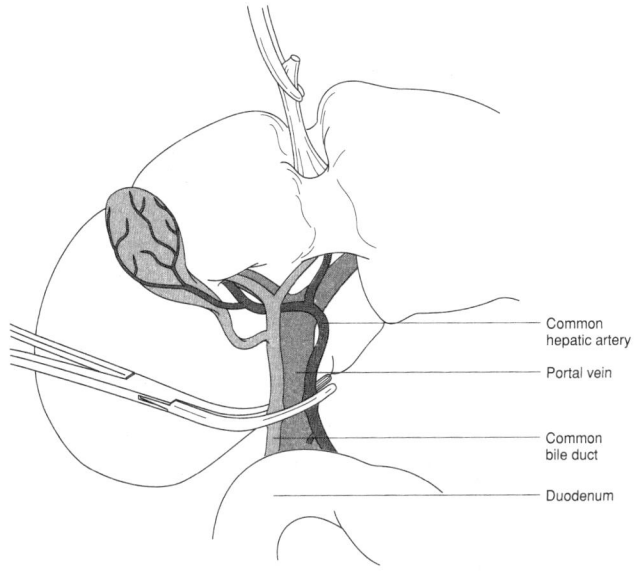

Pringle maneuver. Portal triad structures are compressed with a noncrushing vascular clamp for hepatic inflow control.

Atriocaval shunt – for retrohepatic IVC injury, allows for control while performing repair
Perihepatic packing – can pack severe penetrating liver injuries if patient becomes unstable in the OR. Go to the ICU and get the patient resuscitated and stabilized. Live to fight another day.
Portal triad hematomas – need to be explored

Common bile duct injury
<50% of circumference – **repair over stent**
>50% or complex injury – **go with choledochojejunostomy**
May need intraoperative cholangiogram to define injury
10% of duct anastamoses leak.

Portal vein injury – need to repair
May need to transect through the pancreas to get to the injury in the portal vein
Will need to perform distal pancreatectomy with that maneuver
Ligation of portal vein associated with 50% mortality

Omental graft – can be placed in liver laceration to help with bleeding and prevent bile leaks
Leave drains with liver injuries.

Conservative management of blunt liver injuries
Has failed if patient becomes unstable despite aggressive resuscitation, including 4 units of PRBCs (HR >120 or SBP <90) or requires >4 units of PRBCs to keep Hct >25. **Go to OR.**

Active blush on abdominal CT or pseudoaneurysm also indication for **OR**
  If <u>posterior</u>, may be better off going to **angiogram** (when in doubt → OR)
  If <u>anterior</u>, **go to OR**
With conservative management, need bed rest for 5 days

Spleen trauma
Fully healed after 6 weeks
Postsplenectomy sepsis most common in 1st 5 years of life; greatest risk within 2 years of splenectomy
Splenic salvage is associated with increased transfusions.
Conservative management of blunt splenic injuries
  Has failed if patient becomes unstable despite aggressive resuscitation, including 2 units of PRBCs (HR >120 or SBP <90) or requires >2 units of PRBCs to keep Hct >25. **Go to OR.**
  Active blush on abdominal CT or pseudoaneurysm also indication for **OR**
  With conservative management, need bed rest for 5 days
  Threshold for splenectomy in **children** is much higher; hardly any children undergo splenectomy.
  Need immunizations after trauma splenectomy

Pancreatic trauma
Penetrating injury – accounts for 80% of all pancreatic injuries
Blunt injury – can result in pancreatic duct fractures, usually perpendicular to the duct

Edema or necrosis of peripancreatic fat usually indicative of injury
Pancreatic contusion – leave if stable, place drain

Distal pancreatic duct injury – distal pancreatectomy, can take up to 80% of the gland
Pancreatic head injury that is not reparable – place drains initially; delayed Whipple may be eventually necessary
May be able to treat pancreatic duct injuries with ERCP and stent as opposed to resection

Whipple vs distal pancreatectomy based on duct injury in relation to the **SMA/SMV**
Injuries to the right of the SMA/SMV treated with drains instead of Whipple initially

Kocher maneuver helps evaluate the pancreas operatively.
Leave drains with pancreatic injury.
Pancreatic hematoma – both penetrating and blunt need to be opened

Persistent or rising **amylase** may indicate missed pancreatic injury.
CT scans poor at diagnosing pancreatic injuries initially
  Delayed signs – fluid, edema, necrosis
Dx: ERCP good at picking up duct injuries and may be able to treat with stent

Vascular trauma
Vascular repair performed before orthopaedic repair
Major signs of vascular injury – active hemorrhage, pulse deficit, expanding or pulsatile hematoma, distal ischemia, bruit, thrill → **go to OR for exploration** (some say angio 1st)
Moderate/soft signs of vascular injury – history of hemorrhage, deficit of anatomically related nerve, large stable/nonpulsatile hematoma → **go to angio**
Saphenous vein graft – will be needed if segment >2 cm missing

Vein injuries that need repair – vena cava, femoral, popliteal, brachiocephalic, subclavian, axillary
Transection of single artery in the calf in otherwise healthy patient → ligate
Coverage of site of anastamoses with viable tissue and muscle important
Consider **fasciotomy** if ischemia >4 hours – prevents compartment syndrome
Compartment syndrome – consider with pressures >20 mmHg or if clinical exam suggests elevated pressures
  Pain → parasthesia → anesthesia → paralysis → poikothermia → pulselessness (late finding)

Chapter 15. Trauma

Most commonly occurs after supracondylar humeral fractures, tibial fractures, crush injuries, or other injuries that result in a disruption and then restoration of blood flow

IVC – primary repair if residual stenosis <50% diameter of IVC; otherwise place saphenous vein or synthetic patch

Bleeding of IVC best controlled with proximal and distal pressure, <u>not</u> clamps → can tear it

Repair posterior wall injury through the anterior wall.

May need to cut through the anterior IVC to get to posterior IVC injuries.

Orthopaedic trauma (see also Chap. 42, Orthopaedics)

Can have **>2 L blood loss from a femur fracture**

Orthopaedic emergencies – pelvic fractures in unstable patients, spine injury with deficit, open fractures, dislocations or fractures with vascular compromise, compartment syndrome

Femoral neck fractures – high risk for avascular necrosis

Orthopaedic Trauma	Concomitant Nerve/Artery Injury
UPPER EXTREMITY	
Anterior shoulder dislocation	Axillary nerve
Posterior shoulder dislocation	Axillary artery
Proximal Humerus	Axillary nerve
Midshaft humerus (or spiral humerus fracture)	Radial nerve
Distal (supracondylar) humerus	Brachial artery
Elbow dislocation	Brachial artery
Distal radius	Median nerve
LOWER EXTREMITY	
Anterior hip dislocation	Femoral artery
Posterior hip dislocation	Sciatic nerve
Distal (supracondylar) femur	Popliteal artery
Posterior knee dislocation	Popliteal artery
Fibula neck	Common peroneal nerve

(Modified from Engelhardt SL, Winchell RJ. Definitive care phase: orthopedic and spinal injuries. In: Greenfield LJ et al, eds. Surgery: scientific principles and practice. Ed 3. Philadelphia: Lippincott Williams & Wilkins, 2001:372.)

Long bone fracture or dislocations with loss of pulse (or weak pulse) → immediate reduction of fracture or dislocation and reassessment of pulse

If pulse does not return → go to OR for vascular bypass or repair (some say proceed to angiography for diagnosis of location of injury and possible intervention)

If pulse is weak → angiography

All knee dislocations need to go to angiogram, unless pulse is absent, in which case some would just go to OR.

Renal trauma

Hematuria is best indicator of renal trauma.

All patients with hematuria need CT scan.

IVP can also be useful if going immediately to OR without abdominal CT scan → will identify presence of functional contralateral kidney, which could affect intraoperative decision making

Left renal vein – can be ligated near IVC; has **adrenal and gonadal vein collaterals**
Right does <u>not</u>.

Anterior → posterior renal hilum structures – **vein, artery, pelvis**

95% of injuries are treated nonoperatively.

Not all urine extravasation injuries require operation.

Indications for operation
 Acutely – ongoing hemorrhage with instability
  After acute phase – major collecting system disruption, unresolving urine extravasation, severe hematuria

With exploration, try to get control of the **vascular hilum 1st**.

Place **drains**, especially if collecting system is injured.

Methylene blue dye can be used at the end of the case to check for leak.

When at exploration for another blunt injury or penetrating trauma
  Blunt renal injury with hematoma – leave unless preop CT/IVP shows no function or significant urine extravasation
  Penetrating renal injury with hematoma – open unless preop CT/IVP shows good function without significant urine extravasation

Trauma to flank and IVP shows no uptake – Tx: angiogram; can stent if flap present

Bladder trauma
Hematuria best indicator of bladder trauma
>95% associated with pelvic fractures
Signs and symptoms – meatal blood, sacral or scrotal hematoma
Dx: cystogram
Extraperitoneal bladder rupture – cystogram shows starbursts
  Tx: Foley 7–14 days
Intraperitoneal bladder rupture – more likely in kids, cystogram shows leak
  Tx: operation and repair of defect, followed by Foley drainage

Ureteral trauma
Hematuria unreliable → IVP and retrograde urethrogram (RUG) best tests

If large ureteral segment is missing (>2 cm) and cannot perform reanastamosis:
  Upper ⅓ injuries and middle ⅓ injuries that won't reach bladder
    Temporize with **urostomy** if patient unstable. Can go with ileal interposition or trans-ureteroureterostomy later
    If stable, most urologists would perform trans-ureteroureterostomy.
  Lower ⅓ injuries – reimplant in the bladder; may need bladder hitch procedure
If small ureteral segment is missing (<2 cm), try to mobilize ends of ureter and perform **primary repair** over stent or reimplant.

One-shot IVP does not evaluate the ureters sufficiently.
IV indigo carmine or methylene blue can be used to check for leaks.
Blood supply is medial in the upper ⅔ of the ureter and lateral in the lower ⅓ of the ureter.
Leave drains for all ureteral injuries.

Urethral trauma
Hematuria or blood at meatus best sign; free-floating prostate gland; usually associated with pelvic fractures
No Foley if this injury is suspected
Urethrogram best test
Membranous portion at risk for transection
Significant tears – Tx: suprapubic cystostomy and repair in 2–3 months (safest method)
  High stricture and impotence rate if repaired early
Small, partial tears – Tx: may get away with bridging urethral catheter across tear area and repair in 2–3 months
Genital trauma – can get fracture in erectile bodies from vigorous sex
  Need to repair the tunica and Buck's fascia
Testicular trauma – get ultrasound to see if tunical albuginea is violated, then repair if necessary

Pediatric trauma
Blood pressure is not a good indicator of blood loss in children – last thing to go.
Heart rate, respiratory rate, mental status, and clinical exam are best indicators of shock.
↑ risk of **hypothermia** (↑ BSA compared with weight)
↑ risk of **head injury**

Normal vital signs by age

Age Group	Pulse (beats/min)	SBP (mmHg)	Respiratory Rate (breaths/min)
Infant (<1 yr)	160	80	40
Preschool (< 5 yr)	140	90	30
Adolescent (>10 yr)	120	100	20

Trauma during pregnancy
At all costs, **save the mother**.
Pregnant patients can have up to a ⅓ total blood volume loss without signs.
Estimate pregnancy based on **fundal height** (20 cm = 20 wk = umbilicus). Place fetal monitor.
Try to avoid CT scan with early pregnancy. If life-threatening and needed, get CT scan.
Ultrasound (FAST scan) may have a role in pregnant patients.
Check for vaginal discharge – blood, amnion. Check for effacement, dilation, fetal station.
Maturity – lecithin:sphingomyelin (LS) ratio >2:1; positive **phosphatidylcholine**

Placental abruption >50% results in 100% fetal death rate.
    Signs of abruption – uterine tenderness, contractions, fetal HR <120
    Can be caused by **shock or mechanical forces**
    Kleihauer-Betke test – test for fetal blood in the maternal circulation → sign of placental abruption

Uterine rupture – more likely to occur in the posterior fundus
    If occurs after delivery of child, aggressive resuscitation even in the face of shock leads to the best outcome. The uterus will eventually clamp down after delivery; just have to aggressively resuscitate until then.

Indications for C-section during exploratory laparotomy for trauma
    Persistent maternal shock
    Pregnancy near term (>34 weeks) and mother with severe injuries
    Pregnancy a threat to the mother's life (hemorrhage, DIC)
    Mechanical limitation to life-threatening vessel injury
    Risk of fetal distress exceeds risk of immaturity
    Direct uterine trauma

Hematomas found intraoperatively

Hematoma	Penetrating Trauma	Blunt Trauma
Pelvic	Open	Leave
Paraduodenal	Open	Open
Portal triad	Open	Open
Retrohepatic	Leave if stable	Leave
Midline supramesocolic	Open	Open
Midline inframesocolic	Open	Open
Pericolonic	Open	Open
Perirenal	Open*	Leave†

*Unless preoperative CT scan or IVP shows no injury.
†Unless preoperative CT scan or IVP shows injury.

Drains – leave drains with pancreatic, liver, biliary system, urinary, and duodenal injuries

CHAPTER 16. CRITICAL CARE

Cardiovascular system
Normal values

Parameter	Value
Cardiac output (CO)	4–8 L/min
Cardiac index (CI)	2.5–4 L/min
Systemic vascular resistance (SVR)	800–1400
Systemic vascular resistance index (SVRI)	1500–2400
Pulmonary capillary wedge pressure (PCWP)	11 ± 4
Central venous pressure (CVP)	7 ± 2
Pulmonary artery (PA)	20–30/6–15
Mixed venous oxygen saturation (SvO_2)	70 ± 5

MAP = CO x SVR, CI = CO/BSA, SVRI = SVR x BSA

Preload – end-diastolic length, linearly related to end-diastolic volume (EDV) and filling pressure
Afterload – resistance against the ventricle contracting (SVR)

Stroke volume determined by LVEDV, contractility, and afterload
 Stroke volume = LVEDV – LVESV
Ejection fraction = stroke volume/EDV

EDV (end-diastolic volume) – determined by preload and distensibility of the ventricle
ESV (end-systolic volume) – determined by contractility and afterload

Cardiac output increases with HR up to 120–150, then starts to go down due to **decreased diastolic filling time**.
Atrial kick – accounts for 15%–30% of LVEDV

Anrep effect – automatic increase in **contractility** secondary to ↑ **afterload**
Bowditch effect – automatic increase in **contractility** secondary to ↑ **HR**

Aortic mean and diastolic pressures slightly greater than radial
Radial systolic pressures slightly higher than aortic

O_2 **delivery** = CO x arterial O_2 content (CaO_2) = CO x (Hgb x 1.34 x O_2 saturation + [O_2 x 0.003])

O_2 **consumption (VO_2)** = CO x (CaO_2 – CvO_2). CvO_2 = venous O_2 content
 Normal O_2 delivery to consumption ratio is **5:1**. CO increases to keep this ratio constant.
 O_2 consumption is usually supply independent → kidney gets 25% of CO, brain gets 15%
 Right shift on oxygen-Hgb dissociation curve (O_2 unloading) – ↑ CO_2, temperature, ATP, 2,3-DPG, or ↓ pH
 Normal p50 (O_2 at which 50% of O_2 receptors are saturated) = 27 mmHg

 ↑ SvO_2 (saturation of venous blood, normally 65%–75%) – occurs with ↑ shunting of blood or ↓ O_2 extraction (sepsis, cirrhosis, cyanide toxicity, hyperbaric O_2, hypothermia, paralysis, coma, sedation)
 ↓ SvO_2 – occurs with ↑ O_2 extraction or ↓ O_2 delivery (↓ O_2 saturation, ↓ CO)

Wedge – may be thrown off by pulmonary hypertension, aortic regurgitation, mitral stenosis, mitral regurgitation, high PEEP, poor LV compliance

Swan-Ganz catheter – should be placed in **zone III** (lower lung)
 Hemoptysis after Swan – pull catheter slightly back and inflate balloon, increase PEEP, which will tamponade the pulmonary artery bleed, mainstem intubate nonaffected side; can try to place Fogarty balloon down affected side; thoracotomy; may need thoracotomy and lobectomy
 Relative contraindications – previous pneumonectomy, left bundle branch block

Chapter 16. Critical Care

Approximate Swan distances – R SCV 45 cm, R IJ 50 cm, L SCV 55 cm, L IJ 60 cm
Pulmonary vascular resistance can be measured only by using a Swan.

↑ **ventricular wall tension and HR** are the primary determinants of <u>myocardial O_2 consumption</u> → can lead to myocardial ischemia

Unsaturated bronchial blood – empties into pulmonary veins; thus, LV blood is 5 mmHg (pO_2) lower than pulmonary capillaries
Alveolar:arterial gradient – 10–15 mmHg normal in nonventilated patient
Blood with the lowest venous saturation → coronary venous blood (30%)

Shock
Adrenal insufficiency
    Acute – cardiovascular collapse; characteristically **unresponsive to fluids and pressors**
    Chronic – hyperpigmentation, weakness, weight loss, GI symptoms, ↑ K, ↓ Na, fever, hypotension
    Steroid potency
        1x – cortisone, hydrocortisone
        5x – prednisone, prednisolone, methylprednisolone
        30x – dexamethasone

Neurogenic shock – loss of sympathetic tone
    <u>Usually have</u> ↓ HR, ↓ BP, warm skin
    Tx: give volume 1st, then phenylephrine after resuscitated; steroids for blunt spinal trauma with deficit

Hemorrhagic shock – initial alteration is ↑ <u>diastolic pressure</u>

Cardiac tamponade
    Causes decreased diastolic ventricular filling and hypotension
    Beck's triad – hypotension, jugular venous distention, and muffled heart sounds
    Echocardiogram shows **impaired diastolic filling of right atrium initially** (1st sign of cardiac tamponade).
    Pericardiocentesis blood does not form clot.
    Tx: fluid resuscitation initially; need pericardial window or pericardiocentesis

Shock	CVP and PCWP	CO	SVRI
Hemorrhagic	↓	↓	↑
Septic (hyperdynamic)*	↓, possibly ↑	↑	↓
Cardiogenic	↑	↓	↑
Neurogenic	↓	↓	↓
Hypoadrenal	↓, possibly ↑	↓	↓

*Severe septic shock that leads to cardiac dysfunction can cause a hypodynamic state, leading to ↓ CO and ↑ SVRI.
(Modified from Maier RV. Shock. In: Greenfield LJ et al, eds. Surgery: scientific principles and practice. Ed 2. Philadelphie: Lippincott-Raven, 1997.)

Early sepsis triad – hyperventilation, confusion, respiratory alkalosis
    Early gram-negative sepsis – ↓ insulin, ↑ glucose (impaired utilization)
    Late gram-negative sepsis – ↑ insulin, ↑ glucose (secondary to insulin resistance)
    Hyperglycemia – often occurs just before patient becomes clinically septic
Activated protein C (Xigris) – used for sepsis; mechanism is <u>fibrinolysis</u>

Emboli
Fat emboli
    Signs include petechia, hypoxia, and confusion (can also be similar to pulmonary embolism [PE]).
    Sudan red stain may show fat in sputum and urine.
    Most common with lower extremity (hip, femur) fractures/orthopaedic procedures
    Pulmonary thromboemboli – echo will show RV strain
        Suspect PE with PA systolic pressures >40, ↓ pO_2 and pCO_2, respiratory alkalosis, chest pain, cough, dyspnea, ↑ HR

Air emboli – place patient head down and roll to left (keeps air in RV and RA), then aspirate out air with central line or PA catheter to RA/RV

Intra-aortic balloon pump (IABP)
Inflates on **T wave (diastole)**; deflates on **P wave or start of Q wave (systole)**
Aortic regurgitation contraindication
Place tip of the catheter just distal to left subclavian.
Used for cardiogenic shock (after CABG, MI) or in patients with refractory angina
Decreases afterload (deflation during ventricular systole)
Improves SBP (inflation during ventricular diastole), which **improves coronary perfusion**

Receptors
Alpha-1 – vascular smooth muscle constriction; gluconeogenesis, glycogenolysis
Alpha-2 – venous smooth muscle constriction
Beta-1 – myocardial contraction and rate
Beta-2 – relaxes bronchial smooth muscle, relaxes vascular smooth muscle; increases insulin, glucagon, renin
Dopamine receptors – relax renal and splanchnic smooth muscle

Cardiovascular drugs
Dopamine (μg/kg/min)
  0–5 – dopamine receptors (renal)
  6–10 – beta-adrenergic (heart contractility)
  >10 – alpha-adrenergic (vasoconstriction and ↑ BP)

Dobutamine
  5–15 – beta-1 (↑ contractility mostly)
  >15 – beta-2 (vasodilation, ↑ HR)

Milrinone
  Phosphodiesterase inhibitor (↑ cAMP)
  Results in ↑ Ca flux and ↑ myocardial contractility
  Also causes vascular smooth muscle relaxation and vasodilation

Phenylephrine
  Alpha-1, vasoconstriction

Norepinephrine
  Low dose – beta-1 (↑ contractility)
  High dose – alpha-1 and alpha-2
  Potent splanchnic vasoconstrictor

Epinephrine
  Low dose – beta-1 and beta-2 (↑ contractility and vasodilation)
    Can ↓ BP at low doses
  High dose – alpha-1 and alpha-2 (vasoconstriction)
    ↑ cardiac ectopic pacer activity and myocardial O_2 demand

Isoproterenol
  Beta-1 and beta-2, ↑ HR and contractility, vasodilates
  Side effects: extremely arrhythmogenic; ↑ heart metabolic demand (rarely used); may actually ↓ BP

Vasopressin
  V-1 receptors – vasoconstriction of vascular smooth muscle
  V-2 receptors (intrarenal) – water reabsorption at collecting ducts
  V-2 receptors (extrarenal) – mediate release of factor VIII and von Willibrand factor

Nipride – arterial and venous dilator
  Cyanide toxicity at doses >3 μg/kg/min for 72 hours; can check **thiocyanate levels** and signs of metabolic acidosis
  Tx: amyl nitrite, then sodium nitrite

Chapter 16. Critical Care

Nitroglycerin – predominately venodilation, modest effect on coronaries; ↓ myocardial wall tension by ↓ preload

Hydralazine – alpha blocker

Pulmonary system
Compliance – (change in volume) / (change in pressure)
  High compliance means lungs easy to ventilate.
  Pulmonary compliance ↓ in patients with ARDS, fibrotic lung diseases, reperfusion injury, pulmonary edema
Aging – ↓ FEV_1 and vital capacity, ↑ functional residual capacity (FRC)
V/Q ratio – highest in upper lobes, lowest in lower lobes

Ventilator
  ↑ PEEP to improve oxygenation (alveoli recruitment) → **improves FRC**
  ↑ rate/volume to ↓ CO_2
  Normal weaning parameters – negative inspiratory force (NIF) >20, FiO_2 <35%, PEEP 5 (physiologic), pressure support 5, RR <24, HR <120, pO_2 >60, pCO_2 <50, pH 7.35–7.45, saturations >93%, off pressors, follows commands, can protect airway

  Pressure support – ↓ the work of breathing (inspiratory pressure is held constant until minimum volume is achieved)
  FiO_2 ≤60% – prevents O_2 radical toxicity
  Barotrauma – high risk if plateaus >30 and peaks >50 → consider prophylactic chest tubes
  PEEP – improves FRC and compliance by keeping alveoli open → best way to improve oxygenation
  Excessive PEEP complications – ↓ RA filling, ↓ CO, ↓ renal blood flow and ↓ urine output, ↑ pulmonary vascular resistance
  High-frequency ventilation – used a lot in kids; tracheoesophageal fistula, bronchopleural fistula
  Inverse ratio ventilation – helps reduce barotrauma (normal 1:2 I:E phase; go to 2:1)

Pulmonary function measurements
  Total lung capacity (TLC) – lung volume after maximal inspiration
    TLC = FVC + RV
  Forced vital capacity (FVC) – maximal exhalation after maximal inhalation
  Residual volume (RV) – lung volume after maximal expiration (20% TLC)
  Tidal volume (TV) – volume of air with normal inspiration and expiration
  Functional residual capacity (FRC) – lung volume after normal exhalation
    FRC = ERV + RV
    Surgery (atelectasis), sepsis (ARDS), and trauma (contusion, atelectasis, ARDS) – all ↓ FRC
  Expiratory reserve volume (ERV) – volume of air that can be forcefully expired after normal expiration
  Inspiratory capacity – maximum air breathed in from FRC
  FEV_1 – forced expiratory volume in 1 second (after maximal inhalation)
  Minute ventilation = TV x RR
  Restrictive lung disease – ↓ TLC, ↓ RV, and ↓ VC
    FEV_1 can be normal or ↑
  Obstructive lung disease – ↑ TLC, ↑ RV, and ↓ FEV_1
    VC can be normal or ↓

Dead space – normally to the level of the bronchiole (150 ml); ↑ with drop in cardiac output, PE, pulmonary HTN, ARDS, excessive PEEP; can lead to high **CO_2 buildup**
  Area of lung that is ventilated but not perfused

COPD – ↑ work of breathing due to prolonged expiratory phase
  Work of breathing normally 2% of total body VO_2

ARDS – mediated by cellular inflammatory processes, ↑ proteinaceous material, ↑ gradient, ↑ shunt
  Most common cause is **sepsis**.

SIRS – mediated by TNF-alpha and IL-1; temperature >38°C or <36°C, RR >20, CO_2 <32, WBC >12 or <4, HR >90
Endotoxin (lipopolysaccharide – lipid A) is the most potent stimulus for **SIRS**.

Aspiration – pH <2.5 and volume >0.4 cc/kg associated with ↑ degree of damage
  Mendelson's syndrome – chemical pneumonitis from aspiration of gastric secretions
  Most frequent site is the posterior portion of RUL and superior portion of RLL.

Atelectasis – bronchial obstruction and respiratory failure main causes
  Most common cause of fever in 1st 48 hours after operation
  Fever, tachycardia
  Increased in patients with COPD, upper abdominal surgery, obesity
  Tx: incentive spirometer

Lots of things can throw off a pulse oximeter → nail polish, dark skin, low-flow states, ambient light, anemia, vital dyes

Pulmonary vasodilation – bradykinin, PGE_1, prostacylin (PGI_2), nitric oxide
Pulmonary vasoconstriction – histamine, serotonin, TXA_2, epinephrine, norepinephrine, **hypoxia**, acidosis
Alkalosis – pulmonary vasodilator
Acidosis – pulmonary vasoconstrictor
Pulmonary shunting – occurs with nipride, nitroglycerin, and nifedipine

Renal system
  Hypotension – most common cause of postoperative renal failure
  70% nephrons need to be damaged before renal dysfunction occurs.
  FeNa = (urine Na/Cr) / (plasma Na/Cr) → best test for azotemia
  Prerenal cause of acute renal failure – FeNa <1%, urine Na <20, BUN/Cr ratio >20, urine osmolality >500 mOsm; otherwise consider renal cause of azotemia
  Oligura
    1st – make sure patient is volume loaded (CVP 11–15)
    2nd – try diuretic trial → Lasix/butanemide
    3rd – dialysis if needed

  Indications for dialysis – fluid overload, ↑ K, metabolic acidosis, uremic encephalopathy, uremic coagulopathy, poisoning
  Hemodialysis – rapid, causes large volume shifts
  CVHD – slower, good for ill patients that cannot tolerate the volume shifts (septic shock, etc)
    Hct increases 5–8 for each liter taken off.

  Renin
    Released in response to ↓ pressure sensed by **juxtaglomerular apparatus** in kidney
    Also released in response to ↑ Na concentrations sensed by the **macula densa**
    Beta-adrenergic stimulation and hyperkalemia also cause release.
    Converts angiotensinogen (synthesized in the liver) to angiotensin I
    Angiotensin-converting enzyme (lung) – converts angiotensin I to angiotensin II
    Adrenal cortex – releases aldosterone in response to angiotensin II
    Distal convoluted tubule – aldosterone acts here to reabsorb more water by ↑ Na/K ATPase on membrane (potassium secreted)
    Angiotensin II – also vasoconstricts, increases HR, contractility, permeability, glycogenolysis, and gluconeogenesis; inhibits renin release

  Atrial natriuretic peptide (or factor)
    Released from atrial wall with atrial distention
    Inhibits Na and water resorption in the collecting ducts
    Also a **vasodilator**

  Antidiuretic hormone (ADH; vasopressin)
    Released by posterior pituitary gland when osmolality is high
    Acts on collecting ducts for water resorption
    Also a **vasoconstrictor**

Efferent limb of kidney controls GFR.
Renal toxic drugs
  NSAIDs – cause renal damage by **inhibiting prostaglandin synthesis**, resulting in renal arteriole vasoconstriction
  Aminoglycosides – direct tubular injury and later renal vasoconstriction
  Myoglobin – direct tubular injury
    Tx: alkalinize urine
  Contrast dyes – direct tubular injury
    Tx: premedicate with N-acetylcysteine and volume

Brain death
Precludes diagnosis – uremia, temperature <30°C, BP <70/40, desaturation with apnea test, drugs (phenobarbital, pentobarbital), metabolic derangements
Must exist for 6–12 hours → unresponsive to pain, absent caloric oculovestibular reflexes, absent oculocephalic reflex, positive apnea test, no corneal reflex, no gag reflex, fixed and dilated pupils
EEG – electrical silence; **MRA** – can be used → will show no blood flow to brain
Apnea test – disconnected from ventilation; CO_2 >60 mmHg or increase in CO_2 by 20 is a positive test for apnea. If arterial pressure drops to <60 or patient desaturates, the test is terminated.
Can still have deep tendon reflexes with brain death

Other conditions
Carbon monoxide
  Can <u>falsely ↑ oxygen saturation reading on pulse oximeter</u>
  Binds hemoglobin directly (creates carboxyhemoglobin)
  Can usually correct with 100% oxygen on ventilator (displaces carbon monoxide); may need hyperbaric O_2 if really high
  Abnormal carboxyhemoglobin >10%; in smokers >20%
Methemoglobinemia (from nitrites like hurricaine spray; nitrites bind Hgb) – **O_2 saturation reads 85%**
  Tx: methylene blue
Critical illness polyneuropathy – motor > sensory neuropathy; occurs with sepsis; can lead to failure to wean from ventilation
Xanthine oxidase – in endothelial cells, forms toxic oxygen radicals with reperfusion, involved in reperfusion injury
  Also involved in the metabolism of purines and breakdown to uric acid
DKA – nausea and vomiting, thirst, polyuria, abdominal pain, ↑ glucose, ↑ ketones, ↓ Na, ↑ K
  Tx: insulin and eventually glucose so patient does not bottom out, isotonic solutions, K^+ (although initial K will be high, it will be driven back into cells by insulin), HCO_3^- for pH <7.25
ETOH withdrawal – HTN, tachycardia, delirium, seizures after 48 hours
  Tx: thiamine, folate, Mg, K, B_{12}, PRN Ativan
ICU (or hospital) psychosis – generally occurs after third postop day and is frequently preceded by lucid interval
  Need to rule out metabolic (hypoglycemia, DKA, hypoxia, hypercarbia, electrolyte imbalances) and organic (MI, CVA) causes

CHAPTER 17. BURNS

Burn classification

Degree	Description
1st	Sunburn (epidermis)
2nd	
Superficial dermis (papillary)	Painful to touch; blebs and blisters; hair follicles intact; blanches
Deep dermis (reticular)	Decreased sensation; loss of hair follicles (need skin grafts)
3rd	Leathery feeling (charred parchment); down to subcutaneous fat
4th	Down to bone, into adjacent adipose or muscle tissue

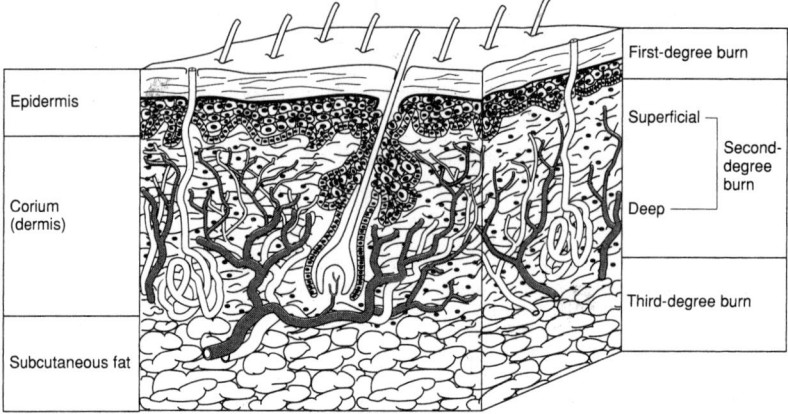

Schematic depiction of the skin.

Admission criteria[1]
- 2nd and 3rd degree burns >10% BSA in patients aged <10 or >50 years
- 2nd and 3rd degree burns >20% BSA in all other patients
- 2nd and 3rd degree burns to significant portions of hands, face, feet, genitalia, perineum, or skin overlying major joints
- 3rd degree burns >5% in any age group
- Electrical and chemical burns
- Concomitant inhalational injury, mechanical traumas, preexisting medical conditions
- Injuries in patients with special social, emotional, or long-term rehabilitation needs
- Suspected child abuse or neglect

Deaths highest in children and elderly (trouble getting away)
Scald burns – most common
Flame burns – more likely to come to hospital and be admitted

Assessing percentage of body surface burned (rule of 9s)
Head = 9, arms = 18, chest = 18, back = 18, legs = 36, perineum = 1
Can also use patient's palm to estimate injury (palm = 1%)

Parkland formula
For burns ≥20% – give 4 cc/kg x % burn in first 24 hours; give ½ in first 8 hours
Use lactated Ringer's solution (LR) in first 24 hours.
    Urine output best measure of resuscitation (0.5–1.0 cc/kg/hr in adults, 2–4 cc/kg/hr in children <6 months)

---

[1] Modified from Feliciano DV et al. Trauma. Ed 3. Stamford, CT, Appleton & Lange, 1996:937.

Parkland formula can grossly underestimate volume requirements with inhalational injury, ETOH, electrical injury, postescharotomy.
Important to use LR in first 24 hours
Colloid (albumin) in 1st 24 hours shown to ↑ pulmonary/respiratory complications
→ can use colloid after 24 hours

Escharotomy indications (perform within 4–6 hours)
Circumferential burns
Low temperature; weak pulse; ↓ capillary refill, ↓ pain sensation, and ↓ neurologic function in extremity → may need fasciotomy if compartment syndrome suspected
Problems ventilating patient with significant chest torso burns

Child abuse

Accounts for 15% of burn injuries in children
Important points of history and exam that suggest abuse or neglect

HISTORY
Delayed presentation for medical care
Conflicting histories
Previous injuries
SUSPICIOUS BURN PATTERNS
Sharply demarcated margins
Uniform depth
Absence of splash marks
Stocking or glove patterns
Flexor sparing
Dorsal location of contact injury of the hands
Very deep localized contact injury

Lung injury

Caused by carbonaceous materials and smoke, <u>not</u> heat
Risk factors for airway injury – ETOH, trauma, closed space, rapid combustion, extremes of age, delayed extrication
Signs and symptoms of possible airway injury – facial burns, wheezing, carbonaceous sputum
Indications for intubation – upper airway stridor or obstruction, worsening hypoxemia, massive volume resuscitation
Pneumonia – most common infection in burn wound patients
Also most common cause of **death** after inhalation injury

Unusual burns

Acid and alkali burns – copious water irrigation
Alkalis produce deeper burns than acid due to <u>liquefaction necrosis</u>.
Acid burns produce <u>coagulation necrosis</u>.
Hydrofluoric acid burns – spread calcium on wound
Powder burns – wipe away before irrigation
Tar burns – cool, then wipe away with a lipophyllic solvent
Electrical burns – cardiac monitoring
Can cause rhabdomyolysis and compartment syndrome
Other complications – polyneuritis, quadraplegia, transverse myelitis, cataracts, liver necrosis, intestinal perforation, gallbladder perforation, pancreatic necrosis
Lightning – cardiopulmonary arrest secondary to electrical paralysis of brainstem

1st week – early excision of burned areas

Cardiac output in severely burned patients – first have ↓ CO for 24–48 hours, then have ↑ CO (ebb and flow phases following burn)
Caloric need: 25 kcal/kg/day + (30 kcal × % burn)
Protein need: 1 g/kg/day + (3 g × % burn)
Glucose – best source of nonprotein calories in patients with burns
Burn wounds use glucose in an obligatory fashion.

Try to excise burn wounds in <72 hours.
Used for deep 2nd and 3rd degree burns
Viability is based on color, texture, punctate bleeding after removal.

Skin grafts contraindicated if culture is positive for **beta-hemolytic strep or bacteria >10^5**.
Autografts (split-thickness [STSG] or full-thickness [FTSG]) – best
  ↓ infection, desiccation, protein loss, pain, water loss, heat loss, and RBC loss
  ↑ granulation tissue and improve survival
Split-thickness grafts should be 12–15 mm (include epidermis and part of the dermis).
Homografts (cadaveric skin) – not as good as autografts; can be a good temporizing material; last 2 weeks
Xenografts (porcine) – not as good as homografts; last 2 weeks
Dermal substitutes – not as good as homografts or xenografts

Wounds to face, palms, soles, and genitals should be deferred for the 1st week.
For each burn wound incision – <1 L blood loss, <20% of skin excised, <2 hours in OR
  Patients can get extremely sick if too much time is spent in OR.
Meshed grafts – back, flank, trunk, arms, and legs
  Reasons to delay autografting – infection, not enough skin, patient septic or unstable, don't want to create any more donor sites with concomitant blood loss
  Most common reason for skin graft loss – seroma or hematoma formation under graft
    Need to apply pressure dressing (cotton balls) to the skin graft to prevent seroma and hematoma buildup underneath the graft
  STSGs are more likely to survive – graft not as thick so easier for imbibition and subsequent revascularization to occur
  FTSGs have less wound contraction – good for areas like the palms and back of hands
Burn scar hypopigmentation and irregularities can be improved with dermal abrasion thin split-thickness grafts.

2nd to 5th weeks – specialized areas addressed, allograft replaced with autograft
  Face – topical antibiotics for 2 weeks, full-thickness grafts for unhealed areas (nonmeshed)
  Hands
    Superficial – ROM exercises, splint in functional position if too much edema
    Deep – immobilize for 7 days after operation, then physical therapy. May need wire fixation of joints if unstable or open. Treat with full-thickness grafts.
  Palms – try to preserve specialized palmar attachments. Splint hand in extension for 1 week. Graft in week 2 with full-thickness nonmeshed autograft graft.
  Genitals – antibiotics for 2 weeks. Graft unhealed areas (can use meshed).

Burn wound infections
Usually apply **bacitracin or Neosporin** immediately after burns
No role for prophylactic IV antibiotics
Pseudomonas is most common organism in burn wound infection, followed by *Staphylococcus, E. coli,* and *Enterobacter.*
Common in burns **>30% BSA**
Topical agents have decreased incidence of burn wound bacterial infections.
Candida infections have increased incidence secondary to topical antimicrobials.
Granulocyte chemotaxis and cell-mediated immunity are impaired in burn patients.

Silvadene (silver sulfadiazene) – can cause neutropenia and thrombocytopenia
  Limited eschar penetration
  Ineffective against some *Pseudomonas* species and other GNRs; effective for *Candida*

Silver nitrate – can cause electrolyte imbalances → hyponatremia and hypochloremia, hypocalcemia and hypokalemia
  Discoloration
  Limited eschar penetration
  Ineffective against some *Pseudomonas* species and GPCs
  Methemoglobinemia – contraindicated in patients with G6PD deficiency

Sulfamylon (mafenide sodium) – painful application
  Metabolic acidosis due to carbonic anhydrase inhibition (↓ renal conversion of H_2CO_3 → $H_2O + CO_2$) – can cause hypersensitivity reactions

Good eschar penetration; good for burns overlying **cartilage**
Broadest spectrum against *Pseudomonas* and GNRs

Signs of burn wound infection – peripheral edema, 2nd to 3rd degree burn conversion, hemorrhage into scar, erythema gangrenosum, green fat, black skin around wound, rapid eschar separation, focal discoloration
Burn wound sepsis – usually due to *Pseudomonas*
HSV – most common viral infection in burn wounds
<10^5 organisms – not a burn wound infection
Best way to detect burn wound infection (and differentiate from colonization) – **biopsy of wound**

Complications after burns
Seizures – usually iatrogenic and related to Na concentration; can also be benzodiazepine withdrawal
Peripheral neuropathy – secondary to small vessel injury and demyelination
Ectopia – from contraction of burned adnexae. Tx: eyelid release
Eyes – fluorescein staining to find injury. Tx: topical fluoroquinolone or gentamycin
Corneal abrasion – Tx: topical antibiotics
Symblepharon – eyelid stuck to conjunctiva. Tx: release with glass rod
Heterotopic ossification of tendons – Tx: physical therapy; may need surgery
Fractures – Tx: often get external fixation to allow for treatment of burns
Curling's ulcer – gastric ulcer that occurs with burns
Marjolin's ulcer – highly malignant squamous cell CA that arises in chronic nonhealing burn wounds or unstable scars
Hypertrophic scar
    Usually occurs 3–4 months after injury secondary to ↑ neovascularity
    More likely to be deep thermal injuries that take >3 weeks to heal, heal by contraction and epithelial spread, or heal across flexor surfaces
    Wait 1–2 years before scar modification
    Tx: grafting, steroids, silicone, compression

Other serious skin injuries
Toxic epidermal necrolysis (TEN; variant of erythema multiforme major) and staphylococcal scalded skin syndrome
    Epidermal-dermal separation seen
    Caused by a variety of drugs (Dilantin, Bactrim, penicillin) and viruses
    Tx: supportive; need to prevent wound dessication with topical antimicrobials and xenografts
    Antibiotics if due to *Staphylococcus aureus*
    No steroids

Stevens-Johnson syndrome (erythema multiforme) – more severe form of TEN
    Hypersensitivity reaction – subepidermal bullae, epidermal cell necrosis, dermal edema
    Caused by a variety of drugs (Dilantin, Bactrim, penicillin) and viruses
    Tx: supportive; need to prevent wound dessication with topical antimicrobials and xenografts
    No steroids

CHAPTER 18. PLASTICS, SKIN, AND SOFT TISSUES

Skin
Epidermis – primarily cellular
- **Keratinocytes** – main cell type in epidermis; originate from basal layer; provide mechanical barrier
- **Melanocytes** – neuroectodermal origin (neural crest cells); in basal layer of epidermis
  - Have dendritic processes that transfer melanin to neighboring keratinocytes via **melanosomes**
  - Density of melanocytes is the same among races; difference is in production.

Dermis – primarily structural proteins for the epidermis

Langerhans cells
- Act as antigen presenting cells (MHC class II)
- Originate from bone marrow
- Have a role in contact hypersensitivity reactions (type IV)

Sensory nerves
- **Pacinian corpuscles** – pressure
- **Ruffini's endings** – warmth
- **Krause's end-bulbs** – cold
- **Meissner's corpuscles** – tactile sense

Eccrine sweat glands – aqueous sweat (thermal regulation, usually hypotonic)

Apocrine sweat glands – milky sweat
- Highest concentration of glands in palms and soles; most sweat is result of sympathetic nervous system via acetylcholine

Lipid-soluble drugs – ↑ skin absorption
Type I collagen – predominant type; 70% weight of dermis; gives tensile strength
Tension – resistance to stretching (collagen)
Elasticity – ability to regain shape (branching proteins that can stretch to 2x normal length)
Cushing's striae – caused by loss of tensile strength and elasticity

Grafts
Split-thickness skin grafts (STSGs)
- Include all of the epidermis and part of the dermis
- Donor site skin regenerated from hair follicles and skin edges on split-thickness grafts

STSGs are more likely to survive → graft not as thick so easier for imbibition and subsequent revascularization to occur

Full-thickness skin grafts – have less wound contraction → good for areas like the palms and back of hands

Imbibition (osmotic) – blood supply to skin graft for days 0–3

Neovascularization – starts around day 3
- Poorly vascularized beds are unlikely to support skin grafting → tendon, bone without periosteum, XRT areas

Pedicled or anastomosed free flap necrosis – **venous thrombosis** most common cause

Tissue expansion occurs by local recruitment, thinning of the dermis and epidermis, mitosis

TRAM flaps
- Complications – flap necrosis, ventral hernia, bleeding, infection, abdominal wall weakness
- Rely on superior epigastric vessels
- **Periumbilical perforators most important determinant of TRAM flap viability**

Pressure sores

Stage	Description	Treatment
I	Erythema and pain, no skin loss	
II	Partial skin loss with yellow debris	Local treatment, keep pressure off
III	Full-thickness skin loss, subcutaneous tissue exposure	Sharp debridement; will likely need myocutaneous flap
IV	Usually involves bony cortex	Myocutaneous flaps

(After Deziel DJ et al. Rush University review of surgery. Ed 3. Philadelphia: WB Saunders, 2000:598.)

UV radiation
- Damages DNA and repair mechanisms
- Both a promoter and initiator
- Melanin single best factor for protecting skin from UV radiation
- **UV-B** – responsible for chronic sun damage

Melanoma
Represents only 3%–5% of skin CA but accounts for 65% of the deaths

Risk factors for melanoma
- **Dysplastic, atypical, or large congenital nevi** – 10% lifetime risk for melanoma
- **Familial BK mole syndrome** – almost 100% risk of melanoma
- **Xeroderma pigmentosum**
- Fair complexion, easy sunburn, intermittent sunburns, previous skin CA

10% of melanomas familial

Most common melanoma site on skin – back in men, legs in women

Prognosis worse for men, ulcerated lesions, ocular and mucosal lesions

Signs of transformation – color change, angulations, indentation/notching, enlargement, darkening, bleeding, ulceration

Originates from **neural crest cells** (melanocytes) in basal layer epidermis

Blue color → most ominous

Lung – most common location for distant melanoma metastases

Most common metastasis to small bowel – **melanoma**

Types
- **Lentigo maligna** – least aggressive, minimal invasion, radial growth 1st usual; elevated nodules
- **Superficial spreading melanoma** – most common, intermediate malignancy; originates from nevus/sun-exposed areas
- **Nodular** – most aggressive; most likely to have metastasized at time of diagnosis; deepest growth at time of diagnosis; vertical growth 1st; bluish black with smooth borders; occurs anywhere on body
- **Acral lentigus** – very aggressive; palms/soles of African-Americans
- **Melanoma in situ or thin lentigo maligna** – 0.5-cm margins OK

Staging – need CXR and LFTs; examine all possible draining lymph nodes

Tx: for all stages, resection of primary tumor with appropriate margins

Alpha-interferon, IL-2, and tumor vaccines can be used for systemic disease

Melanoma staging

Stage	Description
IA	0–0.75 mm
IB	0.75–1.5 mm
IIA	1.5–4 mm
IIB	>4 mm or satellite lesions within 2 cm of primary
III	Regional nodes <5 mm in size or satellite lesions farther than 2 cm
IV	Nodes >5 mm in size, >1 nodal station, >5 intransit metastases, distant metastases

(Melanoma staging and margin tables adapted from Chang AE et al. Cutaneous neo-plasms. In: Greenfield LJ et al, eds. Surgery: Scientific principles and practice. Ed 3. Philadelphia: Lippincott Williams & Wilkins, 2001)

Clark's levels for melanoma

Level	Description
I	Epidermis basement membrane intact
II	Papillary dermis through basement membrane
III	Juntional dermis between papillary and reticular dermis
IV	Reticular dermis
V	Fat

Melanoma margins

Depth	Margin Needed
<1 mm	1 cm
1–4 mm	2 cm
>4 mm	3 cm

Nodes
- Always need to resect clinically positive nodes with melanoma
- Perform sentinel lymph node biopsy if nodes clinically negative and tumor ≥1mm deep.
- **Involved nodes** usually nontender, round, hard, 1–2 cm
- All stage III tumors need full lymph node dissection.

Axillary node melanoma with no other primary – Tx: complete axillary node dissection
Resection of metastases has provided some patients with long disease-free interval and is the best chance for cure.
Isolated metastases (i.e., lung or liver) that can be resected with a low-risk procedure should probably undergo resection.

Survival of AJC clinical stage I and II melanoma patients relative to tumor location

Thickness (mm)	7.5-Year Survival Rate (%)				
	Extremities	Hands or Feet	Head and Neck	Trunk	BANS
<0.85	100	100	100	100	98
0.85–1.69	100	100	100	97	78
1.7–3.64	86	60	64	77	58
≥3.65	83	0	65	12	33

BANS = upper back, posterolateral arm, posterior and lateral neck, and posterior scalp.
(Modified from Chang AE et al. Cutaneous neoplasms. In: Greenfield LJ et al, ed. Surgery: scientific principles and practice. Ed 3. Philadelphia: Lippincott Williams & Wilkins, 2001)

Basal cell carcinoma
Most common malignancy in US; 4x more common than squamous cell skin CA
80% on head and neck
Originates from epidermis – basal epithelial cells and hair follicles
Pearly appearance, rolled borders
Pathology – **peripheral palisading of nuclei and stromal retraction**
Slow, indolent growth
Ulcerative, no metastases, deep invasion, occasionally dark
Regional adenectomy for clinically positive nodes
Morpheaform type – most aggressive; has **collagenase** production
Tx: 0.3–0.5 cm margins

Squamous cell carcinoma
Overlying erythema, papulonodular with crust and ulceration
May have surrounding induration and satellite nodules
Usually red-brown; can have a pearly appearance
Metastasizes more frequently than basal cell CA but less common than melanoma
Can develop in postradiation areas or in old burn scars
Risk factors – actinic keratoses, xeroderma pigmentosum, Bowen's disease, atrophic epidermis, arsenics, hydrocarbons (coal tar), chlorophenols, nitrates, HPV, immunosuppression, sun exposure, fair skin, XRT exposure, previous skin CA
Risk factors for metastasis – poorly differentiated, greater depth, recurrent lesions, immunosuppression
Tx: 0.5–1.0-cm margins for low risk
 Can treat high risk with Mohs surgery (margin mapping using conservative slices; not used for melanoma) when trying to minimize area of resection (i.e., lesions on face)
 Regional adenectomy for clinically positive nodes
 XRT and chemotherapy – may be of limited benefit for inoperable disease or metastases

Soft tissue sarcoma
Most commmon soft tissue sarcomas – **#1 malignant fibrous histiosarcoma**, #2 liposarcoma
50% arise from extremities; 50% in children (arise from embryonic mesoderm)
Most sarcomas are large, grow rapidly, and are painless.
Symptoms: asymptomatic mass (most common presentation), GI bleeding, bowel obstruction, neurologic deficit
Biopsy
 Excisional biopsy if mass <4 cm
 Longitudinal incisional biopsy for masses >4 cm (may need to eventually resect biopsy skin site if biopsy shows sarcoma)
Hematogenous spread, not to lymphatics → metastasis to nodes is rare
 Lung – most common site for metastasis
Staging based on grade, not size or nodes

Tx: Want at least **3-cm margins and at least 1 univolved fascial plane** → try to perform limb-sparing operation
Place clips to mark site of likely recurrence → will XRT these later
Postop XRT – for high-grade tumors, close margins, or tumors >5 cm
Chemotherapy is doxorubicin based.
Tumors >10 cm may benefit from preop XRT and chemotherapy → may allow limb-sparing resection
Isolated sarcoma metastases without other evidence of systemic disease (i.e., lung or liver) can be resected and are the best chance for survival; otherwise can palliate with XRT
Midline incision favored for pelvic and retroperitoneal sarcomas

Poor prognosis overall
Delay in diagnosis
Difficulty with total resection
Difficulty getting XRT to pelvic tumors
40% 5-year survival rate with complete resection

Head and neck sarcomas – can occur in the pediatric population (usually rhabdomyosarcoma)
Hard to get margin because of proximity to vital structures
Postop XRT for positive or close margins as negative margins may be impossible to obtain

Visceral and retroperitoneal sarcomas – most commonly are leiomyosarcomas and liposarcomas
Ability to completely remove the tumor the most important prognostic factor in visceral and retroperitoneal sarcomas

Risk factors
Asbestos – mesothelioma
PVC and arsenic – angiosarcoma
Other risk factors – XRT, chlorophenols, pesticides
Chronic lymphedema – associated with lymphangiosarcoma

Kaposi's sarcoma – vascular sarcoma
Can involve skin, mucous membranes, or GI tract
Associated with immunocompromised state
Rarely a cause of death in AIDS;15–20-year survival; slow growing
Tx: XRT or intralesional vinblastine for local disease; systemic chemotherapy for disseminated disease
Surgery for intestinal hemorrhage

Childhood rhabdomysarcoma
#1 soft tissue sarcoma in kids
Head/neck, genitourinary, extremities and trunk (poorest prognosis)
Embryonal subtype – most common
Alveolar subtype – worst prognosis
Tx: surgery; doxorubicin-based chemotherapy

Bone sarcomas
Most are metastatic at the time of diagnosis.
Osteosarcoma
Increased incidence around the knee
Originates from **metaphyseal cells**
Usually in children
Usually need to take the joint, followed by reconstruction; may require amputation

Genetic syndromes for soft tissue tumors
Neurofibromatosis – CNS tumors, peripheral sheath tumors, pheochromocytoma
LiFraumeni syndrome – childhood rhabdomyosarcoma, many others
Hereditary retinoblastoma – also includes other sarcoma
Tuberous sclerosis – angiomyolipoma
Gardner's syndrome – familial adenomatous polyposis and intra-abdominal desmoids

Other conditions
Xanthoma – yellow, contain histiocytes. Tx: excision
Warts (verruca vulgaris) – viral origin, contagious, autoinocuable, can be painful
   Tx: liquid nitrogen initially
Lipomas – common but rarely malignant; back, neck, between shoulders
Neuromas – can be associated with neurofibromatosis and von Recklinghausen's disease
   Café-au-lait spots, axillary freckling, optic nerve gliomas, CNS tumors
Keratoses
   Actinic keratosis – premalignant, in sun damaged areas; need excisional biopsy if suspicious
   Seborrheic keratosis – <u>not</u> premalignant; trunk on elderly; can be dark
   Arsenical keratosis – associated with squamous cell carcinoma
Merkel cell carcinoma – are **neuroendocrine**
   Aggressive regional and systemic spread; patients have red to purple papulonodule/indurated plaque
   Have **neuron-specific enolase (NSE), cytokeratine, and neurofilament protein**
Glomus cell tumor
   Painful tumor composed of blood vessels and nerves
   Benign; most common in the terminal aspect of the digit
   Tx: tumor excision
Hutchinson's freckle – in elderly, often on face; premalignant, not aggressive
Lip lacerations – important to line up vermillion border
Desmoid tumors – usually benign; occur in fascial planes
   Anterior abdominal wall (most common location) desmoids can occur during or following pregnancy; can also occur after trauma or surgery
   Intra-abdominal desmoids associated with Gardner's syndrome and retroperitoneal fibrosis
   High risk of local recurrences; no distant spread
   Tx: surgery or chemotherapy/XRT if vital structure involved
Bowen's disease – SCCA in situ; 10% turn into invasive SCCA
   Tx: excision with negative margins
Keratoacanthoma
   Rapid growth, rolled edges, crater filled with keratin
   Is not malignant but can be confused with SCCA
   Involutes spontaneously over months
   Always biopsy these to be sure.
   If small, excise; if large, biopsy and observe.
Hyperhydrosis – ↑ sweating, especially noticeable in the palms. Tx: sympathectomy
Hidradenitis – infection of the apocrine sweat glands, usually in axilla and groin regions
   Staph/strep most common organisms
   Tx: antibiotics, improved hygiene 1st; may need surgery
Benign cysts
   Epidermal inclusion cyst – most common; have completely mature epidermis with creamy keratin material
   Trichilemmal cyst – in scalp, no epidermis
   Ganglion cyst – over tendons, usually over wrist; filled with collagenous material
   Dermoid cyst – midline abdominal and sacral lesions, occiput and nose; found along body fusion planes
   Pilonidal cyst – congenital coccygeal sinus with ingrown hair; gets infected and need to be excised
Keloids – autosomal dominant; dark skin
   <u>Collagen goes beyond original scar.</u>
   Tx: XRT, steroids, silicone, pressure garments
Hypertrophic scar tissue – dark skin; flexor surfaces of upper torso
   <u>Collagen stays within confines of scar.</u>
   Often occurs in burns or wounds that take a long time to heal
   Tx: steroids, silicone, pressure garments

CHAPTER 19. HEAD AND NECK

Anatomy and physiology
Anterior neck triangle – sternocleidomastiod muscle, sternal notch, inferior border of the digastric muscle; contains the **carotid sheath**
Posterior neck triangle – posterior border of the sternocleidomastoid muscle, trapezius muscle, and the clavicle; contains the **spinal accessory nerve and the brachial plexus**
Phrenic nerve – on anterior scalene muscle
Parotid glands – secrete mostly serous fluid
Sublingual glands – secrete mostly mucin
Submandibular glands – 50/50
In larynx, the false vocal cords are superior to the true vocal cords.
Trachea has U-shaped cartilage and a posterior portion that is membranous.

Vagus nerve – runs between IJ and carotid arteries
Phrenic nerve – runs on top of the anterior scalene muscle
Trigeminal nerve – ophthalmic, maxillary, mandibluar branches
    Gives sensation to most of face
    Mandibular branch – taste to anterior ⅔ of tongue, floor of mouth, and gingiva
Facial nerve – temporal, zygomatic, bucal, marginal mandibular, and cervical branches
    Motor function to face
Glossopharyngeal nerve – sensory to posterior tongue
    Motor to stylopharyngeus
    Injury affects swallowing.
Hypoglossal nerve – motor to all of tongue except palatoglossus
    Tongue deviates to side of injury.
Recurrent laryngeal nerve – innervates all of larynx except cricothyroid muscle
Superior laryngeal nerve – innervates the cricothyroid muscle
Frey's syndrome – occurs after parotidectomy; injury of **auriculotemporal nerve** that then cross-innervates with sympathetic fibers to sweat glands of skin
    Symptom: gustatory sweating

Thyrocervical trunk – "STAT": suprascapular artery, transverse cervical artery, ascending cervical artery, inferior thyroid artery
External carotid artery – 1st branch is superior thyroid artery
Trapezius flap (spinal accessory nerve, shoulder shrug) – based on transverse cervical artery
Pectoralis major – based on thoracoacromial artery

Torus palatini – congenital bony mass on upper palate of mouth. Tx: nothing
Torus mandibular – similar to above but on the anterior lingual surface of the mandible

Radical neck dissection (RND) – takes accessory nerve (CN XII), sternocleidomastoid, internal jugular, omohyoid, submandibular gland, sensory nerves C2–C5, cervical branch of facial nerve, and ipsilateral thyroid
    Most morbidity occurs from accessory nerve resection.
Modified radical neck dissection (MRND) – takes omohyoid, submandibular gland, sensory nerves C2–C5, cervical branch of facial nerve, ipsilateral thyroid
    No mortality difference compared with RND

Oral cavity cancer
    Most common cancer of the oral cavity, pharynx, and larynx – squamous cell CA
        Biggest risk factors – tobacco and ETOH
        Erythroplakia – considered more premalignant than leukoplakia

    Oral cavity includes mouth floor, anterior ⅓ of tongue, gingiva, hard palate, anterior tonsillar pillars, and lips.
    SCCA – most common cancer of oral cavity
    Lower lip – most common site for oral cavity CA
    Nodal spread <u>unusual</u> for oral cavity CA; <u>submental and submandibular</u> chains 1st
    Notable exception is **anterior tongue tumors**, which spread to anterior <u>cervical chain early</u>.

Survival rate lowest for hard palate tumors – hard to resect

Oral cavity CA increased in patients with Plummer-Vinson syndrome (glossitis, cervical dysphagia from esophageal web, spoon fingers, iron-deficiency anemia)

Treatment
    Wide resection of tumor if ≤2 cm (T1), need 1–2 cm margins
    MRND (modified radical neck dissection) for tumors >2 cm or if clinically positive nodes
    Postop XRT for advanced lesions (>2 cm, positive margins, nerve/vascular/lymphatic invasion)
        Lip CA – lower lip CA more common than upper due to sun exposure
            May need **flaps** if more than ½ of the lip is removed
            Lesions along the **commissure are most aggressive**.
        Tongue CA – can still operate with jaw invasion
        Verrucous ulcer – well-differentiated tumor of the cheek
            Not aggressive
    Tx: full cheek resection +/– flap; no MRND
    Cancer of maxillary sinus – Tx: maxillectomy

Pharyngeal cancer

    Nasopharyngeal SCCA – EBV; Chinese; presents with nose bleeding or obstruction
        Goes to **posterior (deep) cervical neck nodes**
        Tx: **XRT primary; MRND** for tumors >2 cm or clinically positive nodes; postop chemo for advanced stage
        Children – lymphoma #1 tumor of nasopharynx. Tx: chemotherapy
        Papilloma – most common benign neoplasm of nose/paranasal sinuses

    Oropharyngeal SCCA – neck mass, sore throat
        Goes to **posterior (deep) cervical neck nodes**
        Tx: **XRT or surgery; MRND** for tumors >2 cm or if clinically positive nodes

    Tonsillar CA – ETOH, tobacco, males; SCCA most common; asymptomatic until large; 80% have lymph node metastases at time of diagnosis
        Tx: tonsillectomy best way to biopsy; XRT mainstay

    Hypopharyngeal SCCA – hoarseness; early metastases
        Goes to **anterior cervical nodes**
        Tx: **usually surgery** (laryngectomy), **MRND, postop XRT**

    Nasopharyngeal angiofibroma – benign tumor
        Presents in males <20 years (obstruction or epistaxis)
        Extremely vascular
        Tx: angiography and embolization (usually internal maxillary artery), followed by resection

Laryngeal cancer

    Hoarseness, aspiration, dyspnea, dysphagia
    Can preserve larynx in some cases of cancer (glottis free of tumor and mobile)
    Take **ipsilateral thyroid lobe** with RND
    Papilloma – most common benign lesion of larynx

    Supraglottic SCCA – early nodal spread to submental/submandibular areas
        Small – Tx: **XRT or conservative surgery**
        Large – Tx: **laryngectomy, MRND, postop XRT**
    Glottic SCCA – nodal spread to anterior cervical chain
        Small – Tx: **XRT or laser**, chordectomy with recurrence
        Large – Tx: **laryngectomy, MRND, postop XRT**
        Fixed cords require laryngectomy.
    Subglottic SCCA – early nodal to anterior cervical chain and metastatic spread
        Small – Tx: **XRT or conservative surgery**
        Large – Tx: **laryngectomy, MRND, postop XRT**

Salivary gland cancers

Parotid, submandibular, sublingual, and minor salivary glands
Mass in <u>large</u> salivary gland → more likely mass is benign
Mass in <u>small</u> salivary gland → more likely mass is malignant, although the parotid gland is the most frequent site for malignant tumor

Malignant tumors
- **Mucoepidermoid CA** – #1 malignant tumor of the salivary glands
  - Wide range of aggressiveness
- **Adenoid cystic CA** – #2 malignant tumor of the salivary glands; #1 malignant salivary tumor of the minor salivary glands
  - Long, indolent course; propensity to invade nerve roots

Often present as a painful mass but can also present with facial nerve paralysis or lymphadenopathy
Lymphatic drainage to the intraparotid nodes and the anterior cervical chain nodes

Tx for both: **resection of salivary gland (parotidectomy); prophylactic MRND and postop XRT if high grade or SCCA**
  If in parotid, need to take whole lobe; try to preserve facial nerve.

Benign tumors
- **Pleomorphic adenoma** (mixed tumor) – #1 benign tumor of the salivary glands
  - **Malignant degeneration in 5%**
  - Tx: superficial parotidectomy
  - If malignant degeneration, need total parotidectomy; if high grade also need MRND
- **Warthin's tumor** – #2 benign tumor of the salivary glands
  - Males, bilateral in 10%
  - Tx: superficial parotidectomy
  - Often present as a painless mass

Most commn injured nerve with parotid surgery – **greater auricular nerve** (numbness over lower portion of auricle)
For submandibular gland resection – need to find <u>mandibular branch of facial nerve, lingual nerve, hypoglossal nerve</u>
Most common salivary gland tumor in children – **hemangiomas**

Ear

- **Cauliflower ear** – undrained hematomas that organize and calcify; need to be drained to avoid this
- **Chemodectomas** – vascular tumor of middle ear (paraganglionoma). Tx: surgery +/– XRT
- **Acoustic neuroma** – CN VIII, tinnitus, hearing loss, unsteadiness; can grow into cerebellar/pontine angle. Tx: craniotomy and resection; XRT is alternative to surgery
- **Cholesteatoma** – epidermal inclusion cyst of ear; slow growing but erode as they grow; present with conductive hearing loss and clear drainage from ear. Tx: surgical excision
- **Pinna lacerations** – need suture through involved cartilage
- **Ear SCCA** – 20% metastasize to parotid gland. Tx: parotidectomy, MRND for positive nodes or large tumors, XRT
- **Rhabdomyosarcoma** – most common childhood aural malignancy (although rare) of the middle or external ear

Nose

- **Nasal fractures** – set after swelling decreases
- **Septal hematoma** – need to drain to avoid infection and necrosis of septum
- **CSF rhinorrhea** – usually a cribiform plate fracture (CSF has **tau protein**)
  - Repair of facial fractures may help leak; may need contrast study to help find leak
  - Tx: conservative 2–3 weeks; try epidural catheter, may need transethmoid repair
- **Epistaxis**
  - 90% anterior and can be controlled with packing
  - Consider internal maxillary artery or ethmoid artery ligation (direct or angiographically) for persistent posterior bleeding despite packing/balloon

Neck and jaw
Radicular cyst – local excision or curettage; lucent on x-ray
Ameloblastoma – slow-growing malignancy; soap bubble appearance on x-ray; can have metastasess. Tx: wide local excision
Osteogenic sarcoma – poor prognosis. Tx: multimodality approach that includes surgery
Maxillary jaw fractures – most treated with wire fixation
TMJ dislocations – treated with closed reduction
Lip numbness – inferior alveolar nerve damage

Stenson's duct laceration – repair over catheter stent
    Ligation can cause painful parotid atrophy and facial asymmetry.
Suppurative parotitis – usually in elderly patients; occurs with dehydration; staph most common organism
    Tx fluids, salivation, antibiotics; drainage if abcess develops or patient not improving
    Can be life-threatening
Sialoadenitis – acute inflammation of the salivary gand related to a stone in the duct; most calculi near orifice
    Recurrent sialoadenitis is thought to be due to ascending infection from the oral cavity.
    Gland excision may eventually be necessary for recurrent disease.
    80% of the time affects the submandibular or sublingual glands
    Tx: incise duct and remove

Abscesses
Peritonsilar abscess – older kids (>10 years)
    Symptoms: trismus, odynophagia; usually does <u>not</u> obstruct airway
    <u>Tx</u>: needle aspiration 1st, then drainage through tonsillar bed if no relief in 24 hours
        May need to intubate to drain; will self-drain with swallowing once opened

Retropharyngeal abscess – younger kids (<10 years)
    Symptoms: fever, odynophagia, drool; is an **airway emergency**
    Can occur in elderly with Pott's disease
    <u>Tx</u>: intubate the patient in a calm setting; drainage through posterior pharyngeal wall; will self-drain with swallowing once opened

Parapharyngeal abscess – all age groups; occurs with dental infections, tonsillitis, pharyngitis
    Morbidity comes from vascular invasion and mediastinal spread via prevertebral and retropharyngeal spaces.
    <u>Tx</u>: drain through lateral neck to avoid damaging internal carotid and internal jugular veins; need to leave drain in

Ludwig's angina – acute infection of the floor of the mouth, involves **myelohyoid muscle**
    Most common cause is dental infection of the mandibular teeth.
    May rapidly spread to deeper structures and cause airway obstruction
    Tx: airway control, surgical drainage, antibiotics

Asymptomatic head and neck masses
Preauricular tumors
    All lumps near ear are parotid tumors until proved otherwise.
    Diagnosis is usually made after superficial lobectomy.
    80% of all salivary tumors are in parotid.
    80% of parotid tumors are benign.
    80% of benign parotid tumors are pleomorhic adenomas – 5% malignant degeneration
    Most common distant metastases for head and neck tumors → lung
        Tx: **chemotherapy**
Posterior neck masses – if no obvious malignant epithelial tumor, considered to have Hodgkin's lymphoma until proved otherwise. Need FNA or open biopsy

Neck mass workup
    1st – exam, layngoscopy, antibiotics if thought to be inflammatory, FNA if hard
    2nd – panendoscopy with multiple random biopsies, neck and chest CT
    3rd – still can't figure it out → perform excisional biopsy; need to be prepared for MRND
    Adenocarcinoma suggests breast, GI, or lung primary.

Chapter 19. Head and Neck

Epidermoid CA found in cervical node without known primary
  1st – panendoscopy with random biopsies
  2nd – CT scan
  3rd – still can't find primary → ipsilateral MRND, ipsilateral tonsillectomy, bilateral XRT

Other conditions
Esophageal foreign body – dysphagia; most just below the cricopharyngeus (95%)
  Dx: **rigid EGD** under anesthesia
  Perforation risk increases with <u>length of time in the esophagus</u>.
Fever and pain after EGD for foreign body→ CXR and gastrograffin followed by barium swallow to rule out perforation
Laryngeal foreign body – coughing; emergent cricothyroidotomy as a last resort may be needed to secure airway
Lip lacerations – apposition of the vermillion border is key. Layered closure is preferred.
Sleep apnea – associated with MIs, arrhythmias, and death
  More common in obese and those with micrognathia/retrognathia → have snoring and excessive daytime somulence
  Tx: CPAP, uvulopalatopharyngoplasty, hyoid suspension, or permanent trach
Prolonged intubation – can lead to subglottic stenosis, which is treated with laser, dilatation, possible excision
Tracheostomy – consider in patients that will require intubation for >7–14 days
  Decreases secretions, provides easier ventilation, decreases pneumonia risk
Tracheo-innominate fistula – occurs after tracheostomy, can have rapid exsanguination
  Tx: place finger in trach hole and hold pressure → median sternotomy, repair innominate with graft usual method
  This complication is avoided by keeping tracheostomy above the 2nd–3rd tracheal ring.
Median rhomboid glossitis – failure of tongue fusion. Tx: none necessary
Cleft lip (primary palate) – involves lip, alveolus, or both
  Repair at 10 weeks, 10 lb, Hgb 10. Repair nasal deformities at same time.
  May be associated with poor feeding
Cleft palate (secondary palate) – involves hard and soft palates; may affect speech and swallowing if not closed soon enough; may affect maxillofacial growth if closed too early → repair at 12 months
Hemangioma – most common benign head and neck tumor in adults
Mastoiditis – infection of the mastoid cells; can destroy bone
  Rare; results as a complication of untreated acute supportive otitis media
  Ear pushed forward
  Tx: antibiotics, may need emergency mastoidectomy
Epiglottitis
  Rare since immunization against *H. influenzae* type B
  Mainly in children aged 3–5
  Symptoms: stridor, drooling, leaning forward position, high fever, throat pain, thumbprint sign on lateral neck film
  Can cause airway obstruction
  Tx: early control of the airway; antibiotics
Kaposi's sarcoma – oral and pharyngeal mucosa are the most common sites
  Can get odynophagia and dysphagia
  Primary goal usually is palliation.
  Most common neoplasm in patients with AIDS
  Tx: XRT, intratumor vinblastine

CHAPTER 20. PITUITARY

Anatomy and physiology
    Hypothalmus – releases TRH, CRH, GnRH, GHRH, and dopamine into median eminence; passes through neurohypohysis on way to adenohypophysis
    Dopamine – inhibits prolactin secretion
    Posterior pituitary (neurohypophysis)
        ADH – supraoptic nuclei, regulated by osmolar receptors in hypothalamus
        Oxytocin – paraventricular nuclei in hypothalamus
    Neurohypophysis does not contain cell bodies.
    Anterior pituitary (80% of gland, adenohypophysis)
        ACTH, TSH, GH, LH, FSH, and prolactin
        Does not have its own direct blood supply; passes through neurohypophysis 1st

    Bitemporal hemianopia – pituitary mass compressing optic nerve (CN III) at chiasm
    Nonfunctional tumors – almost always macroadenomas; present with mass effect and decreased ACTH, TSH, GH, LH, FSH. Tx: transphenoid resection
    Contraindications to transsphenoid approaches – supracellar extension, massive lateral extension, dumbbell-shaped tumor
    TSH- and FSH-/LH-secreting tumors may respond to **bromocriptine**.

Prolactinoma
    Most common pituitary adenoma
    Mostly microadenomas
    Most patients do not need surgery. Prolactin is usually >150 in these patients.
    Symptoms: galactorrhea, irregular menses, ↓ libido, infertility, ↓ vision
    Tx: bromocriptine for most, or transsphenoidal resection for failure of medical management
        Macroadenomas – resection with hemorrhage, visual loss, wants pregnancy, CSF leak
        Microadenomas – resection if bromocriptine unsafe or ineffective (is OK in pregnancy)

Acromegaly (growth hormone)
    Symptoms: HTN, DM, giganticism
    GH >10 in 90%, usually macroadenomas
    Preoperative octreotide may be helpful (inhibits release of GH).
    Can be life-threatening secondary to cardiac symptoms (valve dysfunction, cardiomyopathy)
    Higher remission rate for microadenomas
    Symptoms: hypertension, diabetes mellitus, gigantism
    Dx: elevated IGF-1, growth hormone >5–10
    Tx: transsphenoidal resection; XRT and bromocriptine can be used for primary or secondary therapy

Other conditions
    Sheehan's syndrome
        Postpartum **trouble lactating – usually 1st sign**
        Can also have amenorrhea, adrenal insufficiency, and hypothyroidism
        Due to **pituitary ischemia** following hemorrhage and hypotensive episode
    Craniopharyngioma – calcified cyst, remnants of Rathke's pouch
        Symptoms: most frequently presents with endocrine abnormalities, visual disturbances, headache, hydrocephalus
        Tx: surgery, XRT
        Diabetes insipidus – frequent complication postoperatively
    Bilateral pituitary masses – check axis; if OK, probably metastases
    Nelson's syndrome
        Occurs after bilateral adrenalectomy; ↑ CRH causes pituitary enlargement, resulting in amenorrhea, visual problems (bitemporal hemianopia)
        Also get hyperpigmentation from **beta-MSH** (melanocyte-stimulating hormone), a peptide byproduct of ACTH
        Tx: steroids
    Waterhouse-Friedrichsen syndrome – adrenal gland hemorrhage that occurs after meningococcal sepsis infection; can lead to adrenal insufficiency

CHAPTER 21. ADRENAL

Superior adrenal – inferior phrenic artery
Middle adrenal – aorta
Inferior adrenal – renal artery
Left adrenal vein goes to left renal vein.
Right adrenal vein goes to inferior vena cava.

Asymptomatic adrenal mass
1%–2% of abdominal CT scans show incidentaloma (5% are metastates or primary adrenal tumors).
Benign adenomas are common.
Adrenals are also common sites for metastases.
Surgery is indicated if mass **has ominous characteristics** or is **>4–6 cm, functioning, or enlarging.**
Need to follow up very 3 months for 1 year, then yearly
Dx: serum K, urine metanephrines/VMA/catecholamines, urinary hydroxycorticosteroids, plasma renin and aldosterone levels if HTN or↓ K; CXR, stool guaiac and colonoscopy, mammogram
Anterior approach for adrenal CA resection

Common metastases to adrenal – breast CA (#1), melanoma, renal CA, lung CA
Cancer history with asymptomatic adrenal mass – need biopsy

Adrenal cortex
From mesoderm – remember GFR = salt, sugar, sex steroids
Glomerulosa – aldosterone; **fasciculata** – glucocorticoids; **reticularis** – androgens/estrogens
Cholesterol → progesterone → androgens/cortisol/aldosterone
All zones have **21- and 11-beta hydroxylase**.
No innervation to the cortex
Medulla receives innervation from the splanchnic nerves.
Lymphatics drain to subdiaphragmatic and renal lymph nodes.
Corticotropin-releasing hormone (CRH) is released from the hypothalamus and goes to anterior pituitary gland.
ACTH is released from the anterior pituitary gland and causes the release of cortisol.
Cortisol has a diurnal peak at 4–6 a.m.
Aldosterone stimulates renal sodium resorption and secretion of potassium, hydrogen ion, and ammonia.
Aldosterone secretion is stimulated by **angiotensin II and hyperkalemia, and to some extent ACTH.**
Excess estrogens and androgens by adrenals – almost always cancer

Congenital adrenal hyperplasia (enzyme defect in cortisol synthesis)
 21-hydroxylase deficiency (90%) – most common; precocious puberty in males, virilization in females
  ↑ 17-OH progesterone leads to ↑ production of testosterone
  Is salt wasting (↓ sodium and ↑ potassium) **and causes hypotension**
  Tx: cortisol, genitoplasty
 11-hydroxylase deficiency – precocious puberty in males, virilization in females
  ↑ 11-deoxycortisone.
  Is salt saving (deoxycortisone acts as a mineralcorticoid) and causes **hypertension**
  Tx: cortisol, genitoplasty
 17-hydroxylase deficiency – ambiguous genitalia in males at birth; salt saving

Hyperaldosteronism (Conn's syndrome)
 Symptoms: HTN secondary to sodium retention without edema; hypokalemia; also have weakness, polydipsia, and polyuria
 Primary disease (low renin) – adenoma (80%–90%) → #1 cause of primary hyperaldosteronism), hyperplasia (10%–20%), ovarian tumors (rare), cancer (rare)

Secondary disease (high renin) – more common than primary disease; CHF, renal artery stenosis, liver failure, pregnancy, diuretics, Bartter's syndrome (renin-secreting tumor)
Dx for primary hyperaldosteronism – urine aldosterone after salt load best (will stay high)
  ↓ serum K, ↑ urine K, ↑ serum Na, metabolic alkalosis
  Plasma renin activity will be low.
Localizing studies – MRI, NP-59 scintography (shows hyperfunctioning adrenal tissue; differentiates adenoma from hyperplasia; 90% accurate); adrenal venous sampling if others nondiagnostic
Tumor vs hyperplasia
  Upright posture
    Tumor (cancer or adenoma) – <u>aldosterone and renin remain suppressed</u>
    Hyperplasia – <u>slight ↑ in aldosterone and renin</u>
  18-OH corticosterone – high (>100 μg/dl) with tumor (cancer or adenoma) and low with hyperplasia
  Adenoma – more sensitive to ACTH
  Hyperplasia – more sensitive to angiotensin II

  Tx: adenoma resection has good results with adrenalectomy
    Hyperplasia – seldom cured (↑ morbidity with bilateral resection)
      Try medical therapy first with hyperplasia using spironolactone, calcium channel blockers, and potassium.
      If bilateral resection is performed (usually done for refractory hypokalemia), patient will need fludrocortisone postoperatively.

Hypocortisolism (adrenal insufficiency, Addison's disease)
#1 cause – **withdrawal of exogenous steroids**
#1 primary disease – **autoimmune disease**
Also caused by pituitary disease, infection, adrenal hemorrhage, adrenal metastasis, surgical resection or injury
Get ↓ cortisol and aldosterone
Dx: ↓ serum Na, ↑ serum K, ACTH stimulation test
Acute adrenal insufficiency – hypotension, fever, lethargy, abdominal pain, ↓ glucose
  ↓ mental status, nausea and vomiting, ↑ K
Tx: dexamethasone, fluids, and ACTH stimulation test (measure cortisol level after test)

Hypercortisolism (Cushing's syndrome)
Most commonly **iatrogenic**
Dx: 1st – 24-hour urine cortisol (most sensitive test)
  2nd – low-dose overnight dexamethasone suppression test; look to see whether it suppresses cortisol production (measure in urine). If cortisol is low, the diagnosis is Cushing's disease (the pituitary adenoma was suppressed). If cortisol remains high, go to 3rd.
  3rd – measure serum ACTH. If high, have either ectopic ACTH or pituitary tumor that was not suppressed with low-dose overnight dexamethasone suppression test, go to 4th. If low ACTH, patient has cortisol-secreting tumor (i.e., adrenal tumor or adrenal hyperplasia).
  4th – if serum ACTH high → high-dose overnight dexamethasone suppression test (positive = pituitary origin, negative = ectopic origin of ACTH). In 20% you still can't tell; go to 5th.
  5th – CRH test → pituitary adenomas will increase ACTH, ectopic producers will have no change in ACTH
MRI useful. NP-59 scintography localizes adrenal tumors and can help differentiate them from hyperplasia.

Pituitary adenoma (Cushing's disease)
#1 noniatrogenic cause of Cushing's syndrome → 70%–80% of cases
Cortisol should be suppressed with either low- or high-dose dexamethasone suppression test.
Mostly **microadenomas**
Need petrosal sampling to figure out which side; MRI can also help
Vertical incisions to find adenoma
Tx: most tumors removed with transsphenoidal approach; unresectable or residual tumors treated with XRT

Chapter 21. Adrenal

Ectopic ACTH
- #2 noniatrogenic cause of Cushing's syndrome
- Most commonly from small cell lung CA
- Cortisol is <u>not</u> suppressed with either low- or high-dose dexamethasone suppression test
- Chest and abdominal CT can help localize.
- Tx: resection of primary if possible; medical suppression or bilateral adrenalectomy for inoperable lesions

Adrenal adenoma
- #3 noniatrogenic cause of Cushing's syndrome
- ↓ ACTH, unregulated steroid production; does not suppress
- Tx: adrenalectomy

Adrenocortical carcinoma – rare cause of Cushing's syndrome
- Tx: radical adrenalectomy; debulking can help patients and prolong survival

Adrenal hyperplasia (macro or micro)
- Tx: bilateral adrenalectomy

Medical therapy for ectopic ACTH production or adrencortical cancer with residual or metastatic disease after resection
- **Ketoconazole and metyrapone** – inhibit steroid formation
- **Aminoglutethimide** – inhibits cholesterol conversion
- **Op-DDD (mitotane)** – adrenal-lytic, used for metastatic disease

Bilateral adrenalectomy – may be needed in patients with ectopic ACTH from tumor that is unresectable or from pituitary adenoma that can't be found
- Need to remember to <u>give steroids postoperatively</u>.

Adrenocortical carcinoma
- Bimodal distribution (before age 5 and in the 5th decade); more common in females
- **50% are functioning tumors** – cortisol, aldosterone, sex steroids
- Children display virilization 90% of the time (precocious puberty in boys, virilization in females)
- Feminization in men; masculinization in women can occur
- Symptoms: abdominal pain, weight loss, weakness
- 80% have advanced disease at time of diagnosis.
- Tx: radical adrenalectomy; mitotane for residual or recurrent disease
- 20% 5-year survival rate

Adrenal medulla
From ectoderm neural crest cells
Catecholamine production – **tyrosine → dopa → dopamine → norepinephrine → epinephrine**
Tyrosine hydroxylase – rate-limiting step (tyrosine to dopa)
PNMT – enzyme that converts norepineprine → epinephrine (requires methylation)
- Enzyme is found only in adrenal medulla (exclusive producers of epinephrine).
Only adrenal pheochromocytomas will produce epinephrine.
MAO (monoamine oxidase) – converts norepinephrine to normetanephrine, epinephrine to metanephrine; VMA produced from these
Extra-adrenal rest of neural crest tissue can exist, usually in the retroperitoneum, most notably in the organ of Zuckerkandl

Pheochromocytoma (chromaffin cells)
- Rare; usually slow growing; arise from sympathetic ganglia or ectopic neural crest cells
- **10% rule** – malignant, bilateral, in children, familial, extra-adrenal
- Can be associated with MEN IIa, MEN IIb, von Recklinghausen's disease, tuberous sclerosis, Sturge-Weber disease
- **Right-sided** predominance
- **Extra-adrenal tumors more likely malignant.**
- Symptoms: HTN (frequently **episodic**), headache, diaphoresis, palpitations
- Dx: **urine metanephrines and VMA** – breakdown products of epi and norepinephrine
  - **VMA most sensitive**
    - **MIBG** scan (norepinephrine analogue) – can help identify location if having trouble finding tumor
    - **Clonidine suppression test** – tumor doses not respond, keeps catecholamines ↑

No venography → can cause hypertensive crisis
CT/MRI can help localize tumors
Not able to localize → still proceed with laparotomy

Preoperatively: volume replacement, alpha-blocker first (phenoxybenzamine → avoids hypertensive crisis); then beta-blocker if patient has tachycardia or arrhythmias
  Need to be careful with beta-blocker and give after alpha-blocker → can precipitate **hypertensive crisis** (unopposed alpha stimulation) and **heart failure** in patients with cardiomyopathy

Tx: check for other tumors at resection; ligate adrenal veins first to avoid spilling catecholamines during tumor manipulation
  Debulking helps symptoms in patients with unresectable disease
  Metyrosine – inhibits tyrosine hydroxylase causing ↓ synthesis of catecholamines

Postop conditions – persistent hypertension, hypotension, hypoglycemia, bronchospasm, arrhythmias, intracerebral hemorrhage, CHF, MI
Other sites of pheochromocytomas – vertebral bodies, opposite adrenal gland, bladder, aortic bifurcation
Most common site of extramedullary tissue – **organ of Zuckerkandl (inferior aorta near bifurcation**
Falsely elevated VMA – coffee, tea, fruits, vanilla, iodine contrast, labatelol, alpha- and beta-blockers
Extramedullary tissue – responsible for **medullary CA of thyroid and extra-adrenal pheochromocytoma**

Ganglioneuroma – rare, benign, asymptomatic tumor of neural crest origin in the adrenal medulla or sympathetic chain

CHAPTER 22. THYROID

Anatomy and physiology
From the 1st and 2nd pharyngeal pouches
Thyrotropin-releasing factor (TRF) – released from the hypothalamus; acts on the anterior pituitary gland and causes release of TSH
Thyroid-stimulating hormone (TSH) – released from the anterior pituitary gland; acts on the thyroid gland to release T3 and T4 (through a mechanism that involves ↑ cAMP)
TRF and TSH release are controlled by T3 and T4 through a negative feedback loop.

Superior thyroid artery – 1st branch off external carotid artery
Inferior thyroid artery – off thyrocervical trunk; supplies inferior and superior parathyroids
Ligate close to thyroid to avoid injury to parathyroid glands with thyroidectomy.
IMA artery – occurs in 1%, arises from the innominate or aorta and goes to the isthmus

Superior and middle thyroid veins – drain into internal jugular vein
Inferior thyroid vein – drains into innominate vein

Nonrecurrent laryngeal nerve – in 2%–3%; more common on the right
Superior laryngeal nerve
  Motor to cricothyroid muscle
  Runs lateral to thyroid lobes
  Tracks close to superior thyroid artery but is variable
  Injury results in **loss of projection and easy voice fatiguablity** (opera singers).
Recurrent laryngeal nerves (RLNs)
  Motor to all of larynx except cricothyroid muscle
  Run posterior to thyroid lobes in the tracheoesophageal groove
  Can track with inferior thyroid artery but are variable
  Left RLN loops around aorta; right RLN loops around right subclavian (or innominate) artery
  Injury results in **hoarseness**; bilateral injury can **obstruct airway** → needs emergency tracheostomy
  The right nerve is more likely <u>not</u> to be recurrent compared with the left.
  Risk of injury for nonrecurrent laryngeal nerve injury during thyroid surgery

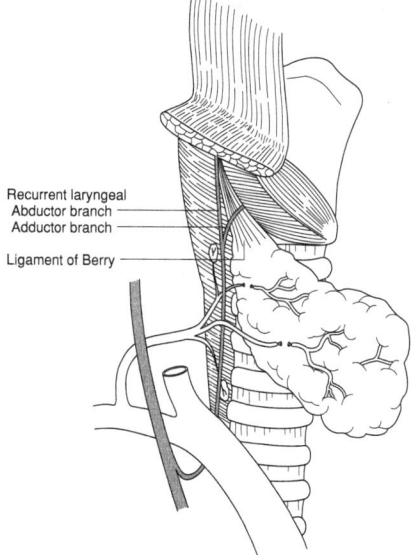

The ligament of Berry and distal recurrent laryngeal nerves.

Ligament of Berry – posterior medial suspensory ligament close to RLNs; careful dissection
Thyroglobulin – stores T3 and T4 in colloid
  Plasma T4:T3 ratio is 15:1; T3 more active form (is tyrosine + iodine)
  Most T3 produced in periphery by T4 to T3 conversion by peroxidases
Peroxidases link (or separate) tyrosine and iodine.
Thyroid-binding globulin – thyroid hormone transport; T3 and T4 also bind albumin
TSH – most sensitive indicator of gland function
Tubercles of Zuckerkandl – most lateral, posterior extension of thyroid tissue
  Rotate medially to find RLNs.
  This portion is left behind with subtotal thyroidectomy because of proximity to RLNs.
Parafollicular C cells – produce **calcitonin**
Resin T3 uptake – measures free T3 by having it bind resin
  ↑ resin uptake → hyperthyroidism or ↓ TBG
  ↓ uptake → hypothyroidism or ↑ TBG
Thyroxine treatment – TSH levels should fall to 50%; osteoporosis long-term side effect
Postthyroidectomy stridor – open neck and remove hematoma emergently → can result in aiway compromise

Thyroid storm
Symptoms: ↑ HR, fever, numbness, irratibility, vomiting, diarrhea, high-output cardiac failure (most common cause of death)
Most common after surgery in patient with undiagnosed **Grave's disease**
Can also be precipitated by anxiety, excessive palpation of the gland, adrenergic stimulants
Tx: beta-blockers, PTU, Lugol's solution (KI), cooling blankets, oxygen, glucose, fluid
  Emergent thyroidectomy rarely indicated
Wolff-Chaikoff effect – very effective for patients in thyroid storm
  Patient given high doses of iodine (Lugol's solution, potassium iodide), which inhibits TSH action on thyroid and inhibits organic coupling of iodide, resulting in less T3 and T4 release

Asymptomatic thyroid nodule
Thyroid function tests
  If elevated, give thyroxine; nodule should regress within 6 months. If not, get FNA.
  If not elevated, proceed with FNA.
Fine-needle aspiration (FNA)
  Determinant in 75%–90% → follow appropriate treatment
    Shows follicular cells → thyroidectomy or lobectomy (5%–10% malignancy risk)
    Shows thyroid CA → thyroidectomy or lobectomy and appropriate treatment (see below)
    Shows cyst fluid → drain fluid
      If it recurs → thyroidectomy or lobectomy
    Shows colloid tissue → most likely colloid goiter; low chance of malignancy (<1%)
      Thyroidectomy or lobectomy if it enlarges
  Indeterminant in 10%–25% → get radionucleide study
Hot nodule → thyroxine for 6 months; if size does not ↓, perform **lobectomy**
Cold nodule → thyroidectomy or lobectomy (more likely malignant than hot nodule)
  85% of thyroid nodules are benign.
  Thyroid nodules have a female predominance.
Goiter
  Any abnormal enlargement
  Most identifiable cause is iodine deficiency.
    Tx: iodine replacement
  Diffuse enlargement without evidence of functional abnormality = colloid goiter
    Tx: try to suppress with thyroxine; ^{131}I (may be ineffective), thionamides, subtotal thyroidectomy or lobectomy on side of goiter if medical treatment ineffective
Substernal goiter
  Usually secondary (vessels originate from superior and inferior thyroid arteries)
  Primary substernal goiter – rare (vessels originate from innominate artery)
    Tx: try to suppress with thyroxine; ^{131}I (may be ineffective), thionamides, subtotal thyroidectomy or lobectomy on side of goiter if medical treatment ineffective
Mediastinal thyroid tissue – most likely from acquired disease with inferior extensions of a normally placed gland

Chapter 22. Thyroid

Abnormalities of thyroid descent
- **Pyramidal lobe** – occurs in 10%, extends from the isthmus toward the thymus
- **Lingual thyroid**
  - Thyroid tissue that persists in the area of the foramen cecum at the base of the tongue
  - Symptoms: dysphagia, dyspnea, dysphonia
  - 2% malignancy risk
  - Tx: thyroxine suppression; abolish with I^{131} or resection if it is enlarged or suggestive of cancer, or if it does not shrink after medical therapy
  - Is the only thyroid tissue in 70% of patients who have it
- **Thyroglossal duct cyst**
  - Classically moves upward with swallowing
  - Susceptible to infection and may be premalignant
  - Tx: resection → need to take midportion or all of hyoid bone along with the thyroglossal duct cyst

Hyperthyroidism treatment
- **Propylthiouracil (PTU) and methimazole** –good for young patients, small goiters, mild T3 and T4 elevation
- **PTU (thionamides)**
  - Inhibits peroxidases and prevents DIT and MIT coupling
  - Side effects: **aplastic anemia or agranulocytosis** (rare)
- **Methimazole**
  - Inhibits peroxidases and prevents DIT and MIT coupling
  - Side effects: **cretinism** in newborns (crosses placenta) and **aplastic anemia or agranulocytosis** (rare)
- **Radioactive iodine (^{131}I)**
  - Good for patients that are poor surgical risks or unresponsive to propylthiouracil
  - ^{131}I should not be used in children or during pregnancy → can traverse placenta
- **Thyroidectomy**
  - Good for large glands, cold nodules in toxic glands, toxic multinodular goiters not responsive to medical therapy, toxic adenomas not responsive to medical therapy, pregnant patients not controlled with medical therapy
  - Best time to operate is 2nd trimester (↓ risk of teratogenic events and premature labor).
  - Subtotal thyriodectomy can leave patient euthyroid.

Causes of hyperthyroidism
- **Grave's disease** (toxic diffuse goiter)
  - Women; exophthalmos, pretibial edema, atrial fibrillation, heart dysfunction, heat intolerance, thirst, ↑ appetite, weight loss, sweating, palpitations
  - Most common cause of hyperthyroidism (80%)
  - Caused by **IgG antibodies to TSH receptor** (long-acting thyroid stimulator, thyroid-stimulating immunoglobulin)
  - If large, can get cervical compression syndromes
  - Dx: ↑ ^{123}I uptake diffusely in thyrotoxic patient with goiter
  - Tx: **thionamides** (70% recurrence), ^{131}I (10% recurrence), **subtotal thyroidectomy** (10% recurrence), or **total thyroidectomy** with thyroxine replacement if medical therapy fails
  - Medical therapy usually manages hyperthyroidism.
  - **Unusual to have to operate** on these patients unless in setting of suspicious nodule
    - **Preop preparation**: PTU or methimazole until euthyroid, beta-blocker, 1 week before surgery, Lugol's solution for 10–15 days to decrease friability and vascularity (start only after euthyroid)
    - **Operation**: bilateral subtotal or total thyroidectomy
    - Indications for surgery: noncompliant patient, recurrence after medical therapy, children, pregnant women not controlled with medical therapy, concomitant suspicious thyroid nodule

- **Toxic multinodular goiter**
  - Most common cause of thyroid enlargement
  - Women; age >50 years, normal thyroid function tests
  - Symptoms: cardiac symptoms, weight loss, insomnia, airway compromise; symptoms can be precipitated by contrast dyes.

Usually nontoxic 1st
Caused by hyperplasia secondary to chronic low-grade TSH stimulation
Tx: ^{131}I and thionamides; ^{131}I can be less effective in some (inhomogeneous uptake by gland); subtotal thyroidecotomy if medical treatment ineffective
Unusual to have to operate on these patients unless in setting of suspicious nodule

Single toxic nodule
Women; younger; can cause cervical compression
>3 cm usually symptomatic
20% of hot nodules eventually cause symptoms
Thought to function autonomously
Tx: ^{131}I and thionamides; lobectomy if medical treatment ineffective

Rare causes of hyperthyroidism – trophoblastic tumors, TSH-secreting pituitary tumors

Causes of thyroiditis
Hashimoto's disease
Most common cause of hypothyroidism in adults
Enlarged gland, painless, chronic thyroiditis
Women; history of childhood XRT
Can cause thyrotoxicosis in the acute early stage
Caused by both **humeral and cell-mediated autoimmune disease** (microsomal and thyroglobulin antibodies)
Goiter secondary to **lack of organification of trapped iodide inside gland**
Pathology shows a **lymphocytic infiltrate**.
Tx: **thyroxine** 1st line; **partial thyroidectomy** if continues to grow despite thyroxine, if nodules appear, or compression symptoms occur
Frequently no surgery is necessary for Hashimoto's disease.

Bacterial thyroiditis (rare)
Usually secondary to **contiguous spread**
Normal thyroid function tests, fever, dysphagia, tenderness
Upper respiratory tract infection (URI) symptoms most common precursor (staph/strep)
Tx: **antibiotics**
May need **lobectomy** to rule out cancer in patients with unilateral swelling and tenderness
May need total thyroidectomy for persistent inflammation

DeQuervain's thyroiditis
Can be associated with hyperthyroidism initially
Viral URI, tender thyroid, sore throat, mass, weakness, fatigue
More common in women
Elevated ESR
Tx: **steroids and ASA**
May need **lobectomy** to rule out cancer in patients with unilateral swelling and tenderness
May need total thyroidectomy for persistent inflammation

Riedel's fibrous struma (rare)
Woody, fibrous component that can involve adjacent strap muscles and carotid sheath
Can resemble thyroid CA or lymphoma (need biopsy)
Disease frequently results in hypothyroidism and compression symptoms.
Associated with sclerosing cholangitis, fibrotic diseases, methysergide treatment, and retroperitoneal fibrosis
Tx: **steroids and thyroxine**
May need isthmectomy or tracheostomy
If resection needed, watch for RLNs.

Thyroid cancer
Most common endocrine malignancy in the US
Follicular cells on FNA – 5%–10% chance of malignancy (unable to differentiate between follicular cell adenoma, follicular cell hyperplasia, normal thyroid tissue, and follicular cell CA on FNA)

Chapter 22. Thyroid

Worrisome for malignancy – solid, solitary, cold, slow growing, hard; male, age >50, previous neck XRT, MEN IIa or IIb
Sudden growth – could be hemorrhage into previously undetected nodule or malignancy
Patients can also present with voice **changes and dysphagia**.
Thyroid adenomas – need to be differentiated from carcinomas → requires lobectomy
Follicular adenomas – colloid, embryonal, fetal → no increase in cancer risk
    Still need lobectomy to prove it is adenoma

Papillary thyroid carcinoma
Most common (80%–90%) thyroid CA
Least aggressive, slow growing, has the best prognosis
Young adults, women, children
Risk factors: childhood XRT (very ↑ risk) → most common tumor following neck XRT
Older age (>40–50 years) predicts a worse prognosis.

Lymphatic spread 1st but is not prognostic
Prognosis based on local invasion
Rare metastases – **lung most common**

Children are more likely to be node-positive (70%–80%) than are adults (10%–20%).
Large, firm nodules in children are worrisome.
Many are **multicentric**.
Pathology – **psammoma bodies** (calcium) and **Orphan Annie nuclei**

Tx: minimal/incidental (<1 cm) → **lobectomy**
    Total thyroidectomy for bilateral lesions, multicentricity, history of XRT, positive margins, tumors >1 cm
    Clinically positive cervical nodes – need ipsilateral MRND
    Extrathyroidal tissue involvement – need ipsilateral MRND
    Metastatic disease, residual local disease, positive lymph nodes, or capsular invasion → ^{131}I 6 weeks after surgery
    XRT only for unresectable disease not responsive to ^{131}I
Do not give thyroid replacement until <u>after</u> treatment with ^{131}I → will suppress uptake
95% 5-year survival rate; death secondary to local disease

Enlarged lateral neck lymph node that shows normal-appearing thyroid tissue is **papillary thyroid CA with lymphatic spread**.
    Tx: total thyroidectomy and MRND

Follicular thyroid carcinoma
Hematogenous spread (**bone** most common) → 50% have metastatic disease at time of presentation
More aggressive than thyroid papillary cell CA
Older adults (50–60s), women
FNA shows just **follicular cells** – 10% chance of malignancy; need thyroidectomy

Tx: **lobectomy** → if pathology shows **adenoma or follicular cell hyperplasia**, nothing else needed
    If follicular CA → total thyroidectomy for lesions >1 cm or extrathyroidal disease
        Clinically positive cervical nodes – need ipsilateral MRND
        Extrathyroidal tissue involvement – need ipsilateral MRND
    Patients with lesions >1 cm or extrathyroidal disease (or capsular invasion) – ^{131}I 6 weeks after surgery
    If microinvasive (<1 cm), has rare nodal spread (<10%), and is usually incidental finding on pathology → as long as margins are negative, lobectomy is probably all that is needed
70% 5-year survival rate; prognosis based on stage

Medullary thyroid carcinoma
Can be associated with MEN IIa or IIb
Usually the 1st manifestation of MEN IIa and IIb
Tumor arises from **parafollicular C cells (which secrete calcitonin)**.
C-cell hyperplasia considered premalignant
Pathology – shows **amyloid** deposition
Gastrin can be used to test for medullary thyroid CA → causes an ↑ in calcitonin

↑ **calcitonin** – can cause <u>flushing and diarrhea</u>
Need to screen for <u>hyperparathyroidism and pheochromocytoma</u>

↑ **lymphatic spread** – most have involved nodes at time of diagnosis
Early metastases to lung, liver, and bone

Tx: **total thyroidectomy with central neck node dissection**
- **MRND** if patient has clinically positive nodes (bilateral MRND if both lobes have tumor) or if extrathyroidal disease present
- Prophylactic thyroidectomy and central node dissection in MEN IIa or IIb patients at age 2
- Liver and bone metastases prevent attempt at cure.
- XRT may be useful for unresectable local and distant metastatic disease.

May be useful to **monitor calcitonin levels for disease recurrence**
More aggressive than follicular and papillary CA
50% 5-year survival rate; prognosis based on presence of regional and distant metastases

Hurthle cell carcinoma
Most are benign (Hurthle cell adenoma); presents in older patients
Early nodal spread if malignant
Metastases go to bone and lung.
Tx: total thyroidectomy; MRND for clinically positive nodes

Anaplastic thyroid cancer
Elderly patients with long-standing goiters
Most aggressive thyroid CA
Rapidly lethal (0% 5-year survival rate); usually beyond surgical management by diagnosis
Tx: total thyroidectomy for the rare lesion that can be resected
Can perform palliative thyroidectomy for compressive symptoms or give palliative chemotherapy or XRT

XRT effective for papillary, follicular, medullary, and Hurthle cell thyroid CA
^{131}**I effective** for papillary and follicular thyroid CA only
- Can cure bone and lung metastases
- Done 6 weeks after surgery
- **Indications**
  - **Recurrent thyroid papillary or follicular CA**
  - **Primary inoperable tumors due to local invasion**
  - **Papillary thyroid CA** with extrathyroidal disease
  - **Follicular thyroid CA >1 cm or with extrathyroidal disease**
  - Patients with papillary or follicular cell CA with metastases → need to perform total thyroidectomy to facilitate uptake of I^{131} to the metastatic lesions
- **Side effects**: sialoadenitis, GI symptoms, infertility, bone marrow suppression, parathyroid dysfunction, leukemia

TSH levels highest 4–6 weeks after thyroidectomy – best time for ^{131}I scan for metastatic disease
Thyroxine – can help suppress TSH and slow metastatic disease
- Administered only after ^{131}I therapy has finished

Lymphoma and squamous cell CA – very rare causes of thyroid CA

CHAPTER 23. PARATHYROID

Anatomy and physiology
Superior parathyroids – 4th pouch; associated with thyroid complex
  Lateral to recurrent laryngeal nerves (RLNs), posterior surface of superior portion of gland, above inferior thyroid artery
Inferior parathyroids – 3rd pouch; associated with thymus
  Medial to RLNs, more anterior, below inferior thyroid artery
  Inferior parathyroids have more variable location and are more likely to be ectopic.
  Occasionaly are found in the **tail of the thymus** (most common ectopic site) and can migrate to the anterior mediastinum
  Other ectopic sites – intrathyroid, posterior mediastinal, near tracheoesophageal groove
90% have all 4 glands.
Inferior thyroid artery – blood supply to **both superior and inferior parathyroid glands**

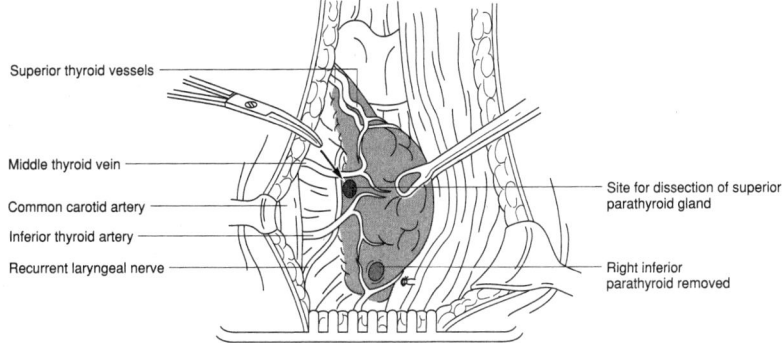

Parathyroid gland. Lateral view of the right side of the neck after rotation of the thyroid lobe, emphasizing the important anatomic landmarks.

PTH – ↑ serum Ca
  ↑ kidney Ca reabsorption in the distal convoluted tubule, ↓ kidney PO_4 absorption
  ↑ osteoclasts in bone to release Ca (and PO_4^-)
  ↑ vitamin D production in kidney (↑ 1-OH hydroxylation) → ↑ Ca-binding protein in intestine → ↑ intestinal Ca reabsorption

Vitamin D – ↑ intestinal Ca and PO_4 absorption by increasing **calcium binding protein**

Calcitonin – ↓ serum Ca
  ↓ bone Ca resorption (osteoclast inhibition)
  ↑ urinary Ca and PO_4 excretion

Normal Ca level: 8.5–10.5 (ionized 4.4–5.5)
Normal PTH level: 5–40 pg/ml
Normal PO_4 level: 2.5–5.0
Normal Cl^- level: 98–107

Most common cause of hypoparathyroidism is **previous thyroid surgery.**

Primary hyperparathyroidism
PRAD-1 oncogene increases risk for adenomas.
Women, older age
Due to autonomously high PTH
Dx: ↑ Ca, ↓ phosphorus; Cl^- to phosphorus ratio >33, ↑ renal cAMP, HCO_3^- secreted in urine
Can get **hyperchloremic metabolic acidosis**

Osteitis fibrosa cystica (brown tumors) – bone lesions from Ca resorption; characteristic of hyperparathyroidism
Most patients **have no symptoms** – ↑ Ca found on routine lab work for some other problem or on checkup
Symptoms: muscle weakness, myalgia, nephrolithiasis, pancreatitis, PUD, depression, bone pain, pathologic fractures, mental status changes, constipation, nausea and vomiting, anorexia
Hypertension can result from renal impairment.

Indications for surgery – symptomatic disease or asymptomatic disease with Ca >13, ↓ Cr clearence, kidney stones, substantially ↓ bone mass

Single adenoma – present in 80% of patients
Multiple adenomas – occur in 4% of the population
Diffuse hyperplasia – occurs in 15%; patients with MEN I or IIa have 4-gland hyperplasia
Parathyroid adenocarcinoma – very rare; can get very high Ca levels

Treatment
    Adenoma – resection; inspect other glands to rule out hyperplasia or multiple adenomas
    Parathyroid hyperplasia
        Don't biopsy all glands → risks hemorrhage and hypoparathyroidism
        Resect 3½ glands or total parathyroidectomy and autoimplantation
    Parathyroid CA → need radical parathyroidectomy (need to take ipsilateral thyroid)
    Pregancy – surgery in 2nd trimester; ↑ risk of stillbirth if not resected

Intraop frozen section → can confirm that the tissue taken was indeed parathyroid
Intraop PTH levels → can help determine if the causative gland is removed (PTH should go to <½ of the preop value); PTH half-life is 18 minutes
Missing gland – check inferiorly in thymus tissue (most common ectopic location), near carotids, vertebral body, superior to pharynx, thyroid
Still can't find gland – close and follow PTH; if PTH still ↑, get parathyroid scan to localize
Some say perform thyroidectomy on the side in which only one gland was found.
At reoperation for missing gland, most common location for the gland is normal anatomic position.

Postop hypocalcemia – caused by bone hunger, hypomagnesemia, failure of parathyroid remnant or graft
Persistent hyperparathyroidism (1%) – most commonly due to missed adenoma remaining in the neck
Recurrent hyperparathyroidism – occurs after a period of hypocalcemia or normocalcemia
    Can be due to new adenoma formation
    Can be due to tumor implants at the original operation that have now grown
    Need to consider recurrent parathyroid CA
Reoperation associated with ↑ risk of recurrent laryngeal nerve injury, permanent hypoparathyroidism

Thallium–technetium scan
    Thallium – both thyroid and parathyroid light up
    Technetium – only thyroid lights up
    Digitally subtract and you find parathyroid tissue.
    Best for trying to find ectopic glands
Sestamibi–^{131}I scan
    Sestamibi – both thyroid and parathyroid light up
    ^{131}I – only thyroid lights up
    Digitally subtract and you find parathyroid tissue.
    Best for trying to find ectopic glands

Secondary hyperparathyroidism
    Seen in patients with renal failure
    ↑ PTH in response to low Ca
    Most do <u>not</u> need surgery (90%).

Chapter 23. Parathyroid

Renal osteodystrophy – **aluminum** accumulation in bones contributes to osteomalacia after several years of dialysis
Ectopic calcification can occur.
Tx: control diet PO$_4$, PO$_4$-binding gel, ↓ aluminum, Ca supplement, vitamin D, Ca in dialysate
  Surgery for bone pain (most common indication; 80%–90% get relief), fractures, or pruritus (80%–90% get relief)
  Surgery involves total parathyroidectomy with autotransplantation or subtotal parathyroidectomy

Tertiary hyperparathyroidism
Renal disease now corrected with transplant but still overproduces PTH
Has similar lab values as primary hyperparathyroidism (hyperplasia)
Tx: subtotal (3½ glands) or total parathyroidectomy with autoimplantation

Familial hypercalcemic hypocalciuria
Patients have ↑ serum Ca and ↓ urine CA (should be ↑ if hyperparathyroidism)
Caused by defect in PTH receptor in distal convoluted tubule of the kidney that causes ↑ resorption of Ca
Dx: Ca 9–11, normal PTH (30–60), ↓ urine Ca
Tx: nothing (Ca generally not that high in these patients); **no parathyroidectomy**

Pseudohyperparathyroidism
Because of defect in PTH receptor in the kidney, does not respond to PTH

Parathyroid cancer
Rare cause of hypercalcemia
50% 5-year survival rate
Mortality is due to hypercalcemia.
↑ Ca, PTH, and alkaline phosphatase (can have extremely high Ca levels)
Lung most common location for metastases
Tx: wide en bloc excision (parathyroidectomy and ipsilateral thyroidectomy)
Recurrence in 50%

Multiple endocrine neoplasia syndromes
Derived from APUD cells
Neoplasms can develop synchronously or metachronously.
Autosomal dominant, 100% penetrance, variable expressivity

MEN I
Parathyroid hyperplasia
  Usually the first part to become symptomatic; urinary symptoms
  Tx: four-gland resection with autotransplantation
Pancreatic islet cell tumors
  Gastrinoma #1
  50% multiple, 50% malignant – major morbidity of syndrome
Pituitary adenoma
  Prolactinoma #1
  Need to correct hyperparathyroidism 1st

MEN IIa
Pheochromocytoma
  Very often bilateral, nearly always benign
Parathyroid hyperplasia
Medullary CA of thyroid
  Nearly all patients; diarrhea most common symptom; often bilateral
  #1 cause of death in these patients
  Usually 1st part to be symptomatic
  Need to correct pheochromocytoma 1st

MEN IIb
- **Pheochromocytoma**
  - Very often bilateral, nearly always benign
- **Medullary CA of thyroid**
  - Nearly all patients; diarrhea most common symptoms; often bilateral
  - #1 cause of death in these patients
  - Usually 1st part to be symptomatic
- **Mucosal neuromas**
- **Marfan's habitus, musculoskeletal abnormalities**
  - Need to correct pheochromocytoma 1st

MEN I – MENIN gene
MEN II – RET protooncogene

Causes of hypercalcemia
- Malignancy
  - Hematologic (25%) – lytic bone lesions
  - Nonhematologic (75%) – cancers that release PTHrp (small cell lung CA, breast CA)
- Hyperparathyroidism
- Hyperthyroidism
- Familial hypercalcemic hypocalciuria
- Immobilization
- Granulomatous disease (sarcoidosis or tuberculosis)
- Excess vitamin D
- Milk–alkali syndrome (excessive intake of milk and calcium supplements)
- Thiazide diuretics

Mithramycin – inhibits osteoclasts (used with malignancies or failure of conventional treatment); has hematologic, liver, and renal side effects
Hypercalcemic crisis – usually secondary to another surgery
  Tx: fluids, furosemide, dialysis
Breast CA metastases to bone – release **PTHrp; can cause hypercalcemia**
  Small cell lung CA and other nonhematologic cancers can do this as well → this is not due to bone destruction
  Associated with ↑ urinary cAMP (from action of PTHrp on kidney)
Hematologic malignancies – these can cause bone destruction; can also ↑ Ca and urinary cAMP will be low

CHAPTER 24. BREAST

Anatomy and physiology
Breast development
Breast formed from ectoderm milk streak
Estrogen – duct development (double layer of columnar cells)
Progesterone – lobular development
Prolactin – synergizes estrogen and progesterone
Cyclic changes
Estrogen – ↑ breast swelling, growth of glandular tissue
Progesterone – ↑ maturation of glandular tissue; withdrawal causes menses
FSH, LH surge – cause ovum release
After menopause, lack of estrogen and progesterone results in atrophy of breast tissue.
Nerves
Long thoracic nerve – innervates **serratus anterior**; injury results in winged scapula
  Lateral thoracic artery to serratus anterior
Thoracodorsal nerve – innervates **latissimus dorsi**; injury results in weak arm pullups and adduction
Thoracodorsal artery to latissimus dorsi
Medial pectoral nerve – innervates pectoralis major and pectoralis minor
Lateral pectoral nerve – pectoralis major only
Intercostobrachial nerve – lateral cutaneous branch of the 2nd intercostal nerve; provides sensation to medial arm and axilla; encountered just below axillary vein when performing axillary dissection
  Can transect without serious consequences
Branches **of internal thoracic artery, intercostal arteries, thoracoacromial artery, and lateral thoracic artery** supply breast.
Batson's plexus – valveless vein plexus that allows direct hematogenous metastasis of breast CA to spine
Lymphatic drainage
97% is to the axillary nodes.
1%–2% is to the internal mammary nodes.
Any quadrant can drain to the internal mammary nodes.
Supraclavicular nodes – considered M1 disease
Primary axillary adenopathy – **#1 lymphoma**
Cooper's ligaments – suspensory ligaments; divide breast into segments
Breast CA involving these strands can dimple the skin.

Benign breast disease
Abscesses – usually associated with breastfeeding. *S. aureus* most common, strep
  Tx: incision and drainage; discontinue breastfeeding; ice, heat, breast pump, antibiotics
Infectious mastitis – most commonly associated with breastfeeding
  S. aureus **most common**; in nonlactating women can be due to chronic inflammatory diseases (actinomyces, tuberculosis, syphilis) or autoimmune disease (SLE)
  May need to rule out necrotic cancer
Periductal mastitis (mammary duct ectasia or plasma cells mastitis)
  Dilated mammary ducts, inspisated secretions, marked periductal inflammation
  Symptoms: noncyclical mastodynia, nipple retraction, creamy discharge from nipple; can have sterile subareolar abscess
  Patients have a history of difficulty with breastfeeding
  Tx: if typical creamy discharge is present that is not bloody and not associated with nipple retraction, may be able to reassure; otherwise need to rule out malignancy
Galactocele – breast cysts filled with milk; occurs with breastfeeding
  Tx: ranges from aspiration to incision and drainage
Galactorrhea – can be caused by ↑ prolactin (pituitary prolactinoma), OCPs, TCAs, phenothiazines, metoclopramide, alpha-methyl dopa, reserpine
  Is often associated with amenorrhea
Gynecomastia – 2-cm pinch; can be associated with cimetidine, spironolactone, marijuana; idiopathic in most
  Tx: will likely regress; may need to resect if cosmetically disforming or causing social problems

Neonatal breast enlargement – due to circulating maternal estrogens; will regress
Accessory breast tissue (polythelia) – can present in axilla (most common location)
Accessory nipples – can be found from axilla to groin (most common breast anomaly)
Breast asymmetry – common
Breast reduction – ability to lactate frequently compromised
Poland's syndrome – hypoplasia of chest wall, amastia, hypoplastic shoulder, no pectoralis muscle
Mastodynia – pain in breast; rarely represents breast CA
    Tx: danazol, OCPs, NSAIDs, evening primrose oil, bromocriptine
    Discontinue caffeine, nicotine, methylxanthines
    Cyclic mastodynia – pain before menstrual period; most commonly from fibrocystic disease
    Continuous mastodynia – continuous pain, most commonly represents acute or subacute infection
        Continuous mastodynia more refractory to treatment than cyclic mastodynia
Mondor's disease – superficial vein thrombophlebitis of breast; feels cordlike, can be painful
    Associated with trauma and strenuous exercise
    Usually occurs in lower outer quadrant
    Tx: NSAIDs

Fibrocystic disease
    Catchall phrase; lots of types: papillomatosis, sclerosing adenosis, apocrine metaplasia, duct adenosis, epithelial hyperplasia, ductal hyperplasia, and lobular hyperplasia
    Symptoms: breast pain, nipple discharge (uncommon, can be yellow to brown), masses, lumpy breast tissue that varies with hormonal cycle
    Only cancer risk is in atypical ductal or lobular hyperplasia (an unusual finding)
        Do not need to get negative margins with atypical hyperplasia; just remove all suspicious areas (i.e., calcifications) that appear on mammogram.
    Sclerosing adenosis can manifest as a cluster of calcifications on mammogram without a mass or pain → can look like breast CA
        Is differentiated from breast CA by regularity of nuclei and absence of mitoses
    Risk factors for benign breast disease – early menarche, late menopause, small breast size, normal or low bodyweight, history of cyclic breast discomfort, irregular menses, history of spontaneous abortions, premenopausal status

Intraductal papilloma
    Most common cause of bloody discharge from nipple
    Are usually small, nonpalpable, and close to the nipple
    These lesions are <u>not</u> premalignant → can get contrast ductogram to find papilloma
    Tx: resection (subareolar resection usually curative)

Fibroadenoma
    Most common breast lesion in adolescents and young women; 10% multiple
    Usually painless, slow-growing, well circumscribed, firm and rubbery
    Often grow to several cm in size and then stop
    Can change in size with menstrual cycle and can enlarge in pregnancy
    Giant fibromas can be >5 cm (treatment is the same)
    Prominent fibrous tissue compressing epithelial cells on pathology
    Can have large, coarse calcifications (popcorns lesions) on mammography from degeneration
    In patients <30 years
        Mass needs to feel clinically benign (firm, rubbery, rolls, not fixed)
        Ultrasound or mammogram needs to be consistant with fibroadenoma
        Need FNA or core needle biopsy showing the lesion (not just normal breast tissue)
    In patients >30 → excisional biopsy to ensure diagnosis
    Avoid resection of breast tissue in teenagers and younger → can affect breast development

Nipple discharge
Most nipple discharge is benign.
    Green discharge – usually due to fibrocystic disease
        Tx: if cyclical and nonspontaneous, reassure patient
    Bloodly discharge – most commonly intraductal papilloma; occasionally ductal CA
        Tx: need galactogram and subareolar resection (see below)
    Serous discharge – worrisome for cancer, especially if coming from only 1 duct or spontaneous
        Tx: excisional biopsy of that ductal area

Chapter 24. Breast

Spontaneous discharge – no matter what the color or consistency is worrisome for cancer
All these patients need some sort of biopsy in the area of the duct causing the discharge.
Nonspontanetous discharge (occurs only with pressure, tight garments, exercise, etc) – not as worrisome but may still need excisional biopsy (i.e., if bloody)

Diffuse papillomatosis
Affects multiple ducts of both breasts
Papillomas are larger than when they occur solitarily.
Usually have serous discharge
Mammogram shows Swiss cheese appearance.
↑ risk of breast CA with diffuse papillomatosis (40% get breast CA)

Ductal carcinoma in situ (DCIS)
Malignant cells of the ductal epithelium without invasion of the basement membrane
50%–60% get cancer if not resected (ipsilateral breast); 5%–10% get cancer in contralateral breast
Considered a **premalignant lesion**
Usually not palpable and presents as a cluster of calcifications on mammography
Need a 2–3 mm margin with excision
Can have solid, cribiform, papillary, and comedo patterns
    Comedo pattern – most aggressive subtype; has necrotic areas
        High risk for multicentricity, microinvasion, and recurrence
        Tx: simple mastectomy
↑ recurrence risk with comedo type and lesions >2.5 cm

Tx: **lumpectomy and XRT**
    Simple mastectomy if high grade (i.e., comedo type, multicentric, multifocal), if a large tumor not amenable to lumpectomy, or if not able to get good margins; **no** **ALND**

DCIS with a small focus (<10%) of microinvasive disease can be treated with lumpectomy and XRT or simple mastectotmy; need negative margins, **no ALND**

Lobular carcinoma in situ (LCIS)
40% get cancer (either breast)
Considered a marker for the development of breast CA, **not premalignant itself**
Has no calcifications; is not palpable.
Primarily found in premenopausal women
Patients that develop breast CA are more likely to develop a **ductal CA (70%)**.
Usually an incidental finding; multifocal disease is common
5% risk of having a synchronous breast CA at the time of diagnosis of LCIS (most likely ductal)
Do not need negative margins
Tx: nothing, tamoxifen, or bilateral subcutaneous mastectomy (no ALND)

Breast cancer
Breast CA decreased in economically poor areas. Japan has lowest rate of breast CA worldwide.
Breast CA risk – **1 in 8 women (12%)**; 4%–5% in women with no risk factors
Screening decreases mortality by 25%.
Untreated breast cancer – median survival 2–3 years
10% of breast CAs have negative mammogram and negative ultrasound.
Clinical features of breast CA – distortion of normal architecture, skin/nipple distortion or retraction, hard, tethered, indistinct borders
Symptomatic breast mass workup
    <30 years old – ultrasound
        If solid → **FNA; excisional biopsy** if FNA is nondiagnostic
            These patients most commonly have fibroadenomas that can be left alone if FNA is diagnostic. However, if the fibroadenoma enlarges, need excisonal biopsy.
    30–50 years – bilateral mammograms and FNA; excisional biopsy if FNA nondiagnostic
    >50 years – bilateral mammograms and excisional or core needle biopsy

Core needle biopsy – gives architecture
FNA – gives cytology (just the cells)
Cyst fluid – if bloody, need cyst excisional biopsy; if clear and recurs, need cyst excisional biopsy.
  If complex cyst, need cyst excisional biopsy

Mammography
Has 90% sensitivity/specificity
Sensitivity increasess with age as the dense parenchymal tissue is replaced with fat.
Mass needs to be ≥5 mm to be detected.
Irregular borders; spiculated; multiple clustered, small, thin, linear, and/or branching calcifications; can have crushed appearance; asymmetric density, ductal asymmetry, distortion of architecture
5% of cancers have sharp margin
Suspicious lesion on mammogram → needle localization and excisional biopsy (core needle biopsy also an option)

Screening
Mammogram every 2–3 years after age 40, yearly after 50
High-risk screening – mammogram 10 years before youngest age of diagnosis of breast CA in first-degree relative
No mammography in patients <30 unless high risk → hard to interpret because of dense parenchyma
  ↓ radiation dose in young patients
Suspicious calcifications or architecture on mammography → perform localized stereotactic needle excisional biopsy
Indeterminate calcifications or architecture on mammography → can perform core needle biopsy; if indeterminate, perform localized stereotactic needle excisional biopsy

Node levels
I – lateral to pectoralis minor muscle
II – beneath pectoralis minor muscle
III – medial to pectoralis minor muscle
Rotter's nodes – between the pectoralis major and pectoralis minor muscles

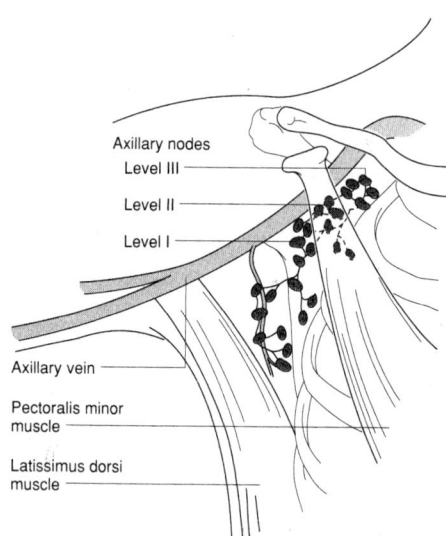

Anatomic classification of axillary lymph nodes into three levels based on their relation to the pectoralis minor muscle. Level I nodes are lateral to the edge of the muscle, level II nodes lie beneath the muscle, and level III nodes are medial to the muscle. Rotter's nodes (*not shown*) are found between the pectoralis major and minor muscles, anterior to the axillary space.

Need to sample only level I nodes.

Nodes are the most important prognostic staging factor. Other factors include tumor size, tumor grade, progesterone, and estrogen receptor status.
Survival is directly related to number of positive nodes.
Larger tumors are more likely to have positive nodes.
30% of nonpalpable nodes are positive at surgery.
  0 nodes positive   75% 5-year survival
  1–3 nodes positive 60% 5-year survival
  4–10 nodes positive 40% 5-year survival

Bone – most common distant metastasis (can also go to lung, liver, brain)
Takes approximately 5–7 years to go from single malignant cell to 1-cm tumor
Central and subareolar tumors have increased risk of multicentricity.

TNM Staging System for Breast Cancer

T1: <2 cm. **T2**: 2–5 cm. **T3**: >5 cm. **T4**: skin or chest wall involvement (does not include pectoral muscles), peau d'orange, inflammatory cancer
N1: ipsilateral axillary nodes. **N2**: fixed ipsilateral axillary nodes. **N3**: ipsilateral internal mammary nodes
M1: distant metastasis (includes ipsilateral supraclavicular nodes)

Stage	TNM Status
I	T1,N0,M0
IIa	T0–1,N1,M0 or T2,N0,M0
IIb	T2,N1,M0 or T3,N0,M0
IIIa	T0–3,N2,M0 or T3,N1–2, M0
IIIb	Any T4 or N3 tumors
IV	M1

(AJCC. Cancer staging handbook. Ed 6. New York: Springer-Verlag, 2002:265–266)

Breast cancer risk
  Greatly increased risk
    BRCA gene in patient with family history of breast CA
    ≥2 primary relatives with bilateral or premenopausal breast CA
    DCIS (ipsilateral breast at risk) and LCIS (both breasts have same high risk)
    Fibrocystic disease with atypical hyperplasia
  Moderately increased risk
    Family history of breast cancer other than above
    Early menarche (<12 years), late menopause (>55)
    Nulliparity or first birth after age 30
    Radiation
    Previous breast CA
    Environmental risk factor – **high-fat diet (obesity)**

  First-degree relative with bilateral, premenopausal breast cancer increases breast CA risk to 50%.
  BRCA gene + family history = 80%–90% chance of breast CA by age 70 (autosomal dominant)
    BRCA I – associated with ovarian (50%), endometrial CA
    BRCA II – associated with male breast CA
  Consider TAH and bilateral oophrectomies in BRCA I families.

Considerations for prophylactic mastectomy
  Family history + BRCA gene
  LCIS
  Also need one of the following: high patient anxiety, poor patient access for follow-up exams and mammograms, difficult lesion to follow on exam or with mammograms, or patient preference for mastectomy

Receptors
Positive receptors – better response to hormones, chemotherapy, surgery, and better overall prognosis
Receptor-positive tumors are more common in **postmenopausal women**.
Progesterone receptor–positive tumors have better prognosis than estrogen receptor–positive tumors.
Tumor that is both both progesterone receptor– and estrogen receptor–positive has best prognosis.
10% of breast CAs negative for both receptors

Male breast cancer
<1% of all breast CAs; usually ductal
Poorer prognosis because of late presentation
Have ↑ pectoral muscle involvement
Associated with steroid use, previous XRT, family history, Klinefelter's syndrome, prolonged hyperestrogenic state
Tx: modified radical mastectomy (MRM)

Ductal CA
85% of all breast CAs
Can have various subtypes
  Medullary breast CA – smooth borders, ↑ lymphocytes, ductal type cancer with bizarre cells
    Vast majority are estrogen– and progesterone receptor–positive
    More favorable prognosis
  Tubular CA – small tubule formations
    Nodes positive in 10%
    More favorable prognosis
  Mucinous CA (colloid) – produces and abundance of mucin
    More favorable prognosis
  Scirrhotic CA – worse prognosis
Tx: MRM or lumpectomy with ALND (or SLNB)

Lobular cancer
10% of all breast CAs
Does not form calcifications; extensively infiltrative; ↑ bilateral, multifocal, and multicentric disease
Signet ring cells confer worse prognosis.
Tx: MRM or lumpectomy with ALND (or SLNB)

Inflammatory cancer
May need chemotherapy and XRT 1st, then mastectomy
Considered T4 disease
Very aggressive → median survival of 36 months
Has **dermal lymphatic invasion**, which causes peau d'orange lymphedema appearance; erythematous and warm

Other histologic types
Metaplastic adenocarcinoma – takes on the appearance of nonglandular cells
  Most common types → squamous and pseudosarcomatous
  Prognosis is the same as the tumor cell line from which it was derived.
Adenoid cystic carcinoma
  Large, well-circumscribed lesions
  Better prognosis than ductal CAs

Preoperative studies
CXR, bilateral mammograms, CBC, LFTs
Abdominal CT if LFTs elevated
Head CT if patient reports headaches
Bone scan if patient has bone pain or abnormal alkaline phosphatase
For patients with more advanced local primary, consider more extensive preop evaluations (head and abdominal CT, bone scan)

Chapter 24. Breast

Surgical options
- **Subcutaneous (simple) mastectomy**
  - Leaves 1%–2% of breast tissue, preserves the nipple
  - Not indicated for breast CA treatment
  - Used for DCIS and LCIS
- **Lumpectomy and SLNB** – need 1-cm margin
  - **Contraindications** – unable to get an acceptable cosmetic result; positive margins
- **SLNB**
  - Fewer complications than ALND
  - Indicated only for malignant tumors >1 cm
  - Not indicated in patients with clinically positive nodes; they need ALND
  - Accuracy best when primary tumor is present (finds the right lymphatic channels).
  - Well suited for small tumors with low risk of axillary metastases
  - Radioactive material or blue dye can be used.
  - Dye or radiotracer is injected directly into the tumor area.
  - Type I hypersensitivity reactions have been reported with Lymphazurin blue dye.
  - Usually find 1–3 nodes; 95% of the time, the sentinel node is found
  - During **SLND** – if no radiotracer or dye is found, need to do a formal ALND
  - **Contraindications** – pregnancy, multicentric disease, neoadjuvant
- **Modified radical mastectomy**
  - Removes all breast tissue including the nipple areolar complex
  - Includes axillary node dissection (level I nodes)
- **Radical mastectomy**
  - Includes MRM and overlying skin, pectoralis major and minor muscles, and level I, II, and III lymph nodes
  - Rarely performed anymore

- **Complications of mastectomy** – infection, flap necrosis, seromas
- **Complications of axillary lymph node dissection**
  - Infection, lymphedema, lymphangiosarcoma
  - **Axillary vein thrombosis** – sudden, early, postop swelling
  - **Lymphatic fibrosis** – slow swelling over 18 months
  - **Intercostal brachiocutaneous nerve** – hyperesthesia of inner arm and lateral chest wall; most commonly injured nerve after mastectomy; no significant sequelae
  - **Drains** – leave in until drainage <40 cc/day

Radiotherapy
- **Complications of XRT** – edema, erythema, rib fractures, pneumonitis, ulceration, sarcoma, contralateral breast CA
- **Contraindications to XRT** – scleroderma (results in severe fibrosis and necrosis), previous XRT, SLE (relative), active rheumatoid arthritis (relative)
- **Indications for XRT after mastectomy**
  - >4 nodes
  - Skin or chest wall involvement
  - Positive margins
  - Tumor >5 cm (T3)
  - Extracapsular nodal invasion
  - Inflammatory CA
  - Fixed axillary nodes (N2) or internal mammary nodes (N3)
- **Lumpectomy with XRT**
  - 10% chance of local recurrence, usually occurs within 2 years of 1st operation
    - These patients often also have distant disease.
  - Need salvage MRM for local recurrence
  - Need to have negative margins following lumpectomy before starting XRT

Chemotherapy
- Cyclophosphamide, methotrexate, and 5FU (CMF) for 3–6 months, or Adriamycin and cyclophosphamide (AC) for 3–6 months
- **Positive nodes** – everyone gets chemo except postmenopausal women with positive estrogen receptors → tamoxifen

>1 cm and negative nodes – everyone gets chemo except patients with <u>positive estrogen receptors</u> → tamoxifen
<1 cm and negative nodes – no further treatment
Alternative hormonal/chemotherapy options – androgenic steroid, aminoglutethimide, bilateral oophorectomy, Megase, aromatase inhibitors (anastrozole, letrozole)
Both chemotherapy (CMF) and hormonal therapy (tamoxifen) have been shown to decrease recurrence and improve survival.
Tamoxifen – decreases short-term risk of breast CA by 50%–60%
1% risk of blood clots; 1% risk of endometrial CA

Almost all women with recurrence die of disease.
Increased recurrences and metastases occur with **positive nodes, large tumors, negative receptors, unfavorable subtype.**

Metastatic flare – pain, swelling, erythema in metastatic areas; XRT can help
XRT is good for bone metastases.

Occult breast CA – breast CA that presents as an axillary metastases with unknown primary
70% are found to have breast CA at mastectomy.

Benign conditions that mimic breast CA
Radial scar – can present as a stellate, irregular, spiculated mass lesion
Fibromatosis – locally invasive spindle cells; can have skin retraction/dimpling
Granular cell tumors (skin retraction/dimpling)
Fat necrosis – poorly defined borders, skin retraction; accompanying fibrosis causes these findings; thought to be related to trauma
Pathology shows macrophages laden with fat or foreign body giant cells (FNA or core needle biopsy)
Malignant tumors with a benign appearance (smooth, rounded masses) – mucinous CA, medullary CA, cystosarcoma phyllodes
Most masses that contain fat are benign – nodes, posttraumatic oil cyst, hamartomas, fibrolipoadenomas

Paget's disease
Scaly skin lesion on nipple; biopsy shows Paget's cells
Patients have DCIS or ductal CA in breast.
Tx: need MRM if cancer present; otherwise simple mastectomy

Cystosarcoma phyllodes
10% malignant, based on mitoses per high-power field (>5–10)
<u>No</u> nodal metastases, hematogenous spread in any (rare)
Resembles giant fibroadenoma; has stromal and epithelial elements (mesenchymal tissue)
Can often be large tumors
Tx: WLE with negative margins; **no ALND**

Stewart-Treves syndrome
Lymphangiosarcoma from chronic lymphedema following axillary dissection (MRM)
Patients present with dark purple nodule or lesion on arm 5–10 years after surgery

Pregnancy with mass
Tends to present late, leading to worse prognosis
Mammography and ultrasound don't work as well during pregnancy.
Try to use ultrasound to avoid radiation.
If **cyst**, drain it and send FNA for cytology.
If **solid**, perform core needle biopsy or FNA.
If core needle and FNA equivocal, need to go to excisional biopsy.
If breast CA
1st trimester – MRM
2nd trimester – MRM
3rd trimester – MRM or if late can perform lumpectomy with ALND and postpartum XRT
May be able to wait until delivery for treatment
No chemotherapy or XRT while pregnant; no breastfeeding after delivery

CHAPTER 25. THORACIC

Anatomy and physiology
Azygos vein runs along right side and dumps into superior vena cava.
Thoracic duct runs along right side, crosses midline, and dumps into left subclavian vein at junction with internal jugular vein.
Left mainstem bronchi longer than right
Right pulmonary artery longer than left before 1st branch
Phrenic nerve – runs anterior to hilum
Vagus nerve – runs posterior to hilum

Right lung volume 55% (3 lobes: RUL, RML, and RLL), left lung volume 45% (2 lobes: LUL and LLL and lingula)
Quiet inspiration – diaphragm 80%, intercostals 20%
Greatest change in dimension superior/inferior
Accessory muscles – sternocleidomastoid muscle (SCM), levators, serratus posterior, scalenes

Type I pneumocytes – gas exchange
Type II pneumocytes – surfactant production

Pores of Kahn – direct air exchange between alveoli
Pleural fluid – 1–2 L/day; parietal pleura produces fluid pleural fluid cleared by **lymphatics** in the visceral pleura

Pulmonary function tests
Need predicted postop **FEV_1 >0.8** (or at least 40% of predicted value)
    If it's close → get qualitative V/Q scan to see contribution of that portion of lung to overall FEV_1 → if low, may still be able to resect
Need predicted postop **DLCO >11–12** ml/min/mmHg CO (at least 50% of predicted value)
    Represents carbon monoxide diffusion capacity
    This value is based on pulmonary capillary surface area, hemoglobin content, and alveolar architecture.
Need predicted postop FVC >1.5 L
No resection if preop **pCO_2 >45** or **pO_2 <50** at rest
No resection if preop VO_2 max **<10 ml/min/kg**

Persistent air leak – most common after segmentectomy/wedge
Atelectasis and arrhythmias – common problems after lobectomy or pneumonectomy

Lung cancer
Symptoms: patients can be asymptomatic with finding on routine CXR or present with atelectasis, PNA, pain, or weight loss
Most common cause of cancer-related death in US
Nodal involvement has strongest influence on survival.
Brain – single most common site of metastasis
    Can also go to supraclavicular nodes, other lung, bone, liver, and adrenals
Recurrence most commonly appears as disseminated metastases (brain most common).
    80% of recurrences are within the 1st 3 years.

Lung CA overall 5-year survival rate 10%; 30% with resection
Stage I and II disease resectable; T3,N1,M0 (stage IIIa) possibly resectable
Lobectomy or pneumonectomy most common; need to sample suspicious nodes
Adenocarcinoma most common lung CA (<u>not</u> squamous)

Non–small cell carcinoma
    80% of lung CA
    Squamous cell carcinoma usually more central
    Adenocarcinoma usually more peripheral
    Local recurrence increased with squamous cell CA
    Distant metastases increased with adenocarcinoma
    Other types of non–small cell CA – undifferentiated large cell and mixed tumors

105

TNM Staging System for Lung Cancer

T1: <3 cm. **T2**: >3 cm but >2 cm away from carina. **T3**: invasion of chest wall, pericardium, diaphragm or <2 cm from carina. **T4**: mediastinum, esophagus, trachea, vertebra, heart, great vessels, malignant effusion (all indicate unresectability)
N1: ipsilateral hilum nodes. **N2**: ipsilateral mediastinal nodes (unresectable). **N3**: contralateral mediastinal or supraclavicular nodes (unresectable)
M1: distant metastasis

Stage	TNM Status
I	T1–2,N0,M0
II	T1–2,N1,M0 or T3,N0,M0
IIIa	T1–3,N2,M0 or T3,N1,M0
IIIb	Any T4 or N3
IV	M1

(Modified from AJCC. Cancer staging handbook. Ed 6. New York: Springer-Verlag, 2002:197–198)

Small cell carcinoma
    20% of lung CA neuroendocrine in origin
        Usually unresectable at time of diagnosis (<5% candidates for surgery)
        Overall 5-year survival rate; very poor prognosis
        Stage T1,N0,M0 5-year survival rate – 50%
        Most get just chemotherapy and XRT

Paraneoplastic syndromes
    Squamous cell CA – PTH-related peptide
    Small cell CA – ACTH, ADH
    Small cell ACTH – most common paraneoplastic syndrome

Mesothelioma
    Most malignant lung tumor
    Aggressive local invasion, nodal invasion, and distant metastases common at the time of diagnosis
    Asbestos exposure

Non–small cell CA chemotherapy (stage II or higher) – carboplatin, Taxol
Small cell lung CA chemotherapy – cisplatin, etoposide
XRT can be used as well.

Mediastinoscopy
    Use for **centrally located tumors** and patients with **suspicious adenopathy** (>0.8 cm or subcarinal >1.0 cm) on chest CT
    Does not assess aortopulmonary (AP) window nodes (left lung drainage)
    Assesses **ipsilateral (N2) and contralateral (N3) mediastinal nodes**
    If positive, tumor unresectable
    Looking into **middle mediastinum with mediastinoscopy**
        Left-sided structures – RLN, esophagus, aorta, main PA
        Right-sided structures – azygous and SVC
        Anterior structures – innominate vein, innominate artery, right PA
Chamberlain procedure – assesses aortopulmonary window nodes; go through left 2nd rib cartilage
Bronchoscopy – needed for centrally located tumors

Pancoast tumor – tumor invades apex of chest wall and patients have Horner's syndrome (invasion of sympathetic chain → ptosis, miosis, anhidrosis) or **ulnar** nerve symptoms
Coin lesion
    Overall 5%–10% are malignant.
    Age <50 → <5% malignant; age >50 → >50% malignant
    No growth in 2 years, smooth contour suggests benign disease
    Core needle biopsy frequently nondiagnostic

Asbestos exposure increases lung CA risk 90x.
Bronchioalveolar CA – can look like pneumonia; grows along alveolar walls; multifocal
Metastases to the lung – if isolated and <u>not</u> associated with any other systemic disease, may be resected for colon, renal cell CA, sarcoma, melanoma, ovarian, or endometrial CA

Carcinoids
Neuroendocrine tumor, usually central
5% have metastases at time of diagnosis; 50% have symptoms
Typical carcinoid – 90% 5-year survival rate; atypical carcinoid – 60% 5-year survival
Tx: resection; treat like cancer
Outcome closely linked to histology; recurrence increased with positive nodes or tumors >3 cm

Bronchial adenomas
Malignant tumors → adenoid cystic adenoma, mucoepidermoid adenoma, mucous gland adenoma
Slow growth, <u>no</u> metastases
Tx: resection
Adenoid cystic adenoma
Submucosal glands; spread along perineural lymphatics, well beyond endoluminal component; XRT sensitive
Slow growing; can get 10-year survival with incomplete resection
Tx: resection; if unresectable, XRT can provide good palliation

Hamartomas
Most common benign adult lung tumor
Have calcifications and can appear as a **popcorn lesion on chest CT**
Diagnosis can be made with CT.
Do not require resection
Repeat chest CT in 6 months to confirm diagnosis

Mediastinal tumors in adults
Most are asymptomatic; can present with chest pain, cough, dyspnea
Neurogenic tumors – most common mediastinal tumor in adults, usually in posterior mediastinum
Location
    Anterior (thymus) – most common site for mediastinal tumor
        T's → Thymoma (#1 anterior mediastinal mass in adults)
            Thyroid CA and goiters
            T-cell lymphoma
            Teratoma (and other germ cell tumors)
            Parathyroid adenomas
    Middle (heart, trachea, ascending aorta)
        Bronchiogenic cysts
        Pericardial cysts
        Enteric cysts
        Lymphoma
    Posterior (esophagus, descending aorta)
        Enteric cysts
        Neurogenic tumors
        Lymphoma

Thymoma
All thymomas require resection.
Thymus too big or associated with refractory myasthenia gravis → resection
50% of thymomas are malignant.
50% of patients with thymomas have symptoms.
50% of patients with thymomas have myasthenia gravis.
10% of patients with myasthenia gravis have thymomas.
Myasthenia gravis – fatigue, weakness, diplopia, ptosis; antibodies to acetylcholine receptors

Tx: anticholinesterase medications, plasmapheresis, steroids
80% get improvement with thymectomy, including patients who do not have thymomas.

Lymphoma
T-cell most common (non-Hodgkin's lymphoma) – lymphoblastic variant most common
Hodgkin's lymphoma – nodular sclerosing most common
Tx: chemotherapy and XRT

Germ cell tumors
Teratoma – most common germ cell tumor in mediastinum
Tx: resection and chemotherapy
Seminoma – most common malignant germ cell tumor in mediastinum
Tx: resection and XRT (extremely sensitive); chemotherapy for positive nodes or residual disease
Nonseminoma – 90% have elevated beta-HCG and alpha-fetoprotein
Tx: resection and cisplatin-based chemotherapy

Cysts
Bronchiogenic – posterior to carina. Tx: resection
Pericardial – at right costophrenic angle. Tx: resection
Neurogenic tumors – have pain, neurologic deficit. Tx: resection
10% have intraspinal involvement that requires simultaneous spinal surgery.
Neurolemoma – most common
Paraganglioma – produce catecholamines
Nerve sheath – associated with von Recklinghausen's disease
Can also get neuroblastomas and neurofibromas
50% of symptomatic mediastinal masses are malignant.
90% of asymptomatic mediastinal masses are benign.

Trachea
Benign tumors – adults: **papilloma**; children: **hemangioma**
Malignant – **squamous cell carcinoma**

Most common late complication after tracheal surgery – granulation tissue formation
Most common early complication after tracheal surgery – laryngeal edema
Tx: reintubation, racemic epinephrine, steroids
Postintubation stenosis – at stoma site with tracheostomy, at cuff site with ET tube
May be able to treat with serial dilatation or with laser
May need resection with end-to-end anastamosis if severe
Tracheoinnominate fistula
Tracheostomy – needs to be 2 or 3 rings below cricoid; not >3 rings → risk tracheoinnominate fistula
Tx: overinflate balloon to plug hole or stick your finger in hole and depress innominate artery. Resect innominate and place graft. Leave trachea alone. Use new tracheostomy site.
Tracheoesophageal fistula (see also Chap. 43, Pediatric Surgery)
Use large-volume cuff below fistula
May need decompressing gastrostomy
Tx: tracheal resection, reanastamosis, sternohyoid flap

Lung abscess
Necrotic area; most commonly associated with aspiration
Most commonly in posterior segment of RUL and superior segment of RLL
Tx: CT-guided drainage, antibiotics 95% successful.
Surgery if this fails or cannot rule out cancer (>6 cm, failure to resolve after 6 weeks)
Chest CT can help differentiate empyema from lung abscess.

Empyema
Usually secondary to **pneumonia and subsequent parapneumonic effusion** (staph, strep)
Can also be due to esophageal, pulmonary, or mediastinal surgery
Symptoms: pleuritic chest pain, fever, cough, SOB
Pleural fluid often has WBCs >500 cells/cc, bacteria, positive Gram stain

Exudative phase (1st week) – Tx: chest tube, antibiotics
Fibroproliferative phase (2nd week) – Tx: chest tube, antibiotics
Organized phase (3rd week) – Tx: likely need decortication; fibrous peel occurs around lung
    May need Eloesser flap (direct opening to external environment) for chronic unresolving empyema
    Can also place a chronic chest tube that is gradually pulled out

Chylothorax
Fluid milky white; has ↑ lymphocytes and TAGs (>110 ml/μl); Sudan red stains fat
Fluid resistant to infection
50% secondary to trauma or iatrogenic injury
50% secondary to tumor (lymphoma most common, due to tumor burden in the lymphatics)
Injury above T5–6 results in left-sided chylothorax.
Injury below T5–6 results in right-sided chylothorax.
3–4 weeks of conservative therapy (chest tube, octreotide, low-fat diet or TPN)
    If that fails, surgery with ligation of thoracic duct on right side low in mediastinum (80% successful) if chylothorax secondary to trauma or iatrogenic injury
    For malignant causes of chylothorax, can perform mechanical or talc pleurodesis (less successful than above

Massive hemoptysis
>600 cc/24 hr; bleeding is from high-pressure **bronchial arteries**
Most commonly secondary to infection, **mycetoma** most common; death due to asphyxiation
Tx: Place bleeding side down if known; rigid bronchoscopy to identify site; mainstem intubation to side opposite of bleeding to prevent drowning in blood; to OR for lobectomy or pneumonectomy; bronchial artery embolization if not suitable for surgery

Spontaneous pneumothorax
Tall, healthy, thin, young, males
Recurrence risk after 1st pneumothorax 20%, after 2nd pneumothorax 60%, after 3rd pneumothorax 80%
Results from rupture of a bleb in the apex of the upper lobe of the lung; can occur in the superior segment of the lower lobe
More common on the right
Tx: **chest tube**
Surgery for recurrence, large blebs on CT scan, air leak >7 days, nonreexpansion
Also need surgery for high-risk profession (airline pilot, diver, mountain climber) or patients who live in remote areas
Surgery consists of thoracoscopy, apical blebectomy, and mechanical pleurodesis.

Other conditions
Bronchiogenic cysts (see also Chap. 43, Pediatric Surgery)
    Most common cysts of the mediastinum
    Abnormal lung tissue outside lung; didn't get connected to bronchial system
    Usually posterior to the carina
    Tx: remove cyst

Sequestration (see also Chap. 43, Pediatric Surgery)
    Lung tissue in lung not connected to bronchial tree.
    Receives blood supply from anomalous systemic arteries → usually off thoracic aorta
    Venous blood supply is either the pulmonary vein or systemic veins.
    Extralobar – more common in <u>children</u>; more likely to have systemic venous drainage
    Intralobar – more common in <u>adults</u>; more likely to have pulmonary vein drainage
    Tx: lobectomy

Solitary pulmonary nodule with history of previous cancer
    Sarcoma/melanoma → nodule more likely metastases
    Head/neck/breast → nodule more likely primary lung CA
    GI/GU → metastases or primary
    In case of primary cancer with a resectable lung metastasis, take out primary 1st, then metastasis.

Tension pneumothorax – most likely to cause arrest after blunt trauma; impaired venous return
Catamenial pneumothorax – occurs in temporal relation to menstruation
    Caused by **endometrial implants** in the visceral lung pleura
Residual hemothorax despite 2 good chest tubes → OR for thoracoscopic drainage
Clotted hemothorax – surgical drainage if >25% of lung, air-fluid levels, or signs of infection (fever, ↑ WBCs); surgery in 1st week to avoid peel
Broncholiths – usually secondary to infection
Mediastinitis – usually after cardiac surgery
Whiteout on chest x-ray
    Midline shift toward whiteout – most likely collapse → need bronchoscopy to remove plug
    No shift – CT scan to figure it out
    Midline shift away from whiteout – most likely effusion → place chest tube
Bronchiectasis – acquired from infection, tumor, **cystic fibrosis**
    Diffuse nature prevents surgery in most patients
Tuberculosis – lung apices; get calcifications, caseating granulomas
    Gohn complex → parenchmal lesion + enlarged hilar nodes
    Tx: INH, rifampine, pyrazinomide
Sarcoidosis – has noncaseating granulomas
Effusions – **exudative**: protein >3, specific gravity >1.016, LDH ratio (pleural fluid:serum) >0.6, ↓ glucose
Recurrent pleural effusions can be treated with mechanical pleurodesis.
    Talc pleurodesis for malignant pleural effusions
Airway fires – usually associated with the laser
    Tx: stop gas flow, remove ET tube, reintubate for 24 hours; bronchoscopy
AVMs – connections between the pulmonary arteries and pulmonary veins; usually in lower lobes; can occur with Osler-Weber-Rendu disease
    Symptoms: hemoptysis, SOB, neurologic events
    Tx: embolization
Chest wall tumors
    Benign – **osteochondroma** most common
    Malignant – **chondrosarcoma** most common

CHAPTER 26. CARDIAC

Congenital heart disease
- **R→L shunts cause cyanosis.**
  - Children squat to ↑ SVRI and ↓ R→L shunts
  - **Cyanosis** – can lead to polycythemia, stokes, brain abscess, endocarditis, hypertrophic osteoarthropathy
  - **Eisenmenger's syndrome** – shift from L→R shunt to R→L
    - Sign of increasing pulmonary vascular resistance and pulmonary HTN
    - This condition is generally irreversible.

- **L→R shunts cause CHF** – can manifest as failure to thrive, ↑ HR, tachypnea, hepatomegaly
  - **CHF in children** – hepatomegaly 1st sign

- **L→R shunts (patients get symptoms of CHF)** – VSD, ASD, PDA
- **R→L shunts (patients have cyanosis)** – tetrology of Fallot, transposition of the great vessels, truncus arteriosus

Ductus arteriosus – connection between descending aorta and left pulmonary artery (PA); blood shunted away from lungs in utero
Ductus venosum – connection between portal vein and IVC; blood shunted away from liver
Fetal circulation to placenta – 2 umbilical arteries
Fetal circulation from placenta – 1 umbilical vein

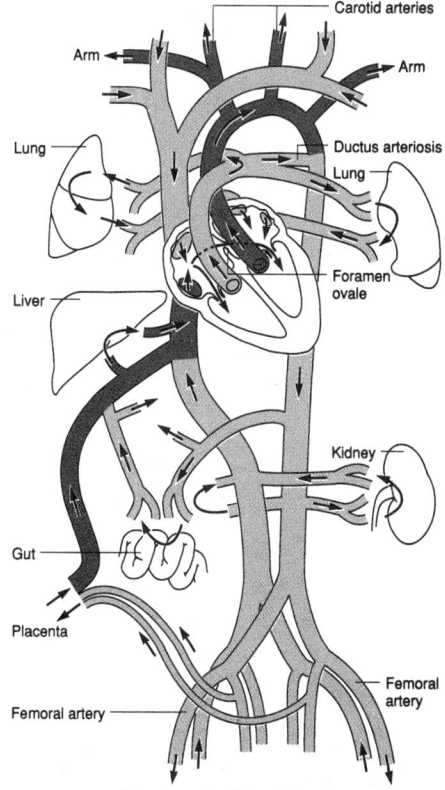

Persistent fetal circulation.

Ventricular septal defect (VSD)
Most common congenital heart defect
L→R shunt – most close spontaneously by age 6 months
Large VSDs – usually cause symptoms after 4–6 weeks of life, as PVR ↓ and shunt ↑
Get CHF, failure to thrive, tachypnea, tachycardia
Medical Tx: diuretics and digoxin
Timing of repair
- **CHF resulting in failure to thrive** – most common reason for repair
- **Before school age if doesn't close spontaneously**
- **PVR >4–6 Woods units** also indication for repair
- PVR >10–2 Woods units contraindication for repair → use vasodilators to see if it's reversible; if so, can repair

Atrial septal defect (ASD)
L→R shunt
Ostium secundum – most common; centrally located, patent foramen ovale (80%)
- Can have anomalous pulmonary venous return (to right atrium or IVC)
- IVC can connect to left atrium

Ostium primum (or atrioventricular septal defects or endocardial cushion defects)
- Defect more inferior
- Can get mitral valve and coronary sinus defects
- Caused by deficiency in remnant of left horn of sinus venosus

Usually symptomatic when Qp/Qs >2 → CHF (fatigue, SOB, recurrent infections)
Rare for ASD to cause increase in PVR before adulthood
Can get paradoxical emboli and arrhythmias in adulthood
Medical Tx: diuretics and digoxin

<u>Timing of repair</u>
- **Volume overload** (occurs with Qp/Qs >1.5)
- **Before school age if doesn't close spontaneously**
- PVR >10–12 Woods units contraindication for repair
- All ostium primum atrioventricular septal defects (ASDs) need repair.

Tetralogy of Fallot
VSD, pulmonic stenosis, overriding aorta, right ventricular (RV) hypertrophy
R→L shunt
Most common congenital heart defect that results in cyanosis
Morphologic abnormality – anterior and superior displacement of the infundibular septum
Medical Tx: beta-blocker
Timing of operation: ↑ cyanosis
Repair: Blalock-Taussig (BT) shunt can be used for palliation to delay repair
Definitive repair: RV outflow tract obstruction division, patch enlargement of outflow tract, and VSD repair

Transposition of the great vessels
Most common cyanotic disorder presenting in the 1st week of life
R→L shunt
Mixing most often occurs through ASD; VSD or PDA can serve as additional mixing conduit.
Medical Tx: atrial septostomy, PGE$_1$
In patients with large VSDs, significant CHF and pulmonary hypertension may occur by 3 months of age.
Repair: optimal – early switch with coronary reimplantation posteriorly (first 2–3 weeks of life) while LV is still getting high resistance
Patients with LVOT obstruction not candidates for early switch
- Most also have large VSDs.
- Palliation with systemic to PA shunting preferred early on (BT shunt)
- Definitive repair at 3–5 years of age

Truncus arteriosus
Usually has associated VSD
R→L shunt
Mixing causes arterial saturations of 85%–90%.
Neonates present with CHF; 80% die in 1st year due to CHF.
CXR shows cardiomegaly.
Medical Tx: diuretics, digoxin, fluid restriction, afterload reduction

Chapter 26. Cardiac

Timing of repair: onset of tachypnea is sign of ↓ PVR
Tx: repair VSD, remove PAs from aorta, and repair aorta; restore RV outflow tract with Dacron graft to PAs

Patent ductus arteriosus (PDA)
L→R shunt
Indomethacin – causes the PDA to close; rarely successful beyond the neonatal period
Usually requires surgical repair through left thoracotomy if persists
PGE_1 – keeps PDA open

Coarctation of the aorta
Usually occurs just distal to the left subclavian artery
Associated with Turner's syndrome
Rib notching from the IMA and intercostal collaterals
Can present with profound CHF
All patients should undergo repair to prevent heart failure.
Try to perform end-to-end repair.

Univentricular heart
Need Fontan procedure to direct all vena cava blood to the PA
Best approach is to attach the right atrium and SVC to the PA directly.
Prerequisites – normal PA pressure (<20 mmHg) and normal PVR (<2 Woods units)

Hypoplastic left heart
Need Norwood procedure
Main PA becomes outlet tract for aorta for what is to become single-ventricle physiology.
Tx: aorta is augmented with large piece of allograft artery and attached to main PA trunk
Distal PAs are separated and supplied through systemic-PA shunt (BT shunt).
Many patients eventually need heart TXP.

Anomalous pulmonary venous return – goes to SVC instead of left atrium
Most often seen in patients with ASDs

Vascular rings – double aortic arch most common
May manifest as recurrent pulmonary infections or dysphagia
Trachea most commonly affected
Tx: divide smaller arch through left thoracotomy

Adult cardiac disease
Coronary artery disease
Most common cause of death in US
Risk factors – smoking, HTN, male gender, family history, hyperlipidemia, diabetes
Medical Tx: nitrates, smoking cessation, weight loss, statin drugs, ASA
Right dominant circulation (most common) – posterior descending artery comes off the right coronary artery
Left dominant circulation – posterior descending artery comes off the circumflex coronary artery
Left main coronary artery branches into left anterior descending and circumflex.
Most atherosclerotic lesions are **proximal**.
Complications of myocardial infarction
VSD (pansystolic murmur), papillary muscle rupture, and free wall rupture
Most likely to occur at 3–7 days post-MI
Post-MI VSD (pansystolic murmur) – **transesophageal echo best test**
Usually occurs **5–7 days after MI**
Step-up in oxygen content between right atrium and pulmonary artery secondary to L→R shunt
LV aneurysm – most commonly occurs after large, transmural, anterior MI
Symptoms: CHF, arrhythmias, angina
Indications for surgery: refractory symptoms, arrhythmias
PTCA – restenosis in 20%–30% in <1 year
Saphenous vein graft – 80%–90% 5-year patency
Internal mammary artery – off subclavian arteries
Best conduit for CABG – >90% 10-year graft patency rate
Collateralizes with superior epigastric **artery**

CABG procedure
Potassium and cold solution cardioplegia – causes arrest of the heart in diastole; keeps the heart protected and still while grafts are placed

Indications[1]
- Left main disease
- Left main equivalent disease (LAD >70% and proximal left complications)
- 3-vessel disease
- 2-vessel disease with:
  - Proximal LAD stenosis and either LVEF <50% or extensive ischemia on noninvasive imaging study
- 1- or 2-vessel disease with:
  - Stable angina, large area of viable myocardium, and high-risk criteria on noninvasive testing *or*
  - Disease causing life-threatening arrythmias *or*
  - Disabling stable angina despite medications when patient has acceptable risk
- Unstable angina – patients with ongoing ischemia despite maximal nonsurgical therapy

High mortality risk factors: emergency operations (#1 risk factor), age, reoperation, and low EF

Valve disease
Aortic stenosis – most common valve lesion
Calcification – produces stenosis
Rheumatic heart disease – most common cause of valve dysfunction
   Mitral most commonly involved valve
Stenosis predominates; see regurgitation with progressive valve degeneration (volcano orifice, sticks open)
Degenerative processes – 3rd or 4th decade of life; **mitral** most commonly affected; **insufficiency** predominates

Tissue valves (do not require anticoagulation)
   For patients who want pregnancy, have contraindication to anticoagulation, are older and unlikely to require another valve in their lifetime, or have frequent falls
   Not as durable as mechanical valves
   Because of rapid calcification in children and young patients, use of tissue valves is contraindicated in these populations.
   Chronic renal dialysis is also a contraindication.

Mitral stenosis
   Leads to signs of pulmonary congestion
   Can develop mural thrombi – 50% go to cerebral circulation
   Indications for operation – when symptomatic (usually have valve area <1 cm^2)

Mitral regurgitation
   LV becomes dilated, wall tension ↑
   Ventricular function – key index of disease progression in patients with MR
   In end-stage disease, left atrium becomes less compliant → pulmonary congestion ensues and can lead to right-sided heart failure. Atrial fibrillation is common.
   Indications for operation – symptoms may not develop until after irreversible heart dysfunction has occurred
      Repair indicated for any functional class II heart failure (SOB on exertion)

Aortic stenosis
   Adequate CO and normal systemic pressures are maintained until late in the disease.
   Eventually, LV hypertrophy leads to ↓ ventricular compliance and pulmonary congestion. LV failure ultimately develops.
   Cardinal symptoms
      Angina – develops in 65%; mean survival is 5 years

---

[1] Eagle KA et al. ACC/AHA guidelines for coronary artery bypass graft surgery: a report of the American College of Cardiology/American Heart Association Task Force on Practice Guidelines. J Am Coll Cardiol 1999;34:1262–347.

Chapter 26. Cardiac

Syncope – develops in 25%, mean survival is 3 years
Heart failure – mean survival is 2 years (strongest prognostic indicator)
Indications for operation – when symptomatic (usually have gradient of 50 mmHg and a valve area <0.4 cm^2/m^2)

Aortic insufficiency
Produces volume loading strain on the LV
LV becomes more dilated, wall tension ↑ (law of LaPlace).
Cardiac output can increase to 30 L/min
Indications for operation – symptoms may not develop until after irreversible heart dysfunction has occurred
Repair indicated for any functional class II heart failure (SOB with exertion)

Endocarditis
Fever, chills, sweats
Aortic valve – most common site of prosthetic valve infections
Mitral valve – most common site of native valve infections
Most commonly left-sided except in drug abusers
Staphylococcus aureus responsible for 50% of cases
Medical therapy first – successful in 75%; sterilizes valve in 50%
Indications for surgery – **failure of antimicrobial therapy, valve failure, perivalvular abscesses, pericarditis**

Periprocedural endocarditis prophylaxis indicated for patients
Prosthetic valves
Rheumatic heart disease
Congenital cardiac malformations
Mitral valve prolapse with mitral regurgitation
Previous history of bacterial endocarditis

1st generation cephalosporins usually used → need to start oral antibiotics 1 day prior

Other cardiac conditions
Most common tumors of heart
Most common benign tumor – **myxoma**; 75% in LA, mitral valve stenosis–type symptoms
Most common malignant tumor – **angiosarcoma**
Most common metastatic tumor to the heart – **lung CA**

Coming off cardiopulmonary bypass and aortic root vent blood is dark and aortic perfusion cannula blood is red.
Tx: **ventilate the lungs**
Coronary veins have the lowest oxygen tension of any tissue in the body due to high oxygen extraction by myocardium.
Superior vena cava (SVC) syndrome – swelling of the upper extremites and face
Most cases secondary to lung CA invading the SVC
These tumors are unresectable since the tumor has invaded the mediastinum.
Tx: XRT
Idiopathic hypertrophic subaortic stenosis
Too much volume can cause pulmonary edema due to stenosis region.
Not enough afterload will cause the aortic outflow tract to collapse, also resulting in pulmonary edema.
Very tricky management
Intra-aortic balloon pump (IABP) – see Chap. 16, Critical Care
Mediastinal bleeding – >500 cc for 1st hour or >250 cc/hr for 4 hours → need to re-explore after cardiac procedure
Risk factors for mediastinitis – obesity, use of bilateral internal mammary arteries, diabetes
Tx: debridement with pectoralis flaps
Postpericardiotomy syndrome – pericardial friction rub, fever, chest pain, SOB
EKG – diffuse ST segment elevation in multiple leads
Tx: **NSAIDs, steroids**
1st sign of cardiac tamponade on echocardiogram – ↓ right atrial diastolic filling

CHAPTER 27. VASCULAR

Most common congenital hypercoagulable disorder – resistance to activated protein C (Leiden factor)
Most common acquired hypercoagulability disorder – smoking

Atherosclerosis stages
  1st – foam cells → macrophages that have absorbed fat and lipids in vessel wall
  2nd – smooth muscle cell proliferation → caused by growth factors released from macrophages; results in wall injury
  3rd – intimal disruption (from smooth muscle cell proliferation) → leads to exposure of collagen in vessel wall and eventual **thrombus formation formation** → fibrous plaques then form in these areas with underlying atheromas
Risk factors: smoking, HTN, hypercholesterolemia, DM, hereditary factors
Atherosclerosis – disease of intima
Hypertension – disease of media

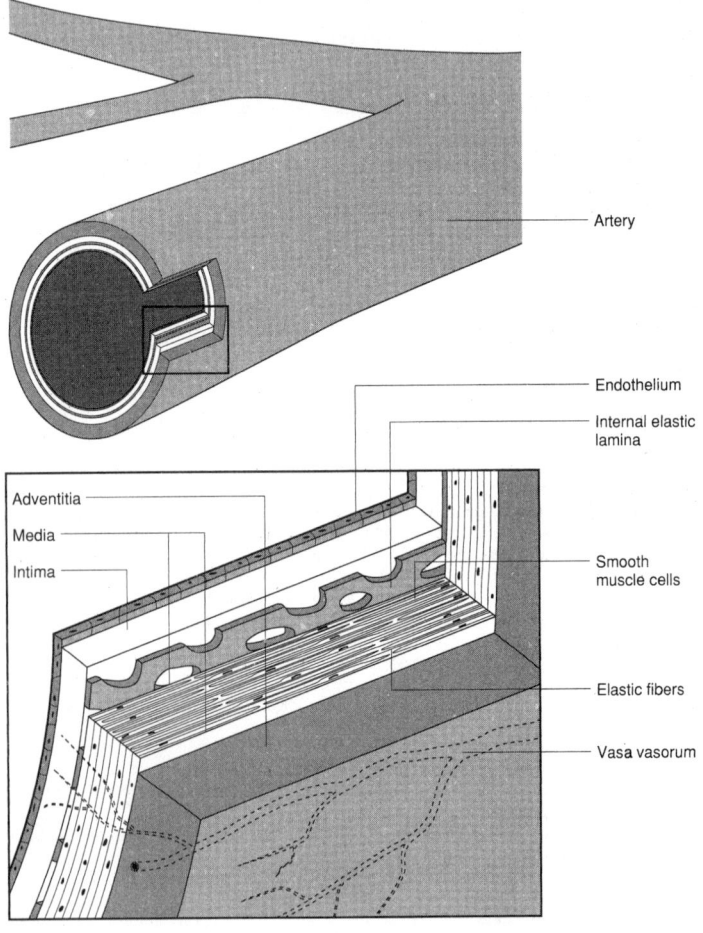

The artery wall.

Cerebrovascular disease

Stroke 3rd most common case of death in the US
HTN – most important risk factor for stroke in asymptomatic patients
Carotids supply 85% of blood flow to brain.
- **Bifurcation** – most common site of stenosis

Normal internal carotid artery has **continuous forward flow.**
Normal external carotid artery has **triphasic flow.**
- 1st branch of external carotid artery – **superior thyroid artery**
- Communication between internal carotid artery and external carotid artery with **ophthalmic artery** (1st branch of ICA) and **internal maxillary artery (off ECA)**

Middle cerebral artery – most commonly diseased <u>intracranial artery</u>
Cerebral ischemic events – most commonly from **arterial embolization** (not thrombosis) from the ICA
- Can also occur from a **low-flow state** through a severely stenotic lesion
- **Heart** 2nd most common source of emboli

Anterior cerebral artery events – mental status changes, release, slowing
Middle cerebral artery events – contralateral motor and speech (if dominant side); contralateral facial droop
Amaurosis fugax – occlusion of the ophthalmic branch of the ICA (visual changes → shade coming down over eyes); visual changes are transient
- See **Hollenhorst plaques** on ophthamologic exam

Carotid traumatic injury with major fixed deficit – do <u>not</u> repair → can exacerbate injury with bleeding

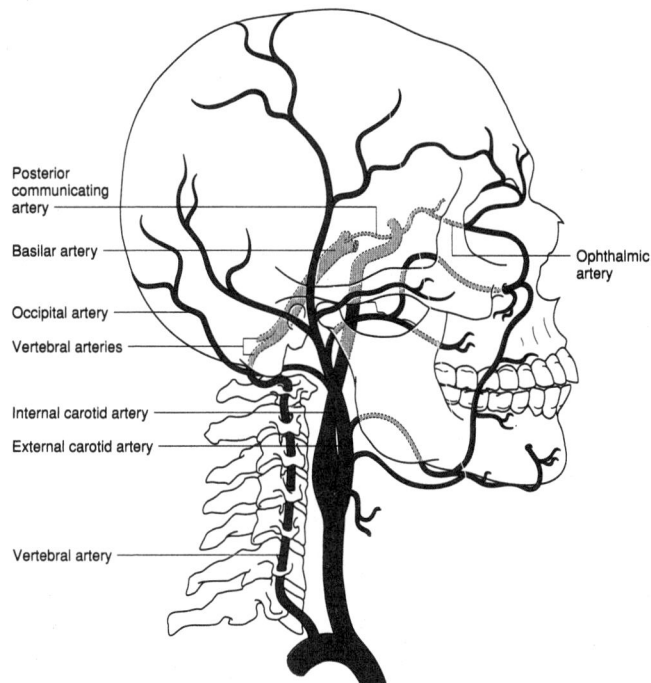

The arterial blood supply to the brain is from the paired carotid and vertebral arteries. Extensive extracranial collaterals between the external carotid and vertebral systems allow antegrade perfusion when either vessel has a proximal occlusion. Likewise, periorbital collateral allows retrograde flow through the ophthalmic artery to the internal carotid artery in the presence of a cervical internal carotid artery occlusion. Extensive side-to-side collateral exists between the right and the left external carotids and the right and left vertebral arteries.

Carotid endarterectomy (CEA)
Should be considered in any patient with >70% stenosis and symptoms
Asymptomatic patients with 70%–80% stenosis more controversial
Any patient with >80%–90% stenosis should have CEA if technically possible.
Recent completed stroke → wait 4–6 weeks and then perform CEA if it meets criteria (bleeding risk if performed earlier)
Emergent CEA may be of benefit with fluctuating neurologic symptoms or crescendo/evolving TIAs.
Shunt during CEA for stump pressures <50

Complications
Vagus nerve – most common cranial nerve injury with CEA → secondary to vascular clamping during endarterectomy; patients get hoarseness
Hypoglossal nerve – tongue deviation to the side of injury → speech and mastication difficulty
Glossopharyngeal nerve – unlikely injury; could occur with really high carotid lesion → causes difficulty swallowing
Ansa cervicalis – strap muscles; no serious deficits
Mandibular branch of facial nerve – affects corner of mouth (smile)

Acute event immediately after CEA → back to OR to check for flap or thrombosis
Pseudoaneurysm – pulsatile, bleeding mass after CEA
  Tx: drape and prep before intubation, intubate, then repair
20% have hypertension following CEA – caused by injury to carotid body
  Tx: nipride to avoid bleeding
Myocardial infarction – most common nonstroke morbidity and mortality following CEA
15% restenosis rate after CEA

Vertebral disease
Usually bilateral, at origins; usually need bilateral disease to have symptoms
Caused by spurs, bands, trauma; get vertebrobasilar insufficiency
Symptoms: diplopia, dysarthria, vertigo, tinnitus, drop attacks, incoordination, binocular vision loss
Tx: PTCA, vertebral artery transposistion to subclavian, transsubclavian endarterectomy, osteophyte resection, unroofing of transverse process foramina, and resection of musculotendinous bands all options

Carotid body tumors
present as a painless neck mass, usually near bifurcation, neural crest cells
Tx: resection

Thoracic aortic disease
Thoracic aortic transection (see also Chap. 15, Trauma)
From trauma, usually a deceleration injury
Address other life-threatening injuries 1st (severe solid organ laceration, pelvic fracture with hemorrhage, etc. → then repair aorta)
Get **mediastinal widening** from bridging veins and arteries, not leaking from aorta itself
Usually tears at the **ligamentum arteriosum**, just distal to the left subclavian
Use left heart bypass with repair.
90% of these patients die at the scene.

Ascending aortic anuerysms
Usually caused by connective tissue disorders; **cystic medial necrosis** most common abnormality – Marfan's syndrome
Dx: chest CT or aortography
Can get aortic insufficiency
Often asymptomatic and picked up on routine CXR
Can also get compression of vertebra (back pain), RLN (voice changes), bronchi (dyspnea or PNA), or esophagus (swallowing trouble)
Symptomatic patients usually have CHF secondary to aortic insufficiency
Indications for repair: acutely symptomatic, ≥7 cm, ≥6 cm with Marfan's, diameter 2x normal, or rapid ↑ in size

Transverse aortic arch aneurysms
From atherosclerosis
Repair indications same as for ascending aortic aneurysms
Patients will likely need to be cooled down and have circulatory arrest to perform repair.

Descending aortic aneurysms (or thoracoabdominal aneurysms)
From atherosclerosis; can become quite large before symptoms occur
Risk of paraplegia 5%–10%
Repair indications same as for ascending aortic aneurysms

Dissections
    Stanford classification – based on the presence or absence of involvement of ascending aorta
        Class A – any ascending aortic involvement
        Class B – descending aortic involvement only

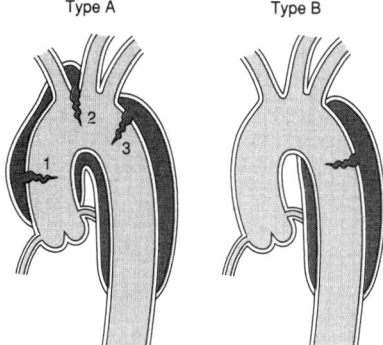

Stanford classification of aortic dissections.

    DeBakey classification – based on site of tear and extent of dissection.
        Type I – ascending and descending
        Type II – ascending only
        Type III – descending only

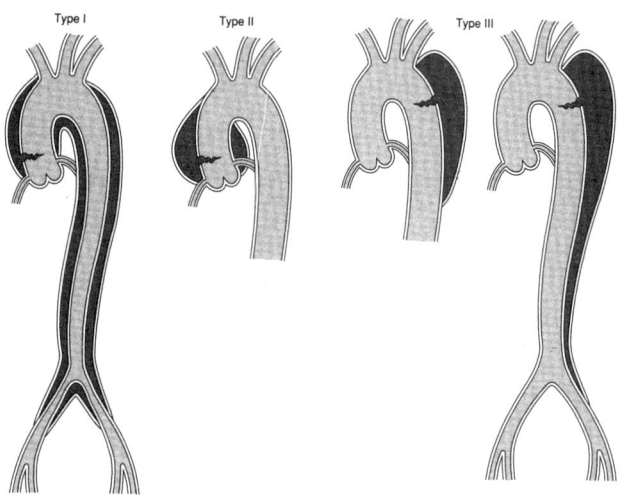

DeBakey classification of aortic dissection.

Most dissections start in **ascending aorta**.
Can mimic myocardial infarction
Symptoms: searing-like chest pain; can have unequal pulses or BP in upper extremities
95% of patients have **severe HTN**
Other risk factors: Marfan's syndrome, previous coarctation repair, atherosclerosis, infection (syphilis)
CXR – usually normal; may have wide mediastinum
Dx: chest CT with contrast
Dissection occurs in **media layer of blood vessel wall**.
Aortic insufficiency occurs in 70% with acute disease, caused by annular dilatation or when aortic valve cusp is sheared off.
Can also have occlusion of the coronaries and major aortic branches
Death with ascending aortic dissections usually secondary to **cardiac failure from aortic insufficiency or tamponade**; can also have **rupture**
Medical Tx if possible → control BP with nipride and beta-blockers
Surgery aims at obliterating the false lumen and placing graft.
> **Operate on all ascending aortic dissections**
> **Operate on descending aortic dissections with visceral, renal, or leg ischemia; persistent pain; large size** (from aortic dilatation after dissection)
> Need to follow these patients with lifetime serial CT scans; 30% will eventually get aneurysm formation requiring surgery

Postop complications for thoracic aortic surgery – MI, renal failure, paraplegia (especially descending thoracic aortic surgery)
Paraplegia caused by ischemia due to occlusion of the intercostal arteries and artery of Adamkiewicz during repair

Abdominal aortic disease
Abdominal aortic aneurysms (AAAs)
Normal aorta 2–3 cm
Aneurysms form from **degeneration of the medial layer**.
Most commonly due to atherosclerosis
Usually found incidentally
Risk factors: HTN, male gender, smoking, elderly age
Can present with rupture, distal embolization (can cause lower extremity ischemic symptoms, compression of adjacent organs

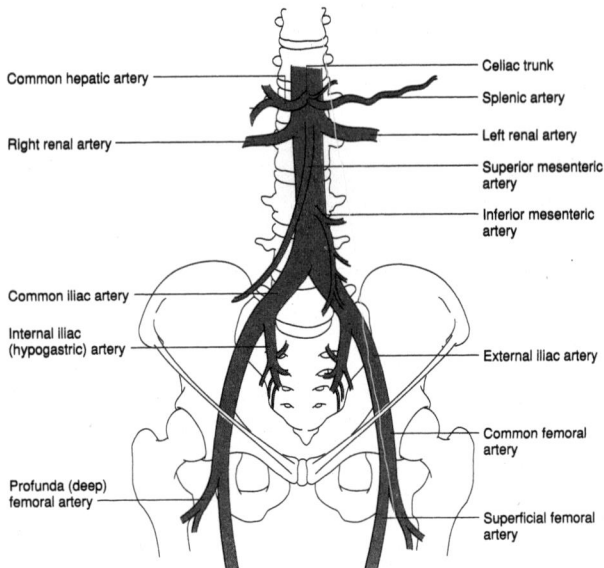

Anatomy of the abdominal aorta and iliac arteries.

Chapter 27. Vascular

Rupture
Leading cause of death without an operation
Patients often have back or abdominal pain; can have profound hypotension
Dx: ultrasound or abdominal CT
AAA rupture risk – starts to rise in AAAs >5 cm (5-cm AAA has 15%–20% 5-year risk of rupture); **>8 cm** → 100% rupture risk within 5 years
CT shows **fluid** in retroperitoneal space, **extraluminal contrast** with rupture
Most likely to rupture on **left posterolateral wall, 2–4 cm below renals**
More likely to rupture in presence of **diastolic HTN or COPD** (thought to be predictors of expansion)
50% mortality with rupture if patient reaches hospital alive
Tx: **repair if symptomatic, >5 cm, or growth >0.5 cm/yr**
Reimplant IMA if backpressure <40 mmHg (poor backbleeding), previous colonic surgery, stenosis at SMA, or flow to left colon appears inadequate
Ligate bleeding lumbar arteries.
Maintain flow to at least **one internal iliac artery** (hypogastric) to avoid **vasculogenic impotence.**
Complications
Major vein injury with proximal cross-clamp – retroaortic renal vein
Impotence in ⅓ secondary to disruption of autonomic nerves and blood flow to the pelvis
5% mortality with elective repair
#1 cause of acute death after surgery – MI
#1 cause of late death after surgery – renal failure
Graft infection rate – 1%
Pseudoaneurysm after graft placement – 1%
Atherosclerotic occlusion – most common late complication after aortic graft placement
Diarrhea (especially bloody) after AAA worrisome for **ischemic colitis**
Inferior mesenteric artery often sacrificed with AAA repair and can cause ischemia of left colon
Dx: endoscopy or abdominal CT; rectum spared from ischemia
If patient has peritoneal signs → take to OR for colectomy and colostomy placement.
Can follow closely if no peritoneal signs

Inflammatory aneurysms
Occurs in 10% of patients with AAA; males
Adhesions to the **3rd and 4th portions of the duodenum**
Ureteral entrapment in 25%
Not secondary to infection
Weight loss, ↑ ESR, thickened rim above calcifications on CT scan
May need to place preoperative ureteral stents
Inflammatory process resolves after aortic graft placement

Mycotic aneurysms
***Salmonella* #1**, *Staphylococcus* #2
Pain, fevers, positive blood cultures in 50%
Periaortic fluid, gas, retroperitoneal soft tissue edema, lymphadenopathy
May need extra-anatomic bypass (axillary bifemoral) and resection of infrarenal abdominal aorta to clear infection
Bacteria infect atherosclerotic plaque, cause aneurysm.

Aortic graft infections
***Staphylococcus* #1**, *E. coli* #2
See fluid, gas, thickening around graft
Blood cultures negative in many patients
Treatment of choice is to resect the graft and bypass through noncontaminated field.
More common with grafts going to groin (aortobifemoral grafts)

Aortoenteric fistula
Usually occurs >6 months after surgery
Herald bleed with hematemesis, then blood per rectum
In 3rd or 4th portion of duodenum near proximal suture line
Tx: axillary bifemoral bypass, resection of graft with aortic stump closure

Stented tube grafts
  Proximal neck – needs to be >1.5 cm in length, <3 cm in diameter (approximately)
  Distal neck – needs to be >1.5 cm in length, <3 cm in diameter (approximately)
    Aneurysm <7 cm (approximately)
  Type I endoleak – proximal, distal, or through the stent
  Type II endoleak– persistent blood flow through lumbars or IMA

Peripheral vascular disease
Leg compartments
  Anterior – deep peroneal nerve (dorsiflexion, sensation between 1st and 2nd toes), anterior tibial artery
  Lateral – superficial peroneal nerve (eversion, lateral foot sensation)
  Deep posterior – tibial nerve (plantarflexion), posterior tibial artery, peroneal artery
  Superficial posterior – sural nerve
Signs of PVD – pallor, hair loss, dependent rubor, abnormal nail growth, slow capillary refill
  Most commonly due to **atherosclerosis**
Statin drugs (lovastatin) – #1 preventive agent for atherosclerosis
Homocysteinuria can ↑ risk of atherosclerosis. Tx: folate, B_6, B_{12}
Claudication – medical therapy 1st → ASA, smoking cessation, exercise until pain occurs to improve collaterals
  2%/yr **gangrene risk** and 1%/yr **amputation risk** with claudication

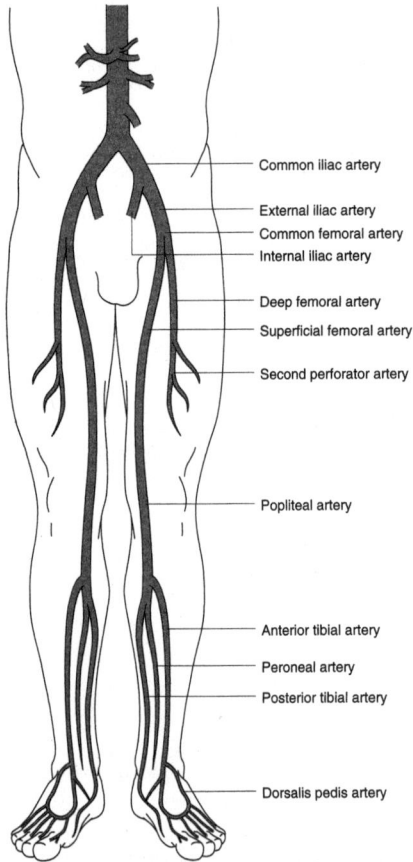

Anatomy of the arterial circulation to the lower extremity.

Symptoms occur one level below occlusion.
    Buttock claudication – aortoiliac disease
    Midthigh claudication – external iliac
    Calf claudication – common femoral artery or proximal superficial femoral artery disease
    Foot claudication – distal superficial femoral artery or popliteal disease
Lumbar stenosis can mimic claudication.
Diabetic neuropathy can mimic rest pain.
Leriche syndrome
    No femoral pulses
    Buttock or thigh claudication
    Impotence (from hypogastirc obstruction and ↓ flow in the internal iliacs)
    Lesion at aortic bifurcation or above
Most common atherosclerotic occlusion in lower extremities – Hunter's canal (distal superficial femoral artery exits here). Sartorius muscle covers Hunter's canal.

Collateral circulation – forms from abnormal pressure gradients
    Circumflex iliacs to subcostals
    Circumflex femoral arteries to gluteal arteries
    Genticulate arteries around the knee
Postnatal angiogenesis – budding from preexisting vessels; angiogenin involved

Ankle-brachial index (ABI)
    <0.9 – start to get claudication (typically occurs at same distance each time)
    <0.6 – start to get rest pain (usually across the distal arch and foot)
    <0.5 – ulcers (usually starts in toes)
    <0.3 – gangrene
    ABIs can be very **inaccurate in patients with diabetes** secondary to incompressibility of vessels; often have to go off Doppler waveforms in these patients.
    In patients with claudication, the ABI in the extremity drops with walking (i.e., resting ABI may be 0.9 but can drop to <0.6 with exercise resulting in pain).
Peripheral vascular resistance studies (PVRs) – to find significant occlusion and at what level
Arteriogram if PVRs suggest significant disease – can also at times treat the patient with angiographic intervention; gold standard for vascular imaging

Surgical indications for PVD – rest pain, ulceration or gangrene, lifestyle limitation, atheromatous embolization
    PTFE (Gortex) – decreases patency when crosses knee
    Dacron – good for aorta and large vessels

    Aortoiliac occlusive disease – most get aortobifemoral repair
        In high-risk patients can perform bilateral axillary-femoral bypasses or an axillary-femoral bypass with a femoral-femoral crossover (keeps you out of the abdomen)
    Isolated iliac lesions – angioplasty with stent 1st choice; if that fails can perform aortobifemoral repair or femoral-to-femoral crossover
    Femoropopliteal grafts
        75% 5-year patency
        Improved patency rate in patients with surgery for claudication as opposed to limb salvage
    Femoral-distal grafts (peroneal, anterior tibial or posterior tibial artery)
        50% 5-year patency; patency not influenced by level of distal anastamosis
        Distal lesions more limb threatening because of lack of collaterals
        Bypasses distal to knee; usually used only for limb salvage
    Synthetic grafts have decreased patency below the knee → need to use saphenous vein
    Extra-anatomic grafts to avoid hostile conditions in the abdomen (aortic graft infections, multiple previous operations)
    Femoral-to-femoral crossover graft – doubles blood flow to donor artery; can get vascular steal in donor leg

Swelling following lower extremity bypass
    Get lower extremity duplex to check for DVT
    2nd most common cause – **edema from reperfusion injury**

Complications of reperfusion of ischemic tissue – **lactic acidosis, hyperkalemia, myoglobinuria, compartment syndrome**
Atherosclerosis – #1 cause of late failure of reversed saphenous vein grafts
Technical problem – #1 cause of early failure of reversed saphenous vein grafts

Patients with heel ulceration to bone → amputation
Dry gangrene – noninfectious; can allow to autoamputate if just toes
  Larger lesions should probably be amputated.
  See if patient has correctable vascular lesion.
Wet gangrene – infectious; amputation to remove infected necrotic material, antibiotics, surgical emergency
Malperforans ulcer
  At metatarsal heads – 2nd MTP most common
  Diabetics; can have osteomyelitis
  Tx: nonweightbearing, debridement of metatarsal head (need to remove cartilage), antibiotics; assess need for revascularization
Percutaneous transluminal angioplasty
  Excellent for common iliac lesions
  Best for short stenoses
  Intima usually ruptured and media stretched, pushes the plaque out
  Requires passage of wire 1st
  Pseudoaneurysm after arteriography – thrombin injection with ultrasound guidance
    Ultrasound duplex best 1st test for this

Compartment syndrome
  Most likely to occur in the **anterior compartment of leg (get footdrop)**
  Pressure >20–30 mmHg abnormal; consider fasciotomies → leave open 5–10 days
  Dx: based on clinical suspicion

Popliteal entrapment syndrome
  Most present with mild intermittent claudication
  Men, 40s; loss of pulses with plantarflexion
  Usually have medial deviation of artery around medial head of gastrocnemius muscle.
  Tx: **resection of medial head of gastrocnemius muscle**; may need arterial reconstruction

Adventitial cystic disease
  Men, 40s; **popliteal most common area**
  Often bilateral – ganglia originate from adjacent joint capsule or tendon sheath
  Symptoms: intermittent claudication; changes in symptoms with knee flexion/extension
  Dx: angiogram
  Tx: vein graft if vessel occluded; otherwise just resection of cyst

Arterial autografts – internal iliac artery for chidren needing renal artery repair, radial grafts for CABG, IMA for CABG

Amputations
For gangrene, nonhealing ulcers, or unrelenting rest pain not amenable to surgery
50% mortality within 3 years of above- (AKA) or below- (BKA) knee amputation
BKA – 80% heal, 70% walk again, 5% die
AKA – 90% heal, 30% walk again, 10% die
Emergency amputation for systemic complications, extensive infection, failure of antibiotics

Acute arterial emboli
Usually don't have collaterals with emboli (do have collaterals with thrombosis)
Usually don't have signs of chronic limb ischemia
Contralateral leg usually has no chronic signs of ischemia and pulses are usually normal.
Usually have no history of claudication
  1st pallor → cyanosis → marbeling
Symptoms: pain, pallor, pulselessness, paresthesia, poikilothermia, paralysis
Most common cause – atrial fibrillation
  Other causes – LV aneurysm with thrombus, prosthetic heart valve, cardiac tumors (myxoma), paradoxical embolus from patent foramen ovale, peripheral arterial or aortic atherosclerotic plaque embolism, aortic or arterial aneurysms with embolism

Common femoral artery most common site of peripheral obstruction from emboli
Tx: **embolectomy**; need to get pulses back; postop angiogram
- Fasiotomy if ischemia >4–6 hours → permanent muscle and nerve damage begins at 4–6 hours
- Aortoiliac emboli (loss of pulses to both feet) can be treated with bilateral femoral artery cutdowns and bilateral embolectomies.

Atheroma embolism – renals most commonly involved; cholesterol clefts in small arteries
- **Blue toe syndrome** – flaking atherosclerotic emboli off abdominal aorta or branches
  Patients typically have good distal pulses.
  Aortoiliac disease most common source
- Dx: need chest/abdomen/pelvis CT scan to look for aneurysmal source, ECHO, angiogram to ruleout atherosclerotic disease
- TX: may need aneurysm repair, endarterectomy, arterial exclusion with bypass

Clinical distinctions between acute arterial embolism and acute arterial thrombosis

Embolism	Thrombosis
Arrhythmia	No arrhythmia
No prior claudication or rest pain	History of claudication or rest pain
Normal contralateral pulses	Contralateral pulses absent
No physical findings of chronic limb ischemia	Physical findings of chronic limb ischemia

<u>**Acute arterial thrombosis**</u>
These patients usually do <u>not</u> have arrhythmias.
Do have a history of claudication and have signs of chronic limb ischemia and poor pulses in the contralateral leg
Tx: threatened limb → give heparin and go to OR for thrombectomy; if limb not threatened can go to angiography for thrombolytics
Thrombosis of PTFE graft → thrombolytics and anticoagulation; if limb threatened → OR

<u>**Renal vascular disease – renovascular hypertension**</u>
Right renal artery runs posterior to IVC.
Accessory renal arteries in 25%
Most renal emboli from heart
Renal atherosclerosis – left side, proximal ⅓, men
  Tx: PTA with stent
Fibromuscular dysplasia – right side, distal ⅓, women
  Tx: PTA with stent
Suggestive of renovascular HTN – bruits, diastolic blood pressure >115, worsening HTN, children, premenopausal women, rapid onset after age 50, HTN resistant to drug therapy
Need to rule out other sources of HTN (pheochromocytoma, etc)
Dx of renal artery stenosis: angiogram
Tx: PTA with stent
Indications for nephrectomy with renal HTN → atrophic kidney <6 cm and minimal collaterals with persistently ↑ renin levels

<u>**Upper extremity**</u>
Occlusive disease – proximal lesions usually asymptomatic secondary to ↑ collaterals
  Subclavian most common site of stenosis
  Tx: PTA with stent; can also perform common carotid to subclavian bypass

Subclavian steal syndrome – proximal subclavian artery stenosis resulting in reversal of flow through ipsilateral vertebral artery into subclavian
  Operate with limb or neurologic (usually vertebrobasilar) symptoms
  Tx: carotid to subclavian bypass or PTA

Thoracic outlet syndrome
  Normal anatomy
    Subclavian vein – passes over the 1st rib anterior to the anterior scalene muscle, then behind clavicle

Brachial plexus and subclavian artery – pass over the 1st rib posterior to the anterior scalene muscle, and anterior to the middle scalene muscle
Dx: CXR, cervical spine x-ray, angiography if thought to be vascular etiology
Can get back and neck symptoms
Adson's test – ↓ radial pulse with head turned ipsilateral side (subclavian artery compression)
Tinsel's test – tapping reproduces symptoms

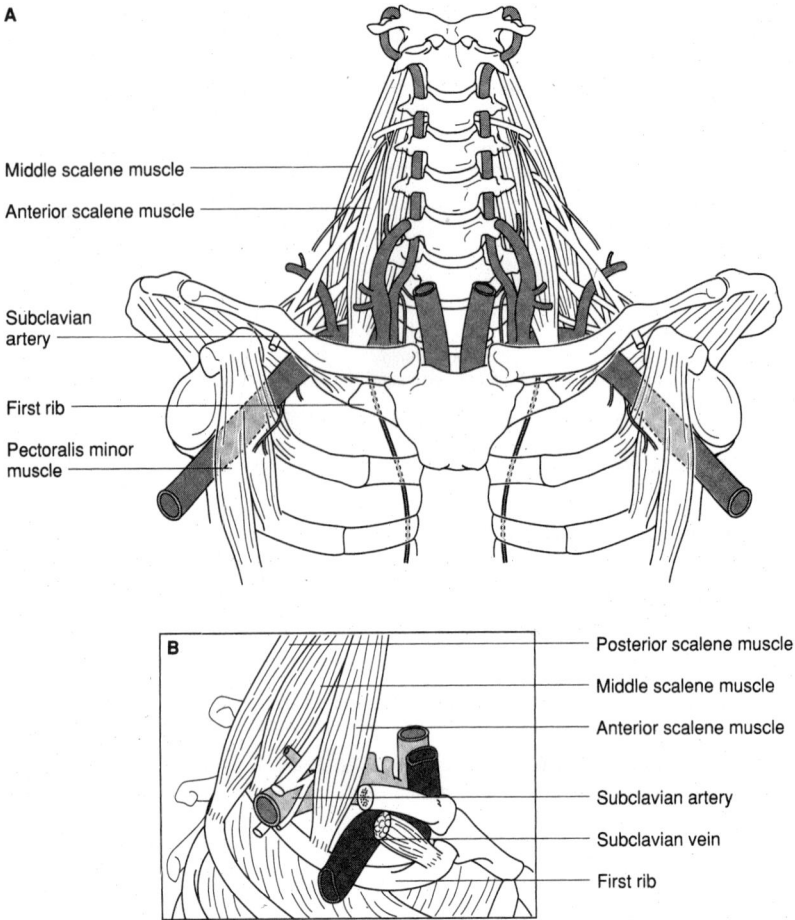

The normal anatomy of the thoracic outlet in anteroposterior (A) and oblique (B) views. The brachial plexus and subclavian artery traverse the narrow traiangle formed by the anterior and middle scalene muscles and the first rib. The subclavian vein lies anteriorly.

Neurologic involvement – much more common than vascular
#1 anatomic abnormality – cervical rib
#1 cause of pain – brachial plexus irritation

Brachial plexus irritation
Usually have normal neurologic exam
↑ back and neck symptoms
Palpation/manipulation – can ↑ symptoms

Ulnar nerve distribution (C8–T1) most common
- Triceps weakness and atrophy, weakness of intrinsic muscles of hand, weak wrist flexion
- Located on inferior portion of brachial plexus

Radial nerve – located on superior portion of brachial plexus
- Finger extensors, wrist extension

Tx: resection of cervical ribs, divide **anterior scalenes** and middle scalenes, +/– 1st rib resection

Subclavian artery
Compression usually secondary to **anterior scalene hypertrophy** (pitchers)
Absent radial pulse with maximal arm abduction
Tx: **surgery** → cervical rib and 1st rib resection, divide anterior scalene muscle, bypass graft

Subclavian vein
Usually presents as effort-induced thrombosis of subclavian vein (Paget–von Schrotter disease)
Venous thrombosis – much more common than arterial
Venography – gold standard for diagnosis
Male gender; pain and swelling ↑ with activity, ↓ with rest
80% have associated thoracic outlet problem.
Tx: **thrombolytics, heparin, warfarin** initial treatment, may eventually need operation for TOS if symptoms continue

Motor function can remain in digits after prolonged ischemia because motor groups are in proximal forearm.

Mesenteric ischemia
Overall mortality 50%–70%
Findings on abdominal CT that suggest intestinal ischemia – bowel wall thickening, intramural gas, portal venous gas, vascular occlusion
Most common causes of visceral ischemia
- **Acute embolic occlusion** – 50%
- **Thrombotic occlusion** – 25%
- **Low flow state** – 15%
- **Venous thrombosis** – 5%

Superior mesenteric artery embolism
Most commonly occurs near origin of SMA – heart #1 source
Pain out of proportion to exam; pain usually of sudden onset; hematochezia; peritoneal signs late finding
May have a history of atrial fibrillation, endocarditis, recent MI, recent angiography
Dx: angiogram or abdominal CT with IV contrast
Tx: volume resuscitation, antibiotics, **embolectomy**, resect infarcted bowel, heparin

Superior mesenteric artery thrombosis
Usually have history of chronic problems (food fear from mesenteric angina), weight loss
May have a history of vasculitis or hypercoagulable state
Symptoms: similar to embolism; may have developed some collaterals
Dx: angiogram or abdominal CT with IV contrast
Tx: **thrombectomy**, usually need **SMA bypass**, resection of infarcted bowel, heparin

Mesenteric vein thrombosis
Usually short segments of intestine involved; bloody diarrhea, crampy abdominal pain
May have a history of vasculitis, hypercoagulable state, portal HTN
Dx: abdominal CT scan or angiogram
Tx: **heparin**, thrombolytics; can try mesenteric vein thrombectomy if diagnosed early; resection of infarcted bowel

Nonocclusive mesenteric ischemia
Spasm, low-flow states, hypovolemia, hemoconcentration, digoxin → final common pathway is low cardiac output state to visceral vessels.
Risk factors: prolonged shock, CHF, prolonged cardiopulmonary bypass

Bloody diarrhea, pain
Watershed areas (Griffith's and Sudak's points) most vulnerable
Tx: volume resuscitation, glucagon, papaverine, nitrates can ↑ visceral blood flow; also need to ↑ cardiac output; resection of infarcted bowel

Median arcuate ligament syndrome
Causes celiac compression
Bruit near epigastrum, chronic pain, weight loss, diarrhea
Tx: transect median arcuate ligament; may need arterial reconstruction
Chronic mesenteric angina
Weight loss secondary to food fear
Visceral angina occurs 30 minutes after meals (food fear).
May need PTA, bypass, or endarterectomy
Get lateral visceral vessel aortography to see origins of celiac and SMA.

Aneurysms
Rupture – most common complication of aneurysms above inguinal ligament
Thrombosis and emboli – most common complications of aneurysm below inguinal ligament
Visceral
Repair all splanchnic aneurysms when diagnosed (50% risk for rupture) except splenic.
Splenic artery aneurysm – most common visceral aneurysm (more common in women, 2% risk of rupture)
Repair splenic artery aneurysms if **symptomatic, if patient is pregnant, or if occurs in women of childbearing age**.
High rate of pregnancy-related rupture – usually occurs in **3rd trimester**
Diameters >2 cm considered aneurysmal
Most visceral aneurysms are treated with exclusion and bypass graft.
Splenic and proximal common hepatic can just be excluded (have good collaterals).
Risk factors: medial fibrodysplasia, portal HTN, arterial disruption secondary to inflammatory disease (i.e., pancreatitis)
Iliac
Surgical indications: symptomatic (thrombosis, emboli, or compression), >3.0 cm, mycotic
Tx: bypass with exclusion
Femoral
Surgical indications: symptomatic (thrombosis, emboli, or compression), >2.5 cm, mycotic
Tx: bypass with exclusion
Popliteal
Most common peripheral aneurysm
Leg exam reveals prominent popliteal pulses
½ are **bilateral**
½ have **another aneurysm elsewhere** (AAA, femoral, etc)
Most likely to get **thrombosis or emboli with limb ischemia**
Can also get leg pain from compression of adjacent structures
Surgical indications: symptomatic, >2 cm, mycotic
Dx: ultrasound
Tx: exclusion and bypass of all popliteal aneurysms; 25% have complication that requires amputation if not treated
Femoral pseudoaneurysm
Collection of blood in continuity with the arterial system but unenclosed by all 3 layers of the arterial wall
Can result from disruption of a suture line between graft and artery or from percutaneous interventions
Tx: if occurs after percutaneous intervention, need ultrasound-guided compression with thrombin injection → if flow remains in the pseudoaneurysm or if pseudoaneurysms is at a suture site, need surgical repair
Renal
Surgical indications: symptomatic, expansion, >1.5 cm; women who want pregnancy
Tx: reconstruction with vein patch; nephrectomy if rupture occurs

Other vascular diseases
Fibromuscular dysplasia
Young women; HTN if renal involved

Renal (right side) most commonly involved vessel, followed by carotid and iliac
String of beads
Medial fibrodysplasia most common variant (80%–90%)
Tx: PTA (1st choice) or bypass

Buerger's disease
Young men, smokers, corkscrew collateral on angiogram and severe distal disease
Severe rest pain with bilateral ulceration
Gangrene of the digits, especially the fingers
Normal arterial tree proximal to popliteal and brachial vessels (small vessel disease)
Tx: stop smoking or will require continued amputations

Cystic medial necrosis syndromes
  Marfan's disease
   Type I collagen defect; Marfanoid habitus, retinal detachment, aortic root dilatation
  Ehlers-Danlos syndrome
   Many types of collagen defects identified
   Easy bruising, hypermobile joints, tendency for **arterial rupture**, especially abdominal vessels
   Get aneuryms and dissections
   No angiograms → risk of laceration to vessel
   Often too difficult to repair and need ligation of vessels to control hemorrhage

Immune arteritis
  Large arteries
   Temporal arteritis
    Giant cell arteritis, granulomatous disease
    Involves inflammation of large vessels
    Long segments of smooth stenosis alternating with segments of larger diameter
    Women, age >55; visual changes (risk of blindness)
    Symptoms: fever, arthralgia, myalgia, anorexia
    Can affect branches of aorta and aorta itself and pulmonary artery
    Tx: **steroids**, bypass of large vessels if needed; no endarterectomy
   Takayasu's arteritis – same pathology, symptoms and treatment as temporal arteritis; affects women <35 years
  Medium arteries
   Polyarteritis nodosa
    Get aneurysms that thrombose or rupture
    Renals most commonly involved
    Tx: **steroids**
   Kawasaki's disease
    Children; get dilated coronaries and brachiocephliac vessels
    Die from arrhythmias
    Tx: **steroids, CABG**
  Small arteries
   Hypersensitivity angiitis
    Often secondary to drug/tumor antigens
    Symptoms: rash, fever, symptoms of end-organ dysfunction
    Tx: **calcium channel blockers, pentoxifylline,** stop offending agent

Radiation arteritis
  Early – sloughing and thrombosis (obliterative endarteritis)
  Late (1–10 years) – fibrosis, scar, stenosis
  Late late (3–30 years) – advanced atherosclerosis

Raynaud's disease – young women; pallor → cyanosis → rubor
  Tx: **calcium channel blockers, warmth**

Venous disease
Greater saphenous vein – joins femoral vein near groin; runs medially
Lesser saphenous vein – joins popliteal vein in lower leg; runs lateral at first
No clamps on IVC → will tear

Left renal vein can be ligated safely because of increased collaterals → left gonadal vein, left adrenal vein

Access grafts
  Most common failure of A-V grafts for dialysis – **venous obstruction secondary to intimal hyperplasia**
  Cimeno – radial artery to cephalic vein; wait 6 weeks to use → allows vein to mature
  Interposition graft – wait 6 weeks to allow fibrous scar to form

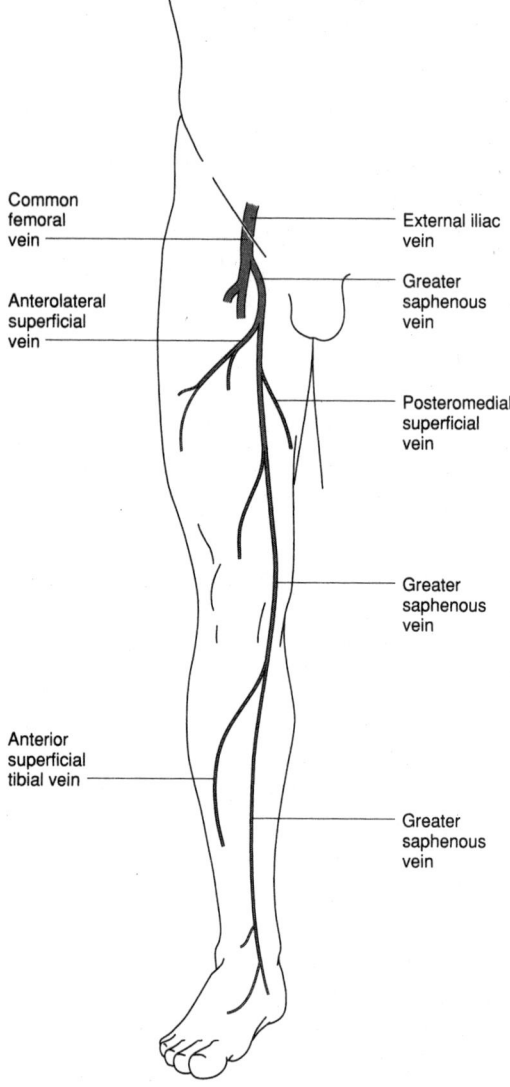

Greater saphenous vein and its branches.

Acquired A-V fistula – usually secondary to trauma; can get peripheral arterial insufficiency, CHF, aneurysm, limb-length discrepancy
  Most need repair → lateral venous suture; arterial side may need bypass graft

Chapter 27. Vascular

Varicose veins
Smoking, obesity, low activity
Tx: stockings, elevation, exercise, sclerotherapy → most do <u>not</u> need surgery
Surgery for severe symptoms, recurrent ulcers, severe varicosities
DVT contraindication to sclerotherapy and vein stripping

Venous ulcers
Secondary to venous valve incompetence (90%)
Unna boot compression cures 90%.
May need to ligate perforators or have vein stripping of greater saphenous vein

Venous insufficiency
Aching, swelling, night cramps, brawny edema
Ulceration occurs above and posterior to malleoli.
Edema – secondary to incompetent perforators
Elevation brings relief.
Trendelenburg test
1st part – elevate leg, occlude greater saphenofemoral vein junction, lower leg → rapid filling of greater saphenous vein suggests incompetent perforators
2nd part – if 1st part did not fill greater saphenous vein, release pressure on saphenofemoral junction → rapid filling of greater saphenous vein suggests incompetent valves in greater saphenous
Tx: leg wraps, ambulation with avoidence of long standing; ulcers <3 cm often heal without surgery
Greater saphenous vein stripping with moderate to severe symptoms, recurrent ulceration despite medical Tx

Superficial thrombophlebitis – nonbacterial inflammation
Tx: NSAIDs, warm packs, ambulation
Suppurative thrombophlebitis – fever, ↑ WBCs, erythema, fluctuance
Tx: resect vein
Migrating thrombophlebitis – pancreatic CA
Mondor's disease – self-limiting thrombophlebitis of the breast

Normal venous Doppler ultrasound – augmentation of flow with distal compression or release of proximal compression

Sequential compression devices (SCDs) – help prevent blood clots by ↓ venous stasis, ↑ AT-III, tPA, and ↑ fibrinolysin

Deep venous thrombosis (DVT)
Most common in calf
Pain, tenderness, calf swelling
Left leg 2x more involved than right (longer left iliac vein compressed by right iliac artery
Risk factors: Virchow's triad → venous stasis, hypercoaguability, venous wall injury
Calf DVT – minimal swelling
Femoral DVT – ankle and calf swelling
Iliofemoral DVT – severe leg swelling
Phlegmasia alba dolens – tenderness, pallor (whiteness), edema
Tx: heparin
Phlegmasia cerulea dolens – tenderness, cyanosis (blueness), massive edema
Tx: heparin; rarely need surgery
Long-term Tx
1st – coumadin 6 months
2nd – coumadin 1 year
3rd or pulmonary embolism – coumadin lifetime
Filter – contraindication to anticoagulation; PE while on coumadin, free-floating ileofemoral thrombi; after pulmonary embolectomy
Pulmonary embolism with filter in place – comes from ovarian veins, inferior vena cava superior to filter, or from upper extremity

Pulmonary embolism
Get ↓ pO_2 and ↓ pCO_2, ↑ RR, respiratory alkalosis, shock if massive
Most PEs arise from above the knee.

Tx: heparin if symptomatic; lifetime coumadin
Some say all of these patients should get a filter.
If patient is in shock, go to OR for emergency pulmonary artery thrombectomy.

Venous thrombosis with central line – pull out if not needed; can try to treat with systemic heparin or TPA down line

Lymphatics
Do not contain a basement membrane
Not found in bone, muscle, tendon, cartilage, brain, or cornea

Lymphedema
Occurs when lymphatics are obstructed, too few in number, or nonfunctional
Leads to woody edema secondary to fibrous tissue in subcutaneous tissue – toes, feet, ankle, leg
Cellulitis and lymphangitis secondary to minor trauma – big problem
Strep most common infection
Deep lymphatics have valves.
Congenital lymphedema L > R
Tx: leg elevation, compression, antibiotics for infection

Lymphangiosarcoma
Raised blue/red coloring; early metastases to lung
Stewart-Treves syndrome – associated with breast axillary dissection

Lymphangiectasia – dilation of preexisting lymphatic channels
Dx: lymphangiography
Tx: resection

Lymphocele following surgery
Usually after dissection in the groin (i.e., for femoral to popliteal bypass)
Leakage clear fluid; need to rule out an infectious source for the fluid (send complications, get CT scan of area)
Small lymphoceles can be observed (may resorb spontaneously).
Large or symptomatic or lying close to graft material – need early excision
Tx: inject **isosulfan blue dye** into foot to identify the lymphatic channels supplying the lymphocele
Resect the lymphocele and ligate the supplying lymphatic channel

CHAPTER 28. GASTROINTESTINAL HORMONES

Gastrin – produced G cells in **antrum**
    Secretion stimulated by amino acids, vagal input (acetylcholine), calcium, ETOH, antral distention, pH > 3.0
    Secretion inhibited by pH <3.0, somatostatin, secretin, CCK, vasoactive intestinal peptide, gastric inhibitory peptide
    Target cells – parietal cells and chief cells
    Response – ↑ HCl, intrinsic factor, and pepsinogen secretion
    Omeprazole blocks H/K ATPase of parietal cell **(final pathway for H^+ release)**.

Somatostatin – produced by D (somatostatin) cells in **antrum**
    Secretion stimulated by acid in duodenum
    Target cells – many; is the great inhibitor
    Response – inhibits gastrin and HCl release; inhibits release of insulin, glucagons, secretin, GIP, motilin, neurotensin, enteroglucagon; ↓ pancreatic and biliary output
    Octreotide (somatostatin analogue) – can be used to ↓ pancreatic fistula output

Gastric inhibitory peptide – produced by K cells in **duodenum**
    Secretion stimulated by amino acids, glucose, long-chain fatty acids, ↓ pH
    Target cells – parietal cells of stomach and beta cells of pancreas
    Response – ↓ HCl secretion and pepsin; ↑ insulin release

CCK – produced by I cells of **duodenum** and jejunum
    Secretion stimulated by amino acids and fatty acid chains
    Response – gallbladder contraction, relaxation of sphincter of Oddi, ↑ pancreatic enzyme secretion, some ↑ in intestinal motility

Secretin – produced by S cells of **duodenum**
    Secretion stimulated by fat, bile, pH <4.0
    Secretion inhibited by pH >4.0, gastrin
    Response – ↑ pancreatic HCO_3^- release, ↑ bile flow, inhibits gastrin release (this is reversed in patients with gastrinoma), and inhibits HCl release
        <u>High</u> pancreatic duct output – ↑ HCO_3^-, ↓ Cl^-
        <u>Slow</u> pancreatic duct output – ↑ Cl^-, ↓ HCO_3^- (carbonic anhydrase in duct exchanges HCO_3^- for Cl^-)

Vasoactive intestinal peptide – produced by cells in **gut and pancreas**
    Secretion stimulated by fat, acetylcholine
    Response – ↑ intestinal secretion (water and electrolytes) and motility
    Inhibits gastrin release

Insulin – released by beta cells of the **pancreas**
    Secretion stimulated by glucose, glucagons, CCK
    Secretion inhibited by somatostatin, pancreatostatin
    Response – cellular glucose uptake; promotes protein synthesis

Glucagon – released by alpha cells of the **pancreas** (also from alpha cells in stomach, intestine)
    Secretion stimulated by ↓ glucose, ↑ amino acids, acetylcholine, gastrin-releasing peptide
    Secretion inhibited by ↑ glucose, ↑ insulin, somatostatin
    Response – glygogenolysis, gluconeogenesis, lipolysis, ketogenesis, ↓ gastric acid secretion, ↓ pancreatic secretion, ↓ intestinal motility, ↓ stomach motility, ↑ LES pressure, ↓ MMCs

Pancreatic polypeptide – secreted by islet cells in **pancreas**
    Secretion stimuated by food, vagal stimulation, other GI hormones
    Response – ↓ pancreatic and gallbladder secretion

Motilin – release by intestinal cells of gut
    Secretion stimulated by duodenal acid, food, vagus input, gastrin-releasing peptide
    Secretion inhibited by somatostatin, secretin, pancreatic polypeptide, duodenal fat
    Response – ↑ intestinal (small bowel) motility → **erythromycin** acts on this receptor

Bombesin (gastrin-releasing peptide) – ↑ intestinal motor activity, ↑ pancreatic enzyme secretion, ↑ gastric acid secretion

Peptide YY – released from terminal ileum following a fatty meal → inhibits acid secretion and stomach contraction; inhibits gallbladder contraction and pancreatic secretion

Anorexia – mediated by hypothalamus

Bowel recovery
    Small bowel 24 hours
    Stomach 48 hours
    Large bowel 3–5 days

CHAPTER 29. ESOPHAGUS

Anatomy and physiology

Squamous epithelium, circular inner muscle layer, outer longitudinal muscle layer; no serosa
Vessels directly off the aorta are the major blood supply to the esophagus.

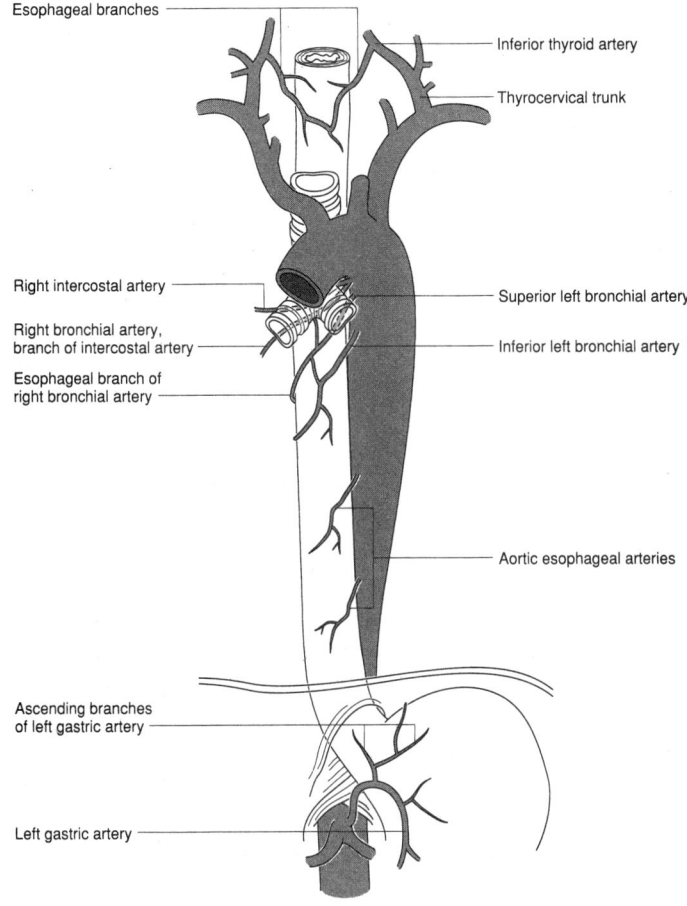

Arterial blood supply of the esophagus.

Cervical esophagus – supplied by the inferior thyroid artery
Abdominal esophagus – supplied by the left gastric artery and inferior phrenic arteries
Lymphatics – upper ⅔ drains cephalad, lower ⅓ caudad
Upper esophagus – **striated muscle**
Lower esophagus – **smooth muscle**
Right vagus nerve – travels on posterior portion of stomach as it exits chest; becomes **celiac plexus**; also has the criminal nerve of Grassi → can cause persistently high acid levels postoperatively if left undivided
Left vagus nerve – travels on anterior portion of stomach; goes to **liver and biliary tree**
Thoracic duct – travels from right to left in chest at upper ⅓ of mediastinum; inserts into left subclavian vein

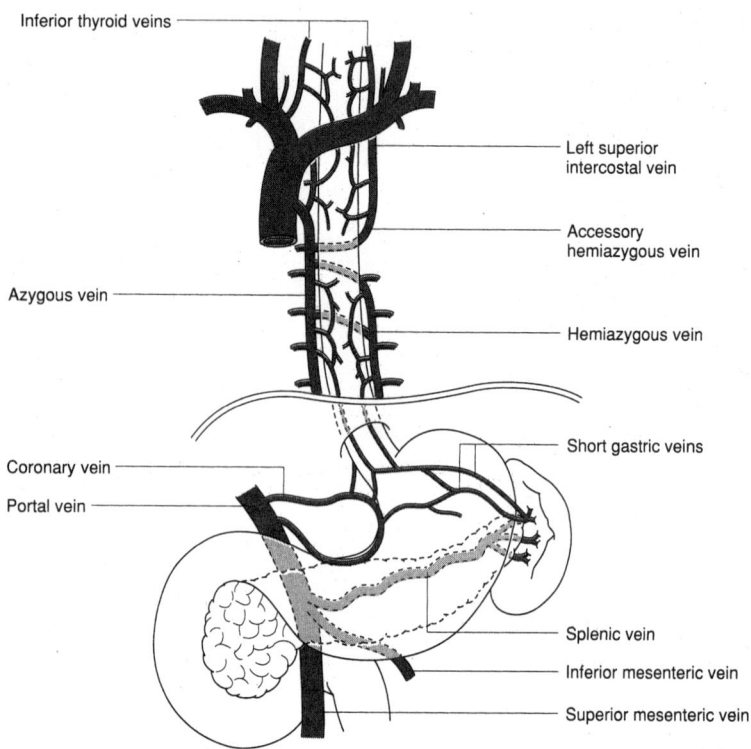

Venous drainage of the esophagus.

Upper esophageal sphincter (15 cm from incisors) – cricopharyngeus muscle (circular muscle, prevents air swallowing); has recurrent laryngeal nerve innervation
Normal UES pressure with food bolus – 12–14 mmHg
Normal UES pressure at rest – 50–70 mmHg
    Cricopharyngeus muscle – most common site of esophageal perforation (usually occurs with EGD)
    Aspiration with brainstem stroke – failure of UES (cricopharyngeus) to relax
Lower esophageal sphincter (40 cm from incisors) – relaxation mediated by inhibitory neurons; muscle is normally contracted at resting state → prevents reflux
Normal LES pressure at rest 10–20 mmHg

Anatomical areas of narrowing
    Cricopharyngeus muscle
    Compression by the left mainstem bronchus and aortic arch
    Diaphragm

Swallowing stages – CNS initiates swallow
    Normal esophageal pressures with food bolus – 70–120 mmHg
    Primary peristasis – occurs with food bolus and swallow initiation
    Secondary peristalsis – occurs with incomplete emptying and esophageal distention, propogating waves
    Tertiary peristalsis – nonpropogating, nonperistalsing (dysfunctional)
    UES and LES are normally contracted between meals.

Swallowing mechanism – soft palate occludes nasopharynx, larynx rises and airway opening is blocked by epiglottis, cricopharyngeus relaxes, pharyngeal contraction moves food into esophagus. **LES relaxes** soon after initiation of swallow.

Chapter 29. Esophagus

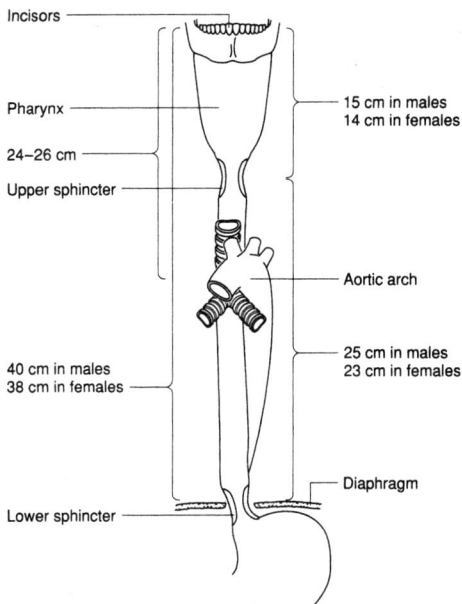

Important clinical endoscopic measurements of the esophagus in adults.

Surgical approach
Cervical esophagus – **left**
Upper thoracic – **right (avoids the aorta)**
Lower thoracic – **left (left-sided course in this region)**

Hiccoughs
Causes – gastric distention, temperature changes, ETOH, tobacco
Reflex arc – vagus, phrenic, sympathetic chain T6–12

Esophageal dysfunction
<u>Primary</u> – unknown cause
<u>Secondary</u> – systemic disease, GERD (most common), scleroderma, polymyositis

Endoscopy – procedure of choice for **heartburn** → can visualize esophagitis, etc
Barium swallow – **procedure of choice for** dysphagia and odynophagia **(better at picking up masses)**
Meat impaction – Dx and Tx: endoscopy

Pharyngoesophageal disorders
Trouble in transferring food from mouth to esophagus
Most commonly neuromuscular disease – myasthenia gravis, Parkinson's disease, polymyositis, muscular dystrophy, Zenker's diverticulum, lye ingestion, stroke
Liquids worse than solids
Cervical esophageal dysphagia – Plummer-Vinson syndrome; usually due to web; Fe-deficient anemia. Tx: **dilation, Fe**

Diverticula
Zenker's diverticulum – caused by ↑ pressure during swallowing
Is a **false diverticulum – posterior**
Symptoms: upper esophageal dysphagia, choking, halitosis
Dx: **barium swallow studies**, manometry; risk for perforation with EGD and Zenker's

Tx: **cricopharyngeal myotomy** (key point); Zenker's itself can either be resected or suspended (removal of diverticula not necessary)
Left cervical incision; leave drains in; esophagogram POD #1

Traction diverticulum
Is a **true diverticula** – usually lies **lateral**
Due to inflammation, granulomatous disease, tumor
Usually found in the mid-esophagus
Symptoms: regurgitation of undigested food, dysphagia
Tx: excision and primary closure, may need palliative therapy (i.e., XRT) if due to invasive CA

Epiphrenic diverticulum
Rare; associated with esophageal motility disorders
Most common in the distal 10 cm of the esophagus
Most are asymptomatic; can have dysphagia and regurgitation
Dx: esophagram and esophageal manometry
Tx: diverticulectomy and long esophageal myotomy on the side opposite the diverticulectomy

Achalasia
Dysphagia, regurgitation, weight loss, respiratory symptoms
Caused by **failure of peristalsis and lack of LES relaxation** after food bolus
Secondary to **neuronal degeneration** in muscle wall
Manometry – ↑ **LES pressure, incomplete LES relaxation, no peristalsis**
Can get tortuous dilated esophagus and epiphrenic diverticula; birdbeak appearance
Tx: calcium channel blocker, LES dilation → effective in 60%; nitrates
  If medical Tx and dilation fail → Heller myotomy – left thoracotomy, transect circular layer of muscle lower esophagus; also need partial Nissen fundoplication
T. cruzi can produce similar symptoms.

Diffuse esophageal spasm
Chest pain; other symptoms can be similar to achalasia. May have psychiatric history
Manometry – frequent strong body contractions of ↑ amplitude and duration, **normal LES tone, strong unorganized contractions**
Surgery better at resolving dysphagia than pain
Nutcracker esophagus has similar symptoms.
Tx: calcium channel blocker, nitrates, antispasmodics, Heller myotomy (transect circular layer of upper and lower esophagus)
Treatment usually less effective for diffuse esophageal spasm than for achalasia

Scleroderma
Causes dysphagia, loss of LES tone; most have strictures, fibrous replacement of smooth muscle
Tx: esophagectomy; Nissen may be effective in some

Gastroesophageal reflux disease (GERD)
Normal anatomic protection from GERD – need LES competence, normal esophageal body, normal gastric reservoir
↑ acid exposure to esophagus from loss of the normal gastroesophageal barrier
Get heartburn symptoms 30–60 minutes after meals
Can also have asthma symptoms (cough), choking, PNA
Symptoms worse lying down
Need to make sure patient does not have another cause for the pain.
  Dysphagia/odynophagia – need to worry about tumors
  Bloating – suggests aerophagia and delayed gastric emptying
  Epigastric pain – suggests peptic ulcer, tumor
Dx: endoscopy, pH probe (best test), manometry (resting LES <6 mmHg), histology
Medical therapy 1st: omeprazole for 12 weeks
Surgical indications: GERD on pH monitoring, failure of medical Tx, complications of GERD (stricture, esophagitis, Barrett's esophagus, cancer)

Chapter 29. Esophagus

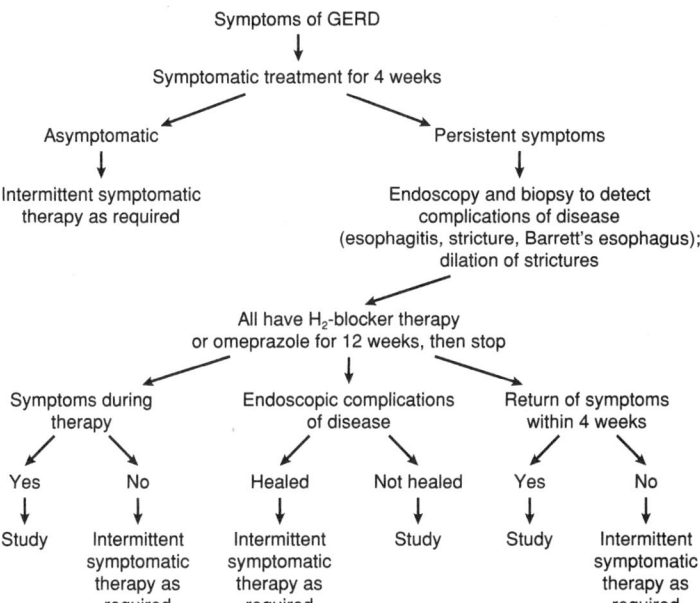

Algorithm for selecting patients with symptoms suggestive of GERD for further study.

Tx: **Nissen** → divide short gastrics, pull esophagus into abdomen, repair defect in phrenoesophageal membrane; 270- (partial) or 360-degree gastric fundus wrap
Phrenoesophageal membrane is an extension of the transversalis fascia.
Key maneuver is identification of the **left crura**.
Complications – injury to spleen, diaphragm, esophagus, or pneumothorax
Belsey – approach is through the chest
Collis gastroplasty – when not enough esophagus exists to pull down into abdomen, can staple along stomach and create a "new" esophagus
Most common cause of dysphagia following Nissen – **wrap is too tight**

Hiatal hernia (also see GERD, above)
Type I – sliding hernia from dilation of hiatus (most common); often associated with GERD
Type II – paraesophageal; hole in the diaphragm alongside the esophagus, normal GE junction. Symptoms: chest pain, dysphagia, early satiety
Type III – combined
Type IV – entire stomach in the chest plus another organ (i.e., colon, spleen)
With type II, still need **Nissen** as diaphragm repair can affect LES; also helps anchor stomach
Paraesophageal hernia (type II) – all need repair → high risk of incarceration
Most patients with type I hiatal hernia <u>do not</u> have reflux.
Most patients with significant reflux <u>do</u> have type I hiatal hernia.

Schatzki's ring
Almost all patients have an associated sliding hiatal hernia
Symptoms: short episodes of dysphagia following rapid swallowing
Tx: dilatation of the ring usually sufficient; may need antireflux procedure

Barrett's esophagus
Squamous metaplasia to columnar epithelium
Occurs with longstanding exposure to gastric reflux

Cancer (adenocarcinoma) risk ↑ 50 times.
Severe Barrett's dysplasia is an indication for esophagectomy.
Uncomplicated Barrett's can be treated like GERD (i.e., Nissen) – surgery will ↓ esophagitis and further metaplasia but will not prevent malignancy or cause regression of the columnar lining
Need careful follow-up with EGD for lifetime, even after Nissen

Esophageal cancer
Esophageal tumors are almost always malignant, early invasion of nodes.
Spreads quickly along **submucosal lymphatic channels**
Symptoms: difficulty swallowing solids, dysphagia, weight loss
Risk factors: achalasia, caustic injury, ETOH, tobacco, nitrosamines
Dx: esophagram diagnostic procedure of choice in patients with dysphagia, odynophagia, or suspected mass lesions
Unresectability – hoarseness (RLN), Horner's syndrome, phrenic nerve involvement, malignant pleural effusion, malignant fistula, airway invasion, vertebral invasion
   Chest/abdominal CT best test for unresectability
Adenocarcinoma #1 esophageal cancer – not squamous
   Adenocarcinoma – most often occurs in lower ⅓ of esophagus
   Squamous cell carcinoma – most often occurs in upper ⅔ of esophagus
Supraclavicular nodes – M1 disease; unresectable
Distant metastases – most go to lung or liver; contraindication to esophagectomy
   Survival <12 months
Nodal disease outside the area of resection (i.e., SMA or celiac nodes) – contraindication to esophagectomy
Preoperative XRT and chemotherapy may down-stage tumors and make them resectable.
Esophagectomy – 5% mortality from surgery; curative in 20%
   Right gastroepiploic artery – primary blood supply to stomach after replacing esophagus (have to divide left gastric and short gastrics)
   Transhiatal approach – abdominal and neck incisions; bluntly dissect intrathoracic esophagus; may have ↓ mortality from esophageal leaks with cervical anastamosis
   Ivor Lewis – abdominal incision and right thoracotomy → exposes all of the esophagus; intrathoracic anastomosis
   3-hole esophagectomy – abdominal, thoracic, and cervical incisions
   Need **pyloromyotomy** with these procedures
   Colonic interposition – may be choice in young patients with benign disease when you want to preserve gastric function; 3 anastamoses required; blood supply depends on marginal vessels
   After esophagectomy → need contrast study on postop day 7 to rule out leak
   Postoperative stricture – most can be dilated
   Palliative esophagectomy may be indicated in some circumstances.
Chemotherapy – 5FU and cisplatin (for node-positive disease or use preop to shrink tumors)
XRT – has been shown to be effective as both preop and postop treatment
Malignant fistulas – most die within 3 months due to aspiration

Leiomyoma
Most common benign tumor of the esophagus; submucosal
Dx: esophagram, endoscopy needed to rule out cancer
Symptoms: dysphagia, pain usually in lower ⅔ of esophagus
Do not biopsy → can form scar and make subsequent resection difficult
Tx: **>5 cm or symptomatic** → excision (enucleation) via thoracotomy

Esophageal polyps
Symptoms: dysphagia, hematemesis
2nd most common benign tumor of the esophagus; usually in the cervical esophagus
Small lesions can be resected with endoscopy; larger lesions require cervical incision.

Caustic esophageal injury
No NG tube. Do **not** induce vomiting. Nothing to drink.
Alkali – causes deep liquefaction necrosis, especially liquid (e.g., Drano)
   Worse injury than acid; also more likely to cause cancer

Acid – causes coagulation necrosis; mostly causes gastric injury
Endoscopy – usually used 1st to diagnose the injury
  Do not use with suspected perforation and do not go past site of injury.
Gastrografin and then barium swallow – used 1st if perforation suspected

Degree of injury
  Primary burn – hyperemia
    Tx: observation and conservative therapy
      Conservative Tx: IVFs, spitting, antibiotics, oral intake after 3–4 days; may need future serial dilation for strictures (usually cervical and near aortic indentation)
      Can also get shortening of esophagus, requiring antireflux procedure
  Secondary burn – ulcerations, exudates, and sloughing
    Tx: prolonged observation; surgery with specifc indications
      Relative indications for surgery – sepsis, peritonitis, persistent back and chest pain, metabolic acidosis, mediastinitis, free air, mediastinal air, crepitance, contrast extravasation, pneumothorax, effusion, air in stomach wall
  Tertiary burn – deep ulcers, charring, and lumen narrowing
    Tx: esophagectomy usually necessary
    Alimentary tract not restored until after patient recovers from the caustic injury

Perforations
  Usually the result of EGD
  Cervical esophagus near **cricopharyngeus muscle** most common site
  Symptoms: pain, dysphagia, respiratory distress, fever, tachycardia
  Dx: gastrograffin swallow followed by barium swallow

  Criteria for nonsurgical management – contained perforation by contrast, self-draining, no systemic effects
    Conservative Tx: IVFs, NPO, spit (some say you can place NGT), broad-spectrum antibiotics
    No NG tube with caustic injuries (see above)

  If free perforation has occurred and quick to diagnose it (<24 hours) or if the area has minimal contamination → try **primary repair** with drains and intercostal muscle pedicle flap if in chest
  For sick patients → cervical esophagostomy for diversion and later placement of a feeding G or J tube
  Esophagectomy – may eventually be needed in patients with <u>intrinsic disease</u>

  If in neck, leave drains; if in chest, leave chest tubes
  Need longitudinal myotomy to see the full extent of injury
  Consider **intercostal muscle flaps** to area of perforation to help the area heal

  Proximal ⅔ of thoracic esophagus – right thoracotomy (may have right effusion)
  Distal ⅓ of thoracic esophagus – left thoracotomy (may have left effusion)

  Use gastrograffin followed by barium swallow 10 days after repair to **rule out leak.**
  Leave drains in until patient taking good oral intake without increase in drainage from drains.
  If patient has a leak without systemic effects, try to let it heal → give patient TPN or place distal feeding tube

  Boerhaave's syndrome
    Forceful vomiting followed by chest pain – perforation most likely to occur in left lateral wall of esophagus at level of T8, 3–5 cm above GE junction
    Hartmann's sign – mediastinal crunching on auscultation
    Early diagnosis and treatment improve survival.
    Dx: gastrograffin swallow
    Tx: left thoracotomy, longitudinal myotomy to see extent of injury, primary repair; leave chest tubes

CHAPTER 30. STOMACH

Anatomy and physiology
   Stomach transit time 3–4 hours
   Peristalsis – occurs only in distal stomach
   Gastroduodenal pain sensed through afferent sympathetic fibers T5–10
   Blood supply
      Celiac trunk – left gastric, common hepatic artery, splenic artery
         Left gastroepiploic and short gastric are branches of splenic artery.
      Greater curvature – right and left gastroepiploics, short gastrics
      Lesser curvature – right and left gastrics
         Right gastric is a branch of the common hepatic artery.
      Pylorus – gastroduodenal artery
   Mucosa – lined with simple columnar epithelium

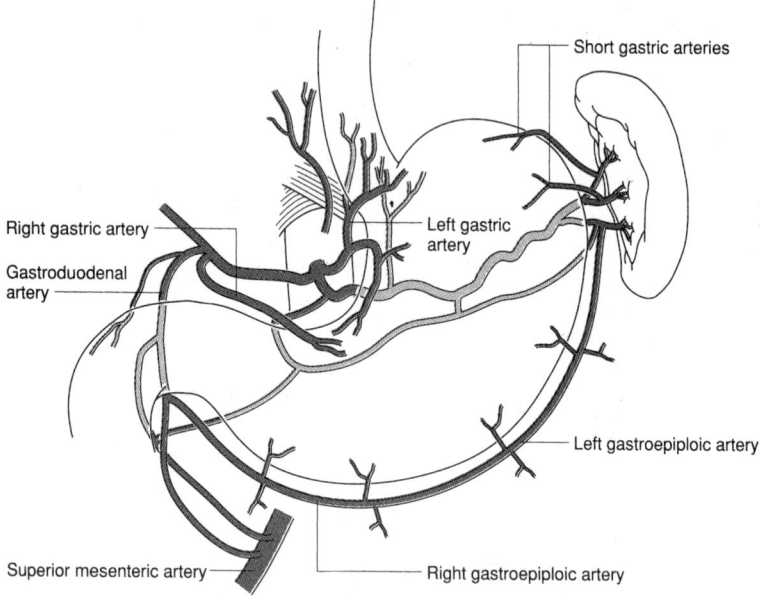

Arterial blood supply of the stomach.

Cardia glands – mucus secreting

Fundus and body (oxynitic) glands
   Chief cells – pepsinogen (1st enzyme in proteolysis)
   Parietal cells – release H^+ and intrinsic factor
      Acetylcholine, gastrin, and histamine cause HCl release.
         Acetylcholine (vagus) and gastrin act on <u>phopholipase</u> → PIP → DAG + IP_3 to ↑ Ca; activates **phophorylase kinase** → ↑ HCl production
         Histamine acts on <u>adenylate cylase</u> → cAMP → **protein kinase A** to ↑ HCl
         Phosphorylase kinase and protien kinase C phosphorylate <u>H/K ATPase</u> to ↑ acid production
            Omeprazole blocks H/K ATPase in parietal cell membrane **(final pathway for H^+ release)**
      Inhibitors of parietal cells – somatostatin, PGE_1, secretin, CCK
      Intrinsic factor – binds B_{12} and the complex is reabsorbed in the terminal ileum

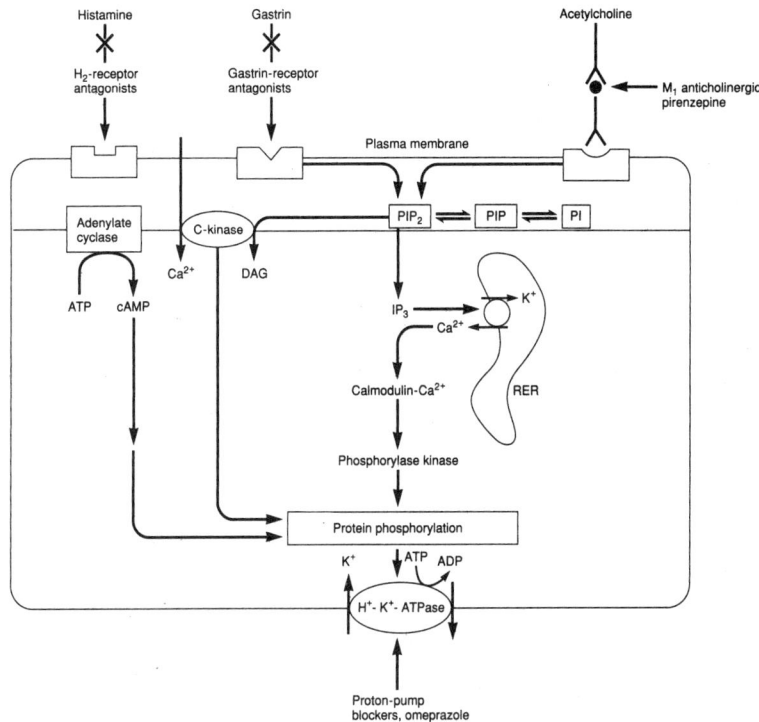

Cellular mechanisms controlling parietal cell acid secretion.

Antrum and pylorus glands
  Mucus and HCO_3^- secreting glands – protect stomach
  G cells release **gastrin** – why antrectomy helpful
    Inhibited by H^+ in duodenum
    Stimulated by amino acids, acetylcholine
  D cells – secrete **somatostatin**; inhibit gastrin and acid release
Brunner's glands – in duodenum; secrete pepsinogen and alkaline mucus
Somatostatin, CCK, and secretin – released with antral and duodenal acidification

↑ **acid and ↑ gastrin** – ZES, antral cell hyperplasia, retained antrum, renal failure, gastric outlet obstruction, short bowel syndrome
↑ **gastrin and normal/↓ acid** – pernicious anemia, chronic gastritis, gastric CA, postvagotomy, medical acid suppression
Rapid gastric emptying – previous surgery (#1), ZES, ulcers
Delayed gastric emptying – opiates, anticholinergics, myxedema, hyperglycemia, diabetes

Billroth I – antrectomy with gastroduodenal anastamosis
Billroth II – antrectomy with gastrojejunal anastamosis

Trichobezoars (hair) – hard to pull out
  Tx: EGD generally inadequate; likely need gastrostomy and removal
Phytobezoars (fiber) – often in diabetics with poor gastric emptying
  Tx: enzymes, EGD, diet changes

↑ **marginal ulceration and diarrhea** with Billroth I and II vs Roux-en-Y gastrojejunostomy
Dieulafoy's ulcer – vascular malformation
Menetrier's disease – mucous cell hyperplasia, ↑ rugal folds

Gastric volvulus
Associated with type II (paraesophageal) hernia
Nausea without vomiting; severe pain; usually organoaxial volvulus
Tx: reduction and Nissen

Mallory-Weiss tear
Secondary to forceful vomiting
Presents as hematemesis following severe retching
Bleeding often stops spontaneously.
Dx/Tx: EGD; tear is usually near lesser curvature of the stomach (near GE junction)
If continued bleeding, may need gastrostomy and oversewing of the vessel

Vagotomies
Vagal denervation – all forms ↑ liquid emptying → **vagally mediated receptive relaxation is removed**
    Results in ↑ gastric pressure that accelerates liquid emptying
Truncal vagotomy – divides vagal trunks at level of esophagus
Selective vagotomy – divides nerves of Latarjet
Highly selective (proximal) vagotomy – divides individual fibers, preserves "crow's foot"
    Complete vagotomy (truncal or selective) – ↓ emptying of solids
    Highly selective vagotomy – normal emptying of solids
    Addition of **pyloroplasty** to either of the above results in ↑ solid emptying.
Other physiologic alterations caused by truncal vagotomy
    Gastric effects – ↓ acid output by 90%, ↑ gastrin, gastrin cell hyperplasia
    Nongastric effects – ↓ exocrine pancreas function, ↓ postprandial bile flow, ↑ gallbladder volumes, ↓ release of vagally mediated hormones
    Diarrhea (30%–50%) – most common problem following vagotomy
        Caused by sustained MMCs forcing bile acids into the colon

Upper gastrointestinal bleeding
Risk factors: previous UGI bleed, peptic ulcer disease, NSAID use, smoking, liver disease, esophageal varicies, splenic vein thrombosis, sepsis, burn injuries, trauma, severe vomiting

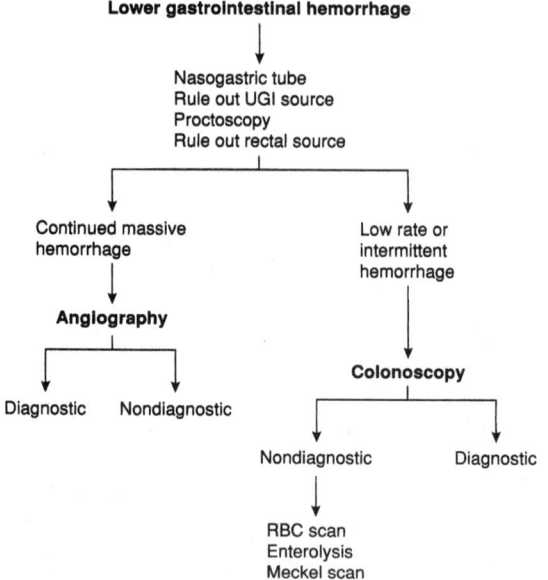

Diagnostic steps in the evaluation of acute upper GI hemorrhage.

1st **NGT and EGD to confirm bleeding is from ulcer**; can potentially treat the ulcer with EGD
　　EGD for bleeding duodenal ulcer – does not change mortality or operative rates; most
　　　　important predictor of continued or recurrent bleeding is bleeding at time of EGD
　　　　If patient hypotensive despite resuscitation and thought to be bleeding from ulcer
　　　　　　→ **go to OR**
　　　　Having trouble localizing bleeding source → **tagged RBC scan**
　　　　Biggest risk factor for rebleeding at time of EGD – #1 spurting blood vessel
　　　　　　(60% chance of rebleed), #2 visible blood vessel (40% chance of rebleed),
　　　　　　#3 diffuse oozing (30% chance of rebleed)
　　　　Patient with liver failure is likely bleeding from esophageal varices, <u>not</u> an ulcer.
　　　　　　Tx: EGD with sclerotherapy or TIPS, not OR

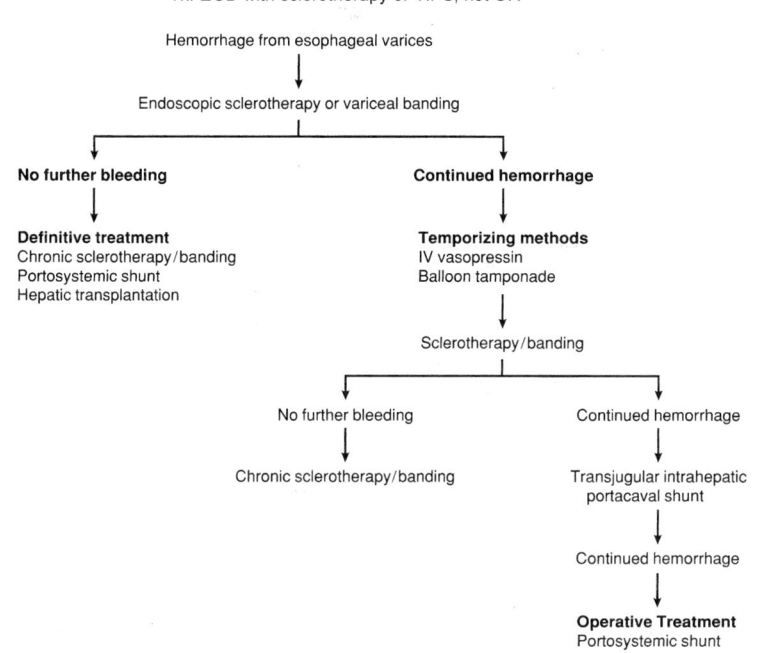

Therapeutic maneuvers in the management of acute hemorrhage from esophageal varices.

Duodenal ulcers
　　↑ acid production and ↓ defense
　　Most frequent peptic ulcer; more common in men
　　Usually in 1st part of the duodenum; **usually anterior**
　　　　Anterior ulcers perforate
　　　　Posterior ulcers <u>bleed from gastroduodenal artery</u>
　　Symptoms: epigastric pain radiating to the back; abates with eating but recurs 30 minutes after
　　Dx: endoscopy
　　Tx: H_2 blockers (cimetidine, ranitidine), H-pump inhibitor (omeprazole), triple therapy for
　　　　patients with *H. pylori* on biopsy → bismuth salts, amoxicillin, metronidazole/tetracycline
　　　　(BAM or BAT)
　　Surgery for ulcer rarely indicated since **introduction of proton pump inhibitors**
　　Surgical indications
　　　　Perforation
　　　　Protracted bleeding despite EGD therapy
　　　　Obstruction
　　　　Intractabilty despite medical therapy
　　　　Inability to rule out cancer (ulcer remains despite treatment) → requires resection of
　　　　　　ulcer

If patient has been on **proton pump inhibitor therapy, acid-reducing surgical procedure is required in addition to surgery for the complication**.
Need to rule out gastrinoma in patients with complicated ulcer disease
Surgical options
- Truncal vagotomy and pyloroplasty
- Truncal vagotomy and antrectomy with Billroth I or Billroth II – best surgery for prevention of recurrence
- Proximal or highly selective vagotomy – lowest rate of postoperative complications, 10% recurrence, no need for antral or pylorus procedure

Bleeding
Most frequent complication of duodenal ulcers
Usually minor but can be life-threatening
Major bleeding – >6 units of blood in 24 hours or patient remains hypotensive despite transfusion
Tx: EGD 1st – sclerose, cauterize; vasopressin, omeprazole
Surgical options
- 1st duodenostomy and **gastroduodenal artery (GDA) ligation**
- Avoid hitting common bile duct with GDA ligation
- If patient has been on H-pump inhibitor therapy, need surgical ulcer procedure as well → **truncal vagotomy and pyloroplasty probably best option** (does not get rid of ulcer)
- Can consider **highly selective vagotomy** as an alternative

Obstruction
Serial dilation initial treatment of choice
Surgical options
- If near ampulla of Vater or if removing ulcer would be very difficult → **gastrojejunostomy (Billroth II, bypasses obstruction), antrectomy, and truncal vagotomy** → probably best option for most patients
- If proximal to ampulla of Vater→ **antrectomy (with ulcer excision) with Billroth II and truncal vagotomy**

Perforation
80% will have free air.
Patients usually have sudden sharp epigastric pain; can have generalized peritonitis
Pain can radiate to the pericolic gutters with dependent drainage of gastric content.
Elderly – some believe that elderly, high-risk patients can be safely observed
- Need to get UGI to make sure that the perforation has sealed

Surgical options
- **Graham patch and highly selective vagotomy** – probably best option for most if patient has been on H-pump inhibitor; otherwise just do Graham patch and place on omeprazole
- Truncal vagotomy and pyloroplasty – need to include ulcer in pyloroplasty
- Truncal vagotomy and antrectomy with Billroth I or II – need to include ulcer

Intractability
>3 months without relief while on H-pump inhibitor therapy or recurrence <1 year after medical therapy
Based in EGD mucosal findings, not symptoms
Surgical options
- **Highly selective vagotomy (does not get rid of ulcer)** – probably best option for most patients
- Truncal vagotomy and pyloroplasty (does not get rid of ulcer)
- Truncal vagotomy and antrectomy with Billroth I or Billroth II

Zollinger-Ellison syndrome
Pancreatic tumors <2 cm can be enucleated.
Secretin test results in high gastrin level.
Can often be multiple and metastatic
Blind pancreatic resections are generally not indicated.
When the tumor is not resectable, **total gastrectomy** best for long-term quality of life
Resection and ablation of metastases are important for **palliation** and decreased need for drug treatment.

Chapter 30. Stomach 147

Gastric ulcers
Older men; slow healing
Risk factors: male, tobacco, ETOH, NSAIDs, *H. pylori*, uremia, stress (burns, sepsis and trauma) steroids, chemotherapy
Most (type I and type IV) have normal acid secretion, due to abnormal mucosal defense
70%–80% on lesser curvature of the stomach
Hemorrhage is associated with higher mortality than duodenal ulcers
Symptoms: epigastric pain radiating to the back; relieved with eating but recurs 30 minutes later; melena or guaiac-positive stools
CLO test – test for *H. pylori* → detects urease released from *H. pylori*
Biopsy for *H. pylori* needs to be from the **antrum**.

Type A blood – associated with type I ulcers
Type O blood – associated with type II–IV ulcers

Surgical indications
  Perforation
  Bleeding
  Obstruction
  Cannot exclude malignancy
  Intractability – >3 months without relief or 2nd recurrence (based on mucosal findings)

Type I – lesser curve along body of stomach; due to ↓ mucosal protection
  Tx: distal gastrectomy including ulcer with Billroth I or Billroth II +/– vagotomy probably best option
    Alternative → ulcer excision +/– highly selective vagotomy or truncal vagotomy and pyloroplasty
Type II – 2 ulcers (lesser curve and duodenal); similar to duodenal ulcer with high acid secretion
  Tx: Distal gastrectomy with Billroth I or Billroth II and truncal vagotomy probably best option
    Alternative → truncal vagotomy and pyloroplasty (does not get rid of ulcers)
Type III – prepyloric ulcer; similar to duodenal ulcer with high acid secretion; ↑ bleeding
  Tx: distal gastrectomy with Billroth I or Billroth II and truncal vagotomy probably best option
    Alternative → truncal vagotomy and pyloroplasty (does not get rid of ulcer)
Type IV – lesser curve high along cardia of stomach; ↑ risk of bleeding due to ↓ mucosal protection
  Tx: **ulcer excision** +/– highly selective vagotomy or truncal vagotomy and pyloroplasty
Type V – ulcer associated with NSAIDs

Stress gastritis
Occurs 3–10 days after event
Lesions appear in fundus 1st
Tx: proton pump inhibitor
Selective angiography with vasopressin injection may help with bleeding.
EGD with cautery of specific bleeding point may be effective.

Chronic gastritis
Type A (fundus) – associated with pernicious anemia, autoimmune disease
Type B (antral) – associated with *H. pylori*

Gastric cancer
Pain unrelieved by eating, weight loss
Antrum has 40% of gastric cancers.
50% of cancer-related deaths in Japan
Dx: EGD
Risk factors – adenomatous polyps, tobacco, previous gastric operations, intestinal metaplasia, atrophic gastritis, pernicious anemia, type A blood, nitrosamines
Adenomatous polyps – 10%–20% risk of cancer. Tx: endoscopic resection
Krukenberg tumor – metastases to ovaries
Virchow's nodes – metastases to supraclavicular node

Intestinal gastric cancer – ↑ in high-risk populations, older men; rare in US
  Associated with chronic atrophy, dyplasia; has blood invasion; glands on histology
  Stage I disease – 85% cure rate; overall 5-year survival rate 10%
  Surgical Tx: Try to perform subtotal gastrectomy (need 5-cm margins)

Diffuse gastric cancer (linitis plastica) – in low-risk populations, women
  Lymphatic invasion; <u>no</u> glands
  Less favorable prognosis than intestinal gastric cancer
    Stage II disease – <50% 5-year survival rate
  Surgical Tx: patients require total gastrectomy because of diffuse nature of linitis plastica
  Chemotherapy (poor response to chemo): 5FU, doxurubicin, mitomycin C

Metastatic disease outside the area of resection – contraindication to resection unless performing surgery for palliation

Palliation of gastric cancer
  Obstruction – proximal lesions can be stented; distal lesion bypasses with gastrojejunostomy
  Low to moderate bleeding or pain – XRT
  If these fail, consider palliative gastrectomy for obstruction or bleeding

Gastric leiomyomas (also called GIST tumors)
Most common benign gastric neoplasm
Symptoms: usually asymptomatic but obstruction and bleeding can occur
Hypoechoic on ultrasound; smooth edges
Dx: biopsy
Tx: resection
Consider chemotherapy if >5 cm or >5–10 mitoses/HPF
Need 1-cm margins
Most are **C-KIT**–positive
Chemotherapy → Gleevec (tyrosine kinase inhibitor)

Gastric leiomyosarcomas
Need en bloc resection
Cancer diagnosis based on mitoses/HPF (>5–10 associated with ↑ risk of metastases)
Hematogenous spread

Gastric lymphomas
Have ulcer symptoms; organ most commonly involved in extranodal lymphoma
Usually non-Hodgkin's lymphoma
Dx: EGD
Chemotherapy and XRT are primary treatment modalities; surgery for complications
Surgery possibly indicated only for stage I disease (tumor confined to stomach mucosa) and then only partial resection is indicated.
Overall 5-year survival rate >50%

Mucosa-associated lymphoproliferative tissue (MALT)
Related to *H. pylori* infection; considered a precursor for **gastric lymphoma**
Should regress after treatment for *H. pylori*
Usually in GI tract; can also occur in lung and Waldeyer's ring
Tx: triple-therapy antibiotics for *H. pylori* and surveillance; if MALT does not regress, need chemotherapy (CHOP)

Morbid obesity
Central obesity – worse prognosis
Surgical eligibility: BMI >40 or BMI >35 with comorbidities
NIDDM, HTN, and sleep apnea often resolve after surgery.
Operative mortality is approximately 1%.

Roux-en-Y gastric bypass
  Better weight loss than just stapling
  Risk of marginal ulcers, leak, necrosis, B_{12} deficiency (intrinsic factor need acidic environment to bind B_{12}), iron-deficiency anemia (bypasses duodenum, where Fe absorbed), gallstones (from rapid weight loss)
  Perform **cholecystectomy** during operation if stones present.
  UGI on postop day 2
  10%–15% failure rate due to high carbohydrate snacking
  Ischemia – most common cause of leak
    Signs of leak – ↑ RR, ↑ HR, pain, fever, elevated WBCs
  Marginal ulcers – develop in 10%. Tx: omeprazole
  Stenosis – usually responds to serial dilation
  Signs of obstruction following surgery – hiccoughs, large stomach bubble

Jejunoileal bypass
  These operations are no longer done.
  Associated with ↑ liver cirrhosis and kidney (stones) problems, osteoporosis (↓ Ca)
  Need to correct these patients and perform Roux-en-Y gastric bypass if ileojejunal bypasses are encountered

Postgastrectomy complications
Dumping syndrome
  Can occur after gastrectomy or after vagotomy and pyloroplasty
  Occurs from rapid entering of carbohydrates into the small bowel
  90% of cases resolve with medical therapy.
  2 phases
    1. Hyperosmotic load causes fluid shift into bowel (diarrhea, dizziness, hypotension)
    2. Reactive ↑ in insulin and ↓ in glucose (2nd phase rarely occurs)
  Can almost always be treated with medical and conservative (dietary changes) therapy
  Tx: small, low-fat, low-carbohydrate, increased-protein meals; no liquids with meals, no lying down after meals
  Octreotide may be effective.
  Surgical options (rarely needed)
    Conversion of Billroth I or Billroth II to Roux-en-Y gastrojejunostomy
    Operations to ↑ gastric reservoir (jejunal pouch) or ↑ emptying time (reversed jejunal loop)

Alkaline reflux gastritis
  Postprandial epigastric pain associated with N/V; pain not relieved with vomiting
  Dx: evidence of bile reflux into stomach, histologic evidence of gastritis
  Tx: H_2 blockers, cholestyramine, metoclopramide
  Surgical option: conversion of Billroth I or Billroth II to Roux-en-Y gastrojejunostomy with afferent limb 60 cm distal to original gastrojejunostomy

Roux stasis
  Stasis of chyme in Roux limb due to loss of jejunal motility
  Dx: EGD, emptying studies
  Tx: metoclopramide, prokinetics
  Surgical option: shorten Roux limb to 40 cm

Chronic gastric atony
  Delayed gastric emptying after vagotomy
  Symptoms: nausea, vomiting, pain, early satiety
  Dx: EGD, gastric emptying study
  Tx: metoclopramide, prokinetics
  Surgical option: near-total gastrectomy with Roux-en-Y

Small gastric remnant (early satiety)
  Actually want this for gastric bypass patients
  Dx: EGD
  Tx: small meals
  Surgical option: jejunal pouch construction

Blind-loop syndrome
With Billroth II or Roux-en-Y
Symptoms: pain, diarrhea, malabsorption, B_{12} deficiency (bacteria use it up), steatorrhea (bacterial deconjugation of bile)
Caused by bacterial (*E. coli*, GNRs) overgrowth and stasis in afferent limb
Tx: tetracycline, Flagyl, metoclopramide
Surgical option: reanastomosis with shorter (40-cm) afferent limb

Afferent-loop obstruction
With Billroth II or Roux-en-Y
Nonbilious vomiting, pain relieved with bilious emesis
Symptoms: RUQ pain, steatorrhea
Caused by obstruction of afferent limb
Risk factors – long afferent limb with Billroth II or Roux-en-Y
Dx: EGD
Tx: balloon dilation may be possible
Surgical option: reanastomosis with shorter (40-cm) afferent limb

Efferent-loop obstruction
Symptoms of obstruction
Dx: UGI, EGD
Tx: balloon dilation
Surgical option: find site of obstruction and relieve it

Postvagotomy diarrhea
Secondary to nonconjugated bile salts in the colon
Caused by sustained postprandial organized MMCs
Tx: cholestyramine, octreotide
Surgical option: reversed interposition jejunal graft

PEG complications – insertion into the liver or colon

CHAPTER 31. LIVER

Anatomy and physiology
Hepatic artery variants
Right hepatic artery off superior mesenteric artery (#1 hepatic artery variant; 20%) courses behind pancreas, posterolateral to the common bile duct
Left hepatic artery off left gastric artery (about 20%) – found in gastrohepatic ligament medially
Common hepatic artery – most common variant is off SMA (2%)
Falciform ligament – separates medial and lateral segments of the left lobe; attaches liver to anterior abdominal wall; extends to umbilicus and carries remnant of the umbilical vein
Ligamentum teres – carries the obliterated umbilical vein to the undersurface of the liver; extends from the falciform ligament
Line drawn from the middle of the **gallbladder fossa to IVC (portal fissure or Cantalies line)** separates the right and left lobes

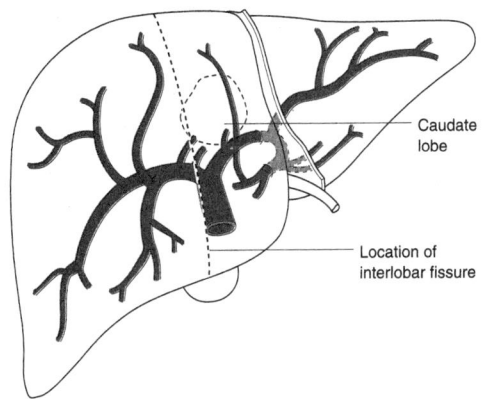

Intrahepatic divisions of the portal vein.

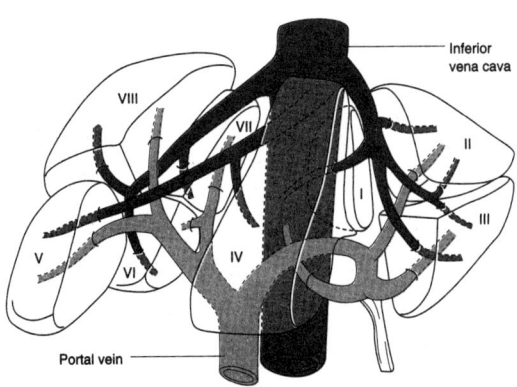

Segments
    I – caudate
    II – superior left lateral segment
    III – inferior left lateral segment
    IV – left medial segment (quadrate lobe)
    V – inferior right anteromedial segment
    VI – inferior right posterolateral segment
    VII – superior right posterolateral segment
    VIII – superior right anteromedial segment

Glisson's capsule – peritoneum that covers the liver
Bare area – area on the posterior-superior surface of liver not covered by Glisson's capsule
Triangular ligaments – lateral and medial extensions of the coronary ligament on the posterior surface of the liver; made up of peritoneum
Portal triad enters segments IV and V.
Gallbladder lies under segments IV and V.

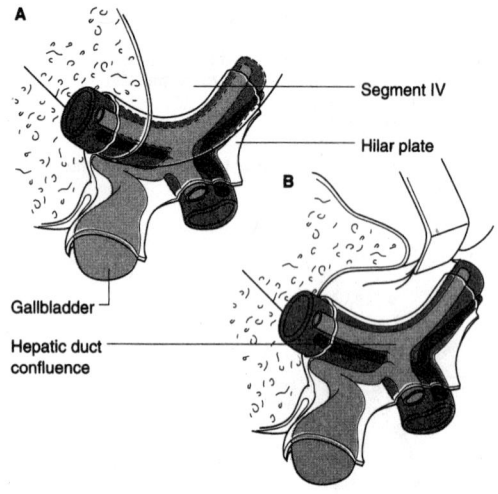

Lowering of the hilar plate. (*A*) The inferior border of segment IV (quadrate lobe) overlies the hepatic duct confluence. (*B*) Division of the connective issue investment allows elevation of segment IV, resulting in a "lower" hilar plate and surgical exposure to the hepatic duct confluence.

Kupffer cells – liver macrophages
Hepatoduodenal ligament – where bile duct, portal vein, and heptic artery meet (portal triad)
Portal triad – **portal vein** posteriorly, **common bile duct** laterally, **hepatic artery** medially
Pringle manuever – porta hepatis clamping; will not stop hepatic vein bleeding

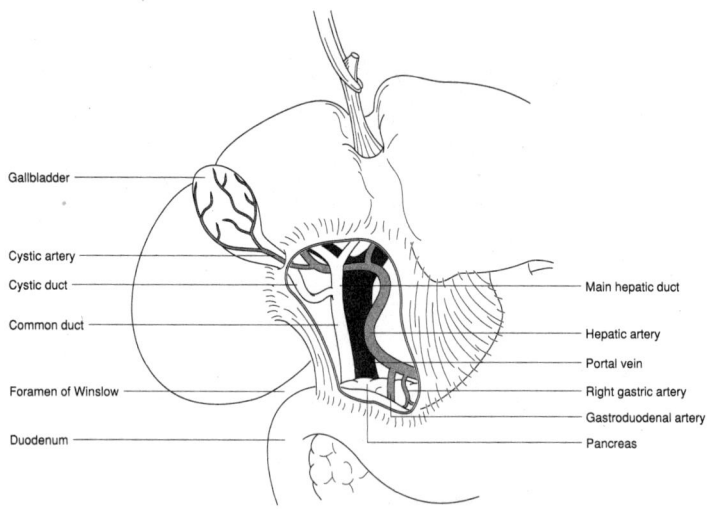

Anatomic relations of structures within the hepatoduodenal ligament.

Portal vein
  Forms from superior mesenteric vein joining splenic vein (no valves)
  Inferior mesenteric vein – enters splenic vein
  Portal veins – 2 in liver; ⅔ of hepatic blood flow
    Left – II, III, and IV
    Right – V, VI, VII, and VIII
Arterial blood supply
  Right, left and middle hepatic arteries (follows hepatic vein system)
  Most primary and secondary tumors of the liver are supplied by the <u>hepatic artery</u>.
Hepatic veins
  3 hepatic veins
    Left – II, III, and superior IV
    Middle – V and inferior IV
    Right – VI, VII, and VIII
  Middle hepatic vein joins left hepatic vein in 80% before going into IVC; other 20% go directly into IVC.
Accessory right hepatic veins – drain medial aspect of right lobe directly into the IVC
Inferior phrenic veins – also drain directly into the IVC
Caudate lobe – receives separate right and left portal and arterial blood flow; drains directly into IVC via separate hepatic veins

Alkaline phosphatase – normally located in canalicular membrane
Nutrient uptake – occurs in sinusoidal membrane
Ketones – usual energy source for liver; glucose converted to glycogen and stored
  Excess glucose converted to fat
Urea – synthesized in the liver
Not made in the liver – von Willebrand factor and factor VIII (endothelium)
Liver stores large amount of **fat-soluble vitamins.**
B_{12} – the only water-soluble vitamin stored in the liver

Bleeding and bile leak – most common problems with hepatic resection
Hepatocytes most sensitive to ischemia – central lobular (acinar zone III)
75% of normal liver can be safely resected.

<u>Bilirubin</u>
  Breakdown product of hemoglobin (Hgb → heme → biliverdin → bilirubin)
  Conjugated to **glucoronic acid (glucoronyl transferase)** in the liver → improves water solubility
  Conjugated bilirubin actively secreted into bile
  Urobilinogen
    Breakdown of bilirubin by bacteria in the terminal ileum
    Is reabsorbed in the blood, and released in the urine
    Excess urobilinogen turns urine dark like cola.

<u>Bile</u>
  Contains bile salts (85%), proteins, phospholipids (lecithin), cholesterol, and bilirubin
  Final bile composition determined by active (Na/K ATPase) reabsorption of water in gallbladder
  Cholesterol – used to make bile acids
  Bile acids conjugated to **taurine or glycine (improves water solubility)**
    <u>Primary bile acids</u> – **cholic and chenodeoxycholic**
    <u>Secondary bile acids</u> – **deoxycholic and lithocolic** (dehydoxylated primary bile acids by bacteria in gut)
  Lecithin – main biliary phospholipid; solubilizes cholesterol and emulsifies fats in the intestine

<u>Jaundice</u>
  Occurs when bilirubin >2.5; <u>1st evident under the tongue</u>
  Maximum bilirubin is 30 unless patient had underlying renal disease, hemolysis, or bile duct–hepatic vein fistula.
  Unconjugated bilirubin – prehepatic causes (hemolysis); hepatic deficiencies of uptake or conjugation
  Conjugated bilirubin – secretion defects into bile ducts; excretion defects into GI tract (stones, strictures, tumor)

Syndromes
Gilbert's disease – abnormal uptake; mildly high unconjugated bilirubin
Crigler-Najjar disease – inability to conjugate; deficiency of glucoronyl transferase; high unconjugated bilirubin → life-threatening disease
Physiologic jaundice of newborn – immature glucoronyl transferase; high unconjugated bilirubin
Rotor's syndrome – deficiency in storage ability; high conjugated bilirubin
Dubin-Johnson syndrome – deficiency in secretion ability; high conjugated bilirubin

Viral hepatitis
All hepatitis viral agents can cause acute hepatitis and fulminant hepatic failure.
Hepatitis B, C, and D can cause chronic hepatitis and hepatoma.

Hepatitis A (RNA) – serious consequences uncommon
Hepatitis B (DNA)
  Infection IgM antibody dominates 1st 6 months.
    Anti-HBc rises 10–12 weeks after infection.
    Anti-Hbe rises 12–14 weeks after infection.
    Anti-HBs rises 14–16 weeks after infection.
  Anti-HBc-IgM (c = core) is elevated in the first 6 months; IgG then takes over.
  Vaccination – have ↑ anti-HBs (s = surface) antibodies only
  ↑ anti-HBc and ↑ anti-HBs antibodies and no HBs antigens (HbsAg) → patient had infection with recovery and subsequent immunity
Hepatitis C (RNA) – can have long incubation period; currently most common viral hepatitis leading to liver TXP
Hepatitis D (RNA) – cofactor for hepatitis B
Hepatitis E (RNA) – fulminant hepatic failure in pregnancy, most often in 3rd trimester

Liver failure
Most common cause of liver failure – cirrhosis
Best indicator of synthetic function in patient with cirrhosis – **prothrombin time (PT)**
Acute fulminant hepatic failure – 80% mortality
  Outcome determined by the course of encephalopathy
Hepatic encephalopathy
  Liver failure leads to inability metabolize – buildup of ammonia, mercatanes, methane thiols, and false neurotransmitters
  Causes other than liver failure for encephalopathy – GI bleeding, infection (spontaneous bacterial peritonitis), electrolyte imbalances, drugs
  May need to embolize previous therapeutic shunts or embolize other major collaterals
  Tx: **lactulose** – cathartic that gets rid of bacteria in the gut and acidifies colon (preventing NH_3 uptake by converting it to ammonium), titrate to 2–3 stools/day
    Limit protein intake (<70 g/day)
      Branched chain amino acids – metabolized by skeletal muscle, may be of some value
    No antibiotics unless for a specific infection
    Neomycin may help.
Cirrhosis mechanism – hepatocyte destruction → fibrosis and scarring of liver → ↑ hepatic pressure → portal venous congestion → lymphatic overload → leakage of splanchnic and hepatic lymph into peritoneum → ascites
Paracentesis for ascites – replace with albumin (1 g for every 100 cc removed)
Ascites – from **hepatic/splanchnic** lymph
  Tx: ↓ NaCl, diuretics, (spironolactone counteracts hyperaldosteronism often seen with liver failure), paracentesis, TIPS, peritoneovenous shunts (Denver, LeVeen shunt → complications include DIC)
↑ aldosterone – secondary to impaired hepatic metabolism and impaired GFR
Hepatorenal syndrome – same appearance as prerenal azotemia
  Tx: stop diuretics, give volume
Neurological changes – asterixis; sign that liver failure is progressing
Peritoneovenous shunts (Denver, LeVeen) – shunt ascites into venous system; can get DIC complications
Postpartum liver failure with ascites – hepatic vein thrombosis
  Dx: SMA arteriogram with venous phase contrast

Spontaneous bacterial peritonitis (SBP)
Fever, abdominal pain, PMNs >250 in fluid, positive cultures
E. coli (#1), pneumococci, streptococci (see Chap. 5, Infection)
Most commonly mono-organism; if not, need to worry about bowel perforation
Risk factors – prior SBP, variceal hemorrhage, low-protein ascites, nephrotic syndrome, SLE in children
Tx: 3rd generation cephalosporins; patients usually respond within 48 hours

Esophageal varices
Bleed by rupture; sclerotherapy 90% effective at treating
Tx: vasopressin (splanchnic artery constriction), octreotide (↓ portal pressure by ↓ blood flow)
Patients with history of CAD should receive NTG while on vasopressin.
Sengstaken-Blakemore (S-B) tube – used to control variceal bleeding, risk of rupture of the esophagus (hardly used anymore)
Propranolol – may help prevent rebleeding; no good role acutely
Can get later strictures from sclerotherapy; usually easily managed with dilatation
TIPS needed for refractory varical bleeding
Bleeding varices have 33% mortality with 1st episode.
50% will rebleed; 50% mortality with each subsequent bleeding episode

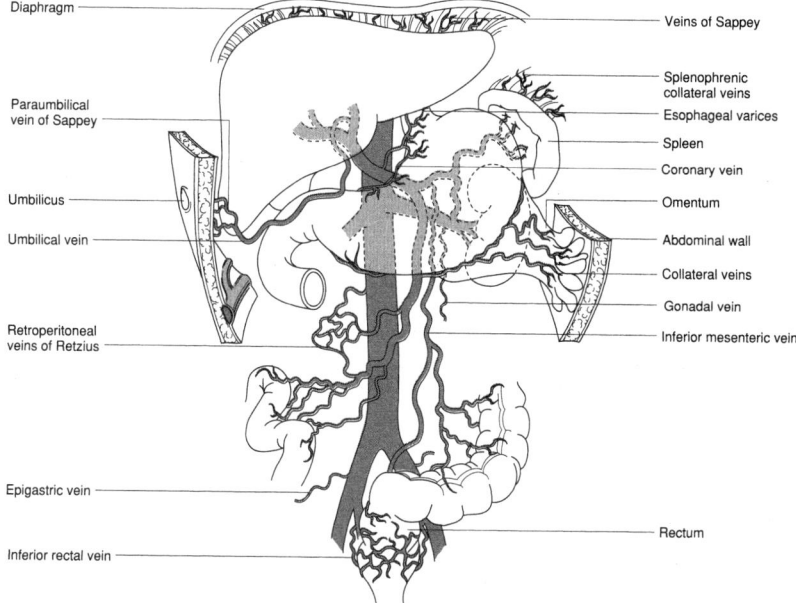

Potential venous collaterals that develop with portal hypertension. The veins of Sappey drain portal blood through the bare areas of the diaphragm and through paraumbilical vein collaterals to the umbilicus. The veins of Retzius form in the retroperitoneum and shunt portal blood from the bowel and other organs to the vena cava.

Portal hypertension
Presinusoidal obstruction – schistosomiasis, congenital hepatic fibrosis, portal vein thrombosis (50% of portal HTN in children)
Sinusoidal obstruction – cirrhosis
Postsinusoidal obstruction – Budd-Chiari syndrome (hepatic vein occlusive disease), constrictive pericarditis, CHF
Normal portal vein pressure <12 mmHg

Coronary veins act as collaterals between the portal vein and the systemic venous system of the lower esophagus.

Portal HTN leads to esophageal variceal hemorrhage, ascites, splenomegaly, and hepatic encephalopathy.

Shunts can decompress portal system.

TIPS – used for protracted bleeding, progression of coagulopathy, visceral hypoperfusion, refractory ascites
Allows antegrade flow
Risk – development of encephalopathy

Splenorenal shunt – low rate of encephalopathy; need to ligate left adrenal vein, left gonadal vein, inferior mesenteric vein, coronary vein, and pancreatic branches of splenic vein
Used only for Child's A cirrhotics who present just with bleeding (rarely used anymore)
Contraindicated in patients with refractory ascites, as splenorenal shunts can worsen ascites

Child's B or C with indication for shunt → **TIPS**
Child's A that just has bleeding as symptom → **consider splenorenal shunt (more durable; otherwise TIPS**

Child's class correlates with mortality after shunt.

	A (2% mortality)	B (10% mortality)	C (50% mortality)
Albumin	>3.5	3–3.5	<3.5
Bilirubin	<2.5	2.5–4	>4
Encephalopathy	None	Minimal	Severe
Ascites	None	Treatable	Refractory
Nutrition	Good	Fair	Poor

(Modified from Wantz, Payne MA. Experience with portacaval shunt for portal hypertension. N Engl J Med 1961;265:721)

Portal HTN in children
Usually caused by **extrahepatic thrombosis of the portal vein**
Most common cause of massive hematemesis in children

Budd-Chiari syndrome
Occlusion of hepatic veins and IVC
RUQ pain, hepatosplenomegaly, ascites, fulminant hepatic failure, muscle wasting, variceal bleeding
Dx: angio, CT scan; liver biopsy shows sinusoidal dilatation, congestion, centrilobular congestion
Tx: portacaval shunt (needs to connect to the IVC above the obstruction)

Splenic vein thrombosis
Can lead to isolated gastric varicies without elevation of pressure in the rest of the portal system
These gastric varices can bleed.
Splenic vein thrombosis is most often caused by pancreatitis.
Tx: splenectomy

Abscesses
Amebic
↑ LFTs; ↑ in **right lobe** of liver, usually single
Primary infection occurs in the colon → amebic colitis
Risk factors – travel to Mexico, ETOH; fecal-oral transmission
Postive serology for *Entamoeba histolytica* – 90% have infection
Symptoms: fever, chills, RUQ pain, ↑ WBCs, jaundice, hepatomegaly
Reaches liver via **portal vein**
Cultures of abscess often sterile → protozoa exist only in peripheral rim
Most do not require aspiration (anchovy paste)
Can usually diagnose based on CT characteristics
Tx: Flagyl; aspiration if refractory or contaminated; surgery only for free rupture

Chapter 31. Liver

Echinococcus
- Forms cyst (hydatid cyst)
- Positive **Casoni skin test**, positive **indirect hemagglutination**
- **Sheep** – carriers; **dogs** – human exposure. ↑ in **right lobe** of the liver
- Do not aspirate → can leak out and cause anaphylactic shock
- Abdominal CT shows ectocyst (calcified) and endocyst.
- Preop ERCP for jaundice, ↑ LFTs, or cholangitis to check for communication with the biliary system
- Tx: preop albendazole, surgical removal (may want to inject cyst with alcohol at time of removal to kill organisms); need to get all of cyst wall

Schistosomiasis
- Maculopapular rash, ↑ eosinophils
- Sigmoid colon – fine granulation tissue, petechiae, ulcers
- Can cause variceal bleeding
- Tx: praziquantel and control of variceal bleeding

Pyogenic abscess
- Account for 80% of all abscesses
- Symptoms: fever, chills, weight loss, RUQ pain, ↑ LFTs, ↑ WBCs, sepsis
- ↑ in right lobe; 15% mortality with sepsis
- GNRs – #1 organism (*E. coli*)
- Commonly secondary to contiguous infection from biliary tract
- Can occur following **bacteremia** from other types of infection (diverticulitis, appendicitis)
- Dx: aspiration
- Tx: CT-guided drainage and antibiotics; surgical drainage for unstable condition and continued signs of sepsis
- May need surgery for biliary obstruction or multiple abscesses

Benign liver tumors
Hepatic adenomas
- Women, steroid use, OCPs, type I collagen storage diseases
- 80% are symptomatic; 10%–20% risk of significant bleeding (rupture)
- Can become malignant
- More common in **right lobe**
- Symptoms: pain, ↑ LFTs, ↓ BP, (from rupture), palpable mass
- Dx: no Kupffer cells in adenomas, thus **no uptake on sulfur colloid scan (cold)**
  - MRI demonstrates a hypervascular tumor.
  - Has peripheral blood supply
- Tx
  - Asymptomatic – stop OCPs; if regression, no further therapy is needed; if no regression, patient needs resection of the tumor
  - Symptomatic – tumor resection for bleeding and malignancy risk; embolization if multiple and unresectable

Focal nodular hyperplasia
- Has central stellate scar that may look like cancer
- No malignancy risk; very unlikely to rupture
- Dx: abdominal CT; has Kupffer cells, so **will take up sulfur colloid on liver scan**
- MRI/CT scan demonstrates a hypervascular tumor.
- Tx: conservative therapy

Hemangiomas
- Most common benign hepatic tumor
- Rupture rare; most asymptomatic; more common in women
- Avoid biopsy → risk of hemorrhage
- Dx: MRI and CT scan show **peripheral to central enhancement**
  - Appears as a **hypervascular** lesion on CT scan/MRI
- Tx: conservative unless symptomatic, then **surgery +/– embolization**;
  - XRT and steroids for unresectable disease
  - **Rare complications of hemangioma** – consumptive coagulopathy (Kasabach-Merritt syndrome) and CHF
  - These complications are usually seen in children.

Solitary cysts
- Congenital; women, right lobe
- Resection needed if bleeding or infected (and cannot be treated percutaneously)
- Complications from these cysts are rare; most can be left alone.
- Walls have a characteristic blue hue.

Malignant liver tumors
Metastases:primary ratio = 20:1
Hepatocellular CA
Most common cancer worldwide
Risk factors – HBV (#1 cause worldwide), HCV, ETOH, hemachromatosis, alpha-1-antitrypsin deficiency, primary sclerosing cholangitis, alfatoxins, hepatic adenoma, steroids, pesticides

Not risk factors – primary biliary cirrhosis, Wilson's disease

Clear cell, lymphocyte infiltrative, and fibrolamellar types (adolescents and young adults) have the best prognosis.

AFP level correlates with tumor size.

30% 5-year survival rate with resection

Few hepatic tumors are resectable secondary to cirrhosis, portahepatic involvement, or metastases.

Need 1-cm margin

Tumor recurrence most likely in the liver after resection

Hepatic sarcoma
Risk factors – PVC, Thorotrast, arsenic → rapidly fatal

Cholangiosarcoma
Risk factors – clonorchiasis infection, ulcerative colitis, hemachromatosis, primary sclerosing cholangitis, choledochal cysts

Intrahepatic associated with worse survival than extrahepatic

Tumor size and satellite nodules correlate with outcome.

Colon CA metastases – can resect if you leave enough liver for the patient to survive
20% 5-year survival rate

Metastatic and primary tumors of the liver are supplied by the **hepatic arteries**.

Primary liver tumors – hypervascular

Metastatic liver tumors – hypovascular

CHAPTER 32. BILIARY SYSTEM

Anatomy and physiology
Gallbladder lies between **segments IV and V**.
Cystic artery branches off right hepatic artery.
  Is found in the triangle of Calot (cystic duct [lateral], common bile duct [medial], liver [superior])
Right hepatic (lateral) and retroduodenal branches of the gastroduodenal artery (medial) supply to the hepatic and common bile duct (9- and 3-o'clock positions when performing ERCP); considered longitudinal blood supply
Cystic veins drain into the right branch of the portal vein and into the liver.
Lymphatics are on the right side of the common bile duct.
Parasympathetic fibers from left (anterior) trunk of the vagus
Sympathetic fibers from T7–T10 coarsing through the splanchnic and celiac ganglions

Gallbladder has **no submucosa**; mucosa is columnar epithelium
Common bile duct and heptic duct **do not have peristalsis**.
Gallbladder normally fills by **contraction of sphincter of Oddi at the ampulla of Vater**
  Morphine – contracts the sphincter of Oddi
  Glucagon – relaxes the sphincter of Oddi

Normal sizes: CBD <8 mm, (<10 mm after cholecystectomy), gallbladder wall <4 mm, pancreatic duct <4 mm
After cholecystectomy, total bile acid pools ↓.
Highest concentration of CCK and secretin cells in the **duodenum**

Rokitansky-Aschoff sinuses – invagination of the epithelium of the wall of the gallbladder; formed from ↑ gallbladder pressure
Ducts of Luschka – biliary ducts that go directly from the liver into the gallbladder; can leak after a cholecystectomy

Bile excretion regulation
  ↑ **bile excretion** – CCK, secretin, and vagal input
  ↓ **bile excretion** – VIP, somatostatin, sympathetic stimulation
  Gallbladder contraction – CCK causes constant, steady tonic contraction

Essential functions of bile
  Fat-soluble vitamin absorption
  Bilirubin excretion
  Cholesterol excretion

Gallbladder – forms concentrated bile by **active resorption of Na and water**

	Na (mEq/L)	Cl (mEg/L)	Bile Salts (mEq/L)	Cholesterol (mEq/dL)
Hepatic bile	140–170	50–120	1–50	50–150
Gallbladder bile	225–350	1–10	250–350	300–700

Bile salt pool (5–7 g) cycles 4–8 times/day
Small amount (5%–10%) of bile salts lost in stool
  Active resorption of conjugated bile acids occurs in the **terminal ileum (50%)**.
  Passive resorption of nonconjugated bile acids can occur in the small intestine (45%) and colon (5%).
Postprandial emptying maximum at 2 hours (80%)
Bile secreted by **bile canalicular cells** (20%) and **hepatocytes** (80%).

Color of bile is mostly due to **conjugated bilirubin**.
  Stercobilin – breakdown product of conjugated bilirubin in gut; gives stool brown color
  Urobilin – breakdown product of conjugated bilirubin in gut; yellow; some gets reabsorbed and released in urine

Cholesterol and bile acid synthesis
HMG CoA → (**HMG CoA reductase**) → cholesterol → (**7-alpha-hydroxylase**) → bile acids
HMG CoA reductase – rate-limiting step in cholesterol synthesis
Stones in obese people – **overactive HMG CoA reductase**
Stones in thin people – **underactive 7-alpha-hydroxylase**

Gallstones
Occur in 10% of the population; most asymptomatic
Only 10% of gallstones are radiopaque

Nonpigmented stones
↑ **cholesterol insolubilization** – caused by stasis, calcium nucleation by mucin glycoproteins, and ↑ water reabsorption from gallbladder
Also caused by ↓ **lecithin and bile acids**
Found almost exclusively in the gallbladder
Most common type of stone found in US (75%)

Pigmented stones – most common worldwide; 25% of stones in US
Caused by solubilization of unconjugated bilirubin with precipitation of **calcium bilirubinate** and insoluble salts
Dissolution agents do not work on pigmented stones (mono-octanoin).

Black stones
Can be caused by **hemolytic disorders or cirrhosis**
Can also occur in patients on **chronic TPN** and in patients with **ileal resection**
Important factors for the development of these stones – ↑ bilirubin load, ↓ hepatic function, and bile stasis
Almost always form in gallbladder
Tx: cholecystectomy

Brown stones (primary CBD stones, formed in ducts)
Infection causing deconjugation of bilirubin
Increased in Asians
E. coli most common – produces beta-glucuronidase, which deconjugates bilirubin, causes formation of **calcium bilirubinate**.
Need to check for ampullary stenosis, duodenal diverticuli, abnormal sphincter of Oddi
Most commonly form in the bile duct (are primary common bile duct stones)
Almost all patients with primary stones need a biliary drainage procedure – sphincteroplasty 90% successful

Cholesterol stones and black stones found in the CBD are considered **secondary common bile duct stones**.

Cholecystitis
Caused by obstruction of the cystic duct by a gallstone
Results in gallbladder wall distention and wall inflammation
Symptoms: RUQ pain, referred pain to the right shoulder and scapula, nausea and vomiting, loss of appetite
  Attacks frequently occur after a fatty meal, and pain is persistent (unlike biliary colic).
Murphy's sign – patient resists deep inspiration with deep palpation to the RUQ secondary to pain
Alkaline phosphatase and WBC are frequently elevated.

Suppurative cholecystits associated with frank purulence in the gallbladder → can be associated with sepsis and shock
Most common organisms in cholecystitis – *E. coli, klebsiella, enterococcus*

Stone risk factors – age >40, female, obesity, pregnancy, rapid weight loss, vagotomy, TPN (pigmented stones), ileal resection (pigmented stones)

Ultrasound – 95% sensitive for picking up stones → hyperechoic focus, posterior shadowing, movement of focus with changes in position

Best initial evaluation test for jaundice or RUQ pain
Findings of suggestive of acute cholecystitis – gallstones, gallbladder wall thickening (>4 mm), pericholecystic fluid
Dilated CBD (>8 mm) suggests CBD stone and obstruction.

HIDA scan – technetium taken up by liver and excreted in the biliary tract
If gallbladder cannot be seen, it is secondary to cystic duct obstruction by stone → needs cholecystectomy
If **<25% of gallbladder volume excreted after CCK over 2 hours** → biliary dyskinesia; although not totally occluded, the excretion is reduced
50% of these patients benefit from cholecystectomy.

Indications for preop ERCP (signs that a common bile duct stone is present) – jaundice, cholangitis, gallstone pancreatitis, ↑ bilirubin (can also be due to primary liver disease), significantly ↑ AST/ALT (can also be due to primary liver disease), stone in CBD on ultrasound
<5% of patients undergoing cholecystectomy will have a retained CBD stone → 95% of these cleared with ERCP

Tx for cholecystitis – cholecystectomy; cholecystostomy tube can be placed in patients who are very ill and cannot tolerate surgery
When patient is subsequently able to tolerate surgery, cholecystectomy performed.

ERCP – best treatment for late common bile duct stone
Sphincterotomy allows for removal of stone.
Grasper and other tools can then be used to remove the stone.
Risks: bleeding, pancreatitis, perforation
Biliary colic – transient cystic duct obstruction caused by passage of a gallstone
Resolves within 4–6 hours
Air in the biliary system most commonly occurs with previous ERCP and sphincterotomy
Can also occur with cholangitis or erosion of the biliary system into the duodenum (i.e., gallstone ileus)
Bacterial infection of bile – dissemination from **portal system** is usual route
Can also get retrograde infection from bacteria in duodenum
Highest incidence of positive bile cultures occurs with **postoperative strictures** (usually *E. coli*, often polymicrobial).

Acalculous cholecystitis
Thickened wall, RUQ pain, ↑ WBCs
Occurs most commonly after severe burns, prolonged TPN, trauma, or major surgery
Primary pathology is **bile stasis** (narcotics, fasting), leading to distention and ischemia.
Also have ↑ **viscosity secondary to dehydration, ileus, transfusions**
Ultrasound shows sludge, gallbladder wall thickening, and pericholecystic fluid.
HIDA scan is positive.
Tx: cholecystectomy; percutaneous drainage if patient too unstable

Emphysematous gallbladder disease
Gas in the gallbladder wall
Can see on plain film
↑ in diabetics; usually secondary to ***Clostridium perfringens***
Symptoms: severe, rapid-onset abdominal pain, nausea, vomiting, and sepsis
Perforation more common in these patients
Tx: emergent cholecystectomy; percutaneous drainage if patient is too unstable

Gallstone ileus
Fistula between gallbladder and duodenum that releases stone, causing small bowel obstruction; elderly
Can see **pneumobilia** (air in the biliary system) on plain film
Terminal ileum – most common site of obstruction
Tx: remove stone with enterotomy proximal to obstruction; perform cholecystectomy and fistula resection if patient can tolerate it.

Common bile duct injuries
Most commonly occur after laparoscopic cholecystectomy
Intraoperative cholangiography does not prevent injuries; may limit severity; ↑ early diagnosis of injury
In 10% of patients, the **right posterior duct** (from segments 6 or 7) **enters the common bile duct separately**.
Risk of injury with cholecystectomy (confused for cystic duct)
If >2 mm, will need to open and perform hepaticojejunostomy

Intraoperative CBD injury – if less than 50% the circumference of the common bile duct, can probably perform primary repair; in all other cases, will likely need hepaticojejunostomy or choledochojejunostomy

Persistent nausea and vomiting or jaundice following laparoscopic cholecystectomy
Ultrasound to look for fluid collection
If fluid collection present, may be bile leak → percutaneous drain into the collection
If fluid is bilious, get ERCP → sphincterotomy and stent if due to cystic duct remnant leak, small injuries to the hepatic or common bile duct, or a leak from duct of Luschka
Larger lesions (i.e., complete duct transection) will require hepaticojejunostomy or choledochojejunostomy

Anastomotic leaks following transplantation or hepaticojejunostomy → usually handled with ERCP and stents

Sepsis following laparoscopic cholecystectomy → fluid resuscitation and stabilize patient
May be due to complete transection of the CBD and cholangitis→ get ultrasound to look for dilated intrahepatic ducts or fluid collections
If no fluid collections but bile ducts are dilated → get ERCP and try to stent the strictured area
If that fails, place a PTC tube.

Common bile duct or hepatic duct strictures
Most commonly occur after laparoscopic cholecystectomy
Ischemia – most important cause of late postoperative biliary strictures
Can also be caused by chronic pancreatitis or stricture of a biliary enteric anastomosis
Dx: ERCP
Symptoms: sepsis, cholangitis, jaundice
Tx: **ERCP with sphincterotomy** and possible stent placement to decompress; **PTC tube if that fails**
For lesions that cause early symptoms (≤7 days) – **hepaticojejunostomy**
For lesions that cause later symptoms (>7 days) – **hepaticojejunostomy** 6–8 weeks after injury
Acute injuries are unlikely to be treated sufficiently with ERCP, stent, and balloon.
Late injuries (years later) – can often be treated with ERCP, sphincterotomy, and stent.

Hemobilia
Fistula between bile duct and hepatic arterial system (most commonly)
Patients classically present with UGI bleed, jaundice, and RUQ pain.
Most commonly occurs with **trauma** (50% of all cases), infections, primary gallstones, aneurysms, and tumors
Dx: angiogram
Tx: resuscitation; angiogram and embolization 1st; operation if that fails

Gallbladder adenocarcinoma
Rare; most common cancer of the biliary tract
Four times more common than bile duct CA; most have stones
Liver – most common site of metastasis
Porcelain gallbladder – risk of gallbladder CA (10%–20%) → these patients need cholecystectomy
1st spreads to **segments IV and V**; 1st nodes are the cystic duct nodes (right side)
Symptoms: jaundice 1st, then RUQ pain

Chapter 32. Biliary System

If limited to the mucosa (stage I), cholecystectomy is all that is needed.
　This scenario usually occurs as an incidental finding following laproscopic cholecystectomy.
If through the muscle (stage II), need wide resection around liver bed at segments IV and V (2–3 cm margins), regional lymphadenectomy, including portal triad; may need Whipple, lobectomy or resection of the CBD
90% of patients present with **stage IV disease**.
High incidence of **tumor implants** in trocar sites when discovered after laparoscopic cholecystectomy
Laparoscopic approach contraindicated for gallbladder CA
5% 5-year survival overall

Bile duct cancer (cholangiocarcinoma)
Occurs in elderly; males
Risk factors: C. sinesis infection, typhoid, ulcerative colitis, choledochal cysts, sclerosing cholangitis, congenital hepatic fibrosis, chronic bile duct infection
Symproms: early – painless jaundice most common; can also get cholangitis; late – weight loss, anemia, pruritus
Persistent ↑ in bilirubin and alkaline phosphatase
Dx: ERCP 1st; MRI may help define the lesion (these tumors can be hard to find)
Invades contiguous structures early
Discovery of a **focal bile duct stenosis** in patients without a history of biliary surgery is highly suggestive of bile duct CA.
Klatskin tumors – upper ⅓
　Most common type, worst prognosis, usually unresectable
　　Tx: can try lobectomy and stenting of contralateral bile duct if localized to either the right or left lobe
Middle ⅓ – hepaticojejunostomy
Lower ⅓ – Whipple
Palliative stenting for unresectable disease
Overall 5-year survival rate – 20%

Choledochal cysts (see also Chap. 43, Pediatric Surgery)
Female gender; Asia, Japan; 90% extrahepatic; 15% cancer risk (cholangiocarcinoma)
Older patients have episodic pain, fever, jaundice, cholangitis.
Most are type I – fusiform or saccular dilatation of extrahepatic ducts (very dilated)
Infants can have symptoms similar to biliary atresia.
Possibly caused by abnormal reflux of pancreatic enzymes during development secondary to bad angle of insertion
Occurs during uterine development
Tx: cyst excision with hepaticojejunostomy and cholecystectomy
Type IV cysts are partially intrahepatic, and type V (Caroli's disease) are totally intrahepatic → will need partial liver resection

Primary sclerosing cholangitis
Men in 4th–5th decade
Can be associated with retroperitoneal fibrosis, Riedel's thyroiditis, pancreatitis, ulcerative colitis, and DM
Symptoms: fatigue, fluctuating jaundice, pruritus, weight loss, RUQ pain
　Pruritus caused by bile acids
Dx: ERCP – multiple strictures and dilatations (beaded appearance)
Antimitochondrial antibodies
Bacterial cholangitis unusual unless biliary tract manipulation has occurred
Does <u>not</u> get better after colon resection for ulcerative colitis
Leads to portal HTN and hepatic failure (scarring and patching with progressive fibrosis of intrahepatic and extrahepatic ducts
Can have isolated intrahepatic or extrahepatic duct inflammation and fibrosis
Complications – cirrhosis, cholangiocarcinoma
Tx: TXP needed long term for most; PTC tube drainage, choledochojejunostomy may be effective for some; balloon dilatation of dominant strictures may provide some symptomatic relief

Cholestyramine – can ↓ pruritus symptoms (↓ bile acids)
UDCA (urodeoxycholic acid) – can ↓ symptoms (↓ bile acids) and improve liver enzymes

Primary biliary cirrhosis
Women; medium-sized hepatic ducts
Cholestasis → cirrhosis → portal hypertension
Symptoms: fatigue, pruritus, jaundice, xanthomas
Antimitochondrial antibodies
No increased risk for cancer
Tx: TXP

Cholangitis
Charcot's triad – RUQ pain, fever, jaundice
Reynolds' pentad – Charcot's triad plus mental status changes and shock (suggests sepsis)
E. coli and *Klebsiella* – most common organisms
Cholovenous reflux occurs at 20 mmHg pressure → systemic bacteremia
Dx: AST/ALT, bilirubin, alkaline phosphatase, and WBC often ↑
Ultrasound – CBD will be dilated (>8 mm, >10 mm after cholecystectomy) on ultrasound if due to obstruction of the biliary system
Stricture and hepatic abscess are late complications of cholangitis.
Renal failure – #1 serious complication; related to **sepsis**
Gallstones most common etiology
Other causes – biliary strictures (iatrogenic), neoplasm, chronic pancreatitis, congenital choledochal cysts, duodenal diverticuli
Tx: fluid resuscitation, antibiotics
Emergent ERCP with sphincterotomy and stone extraction; if ERCP fails, go to PTC tube
If the patient has cholangitis due to infected PTC tube, change the PTC tube.

Oriental cholangiohepatitis
Asia; recurrent cholangitis from primary CBD stones
Caused by *C. sinensis*, *A. lumbricoides*, *T. trichiura*, and *E. coli* infections
Tx: hepaticojejunostomy and antiparasitic medications

Shock following laparoscopic cholecystectomy
Early (1st 24 hours) – hemorrhagic shock from clip that fell off cystic artery
Late (after 1st 24 hours) – septic shock from accidental clip on CBD with subsequent cholangitis

Other conditions
Adenomyomatosis – thickened nodule of mucosa and muscle associated with Rokitansky-Aschoff sinus
  Not premalignant; does not cause stones, can cause RUQ pain
  Tx: cholecystectomy
Granular cell myoblastoma – benign neuroectoderm tumor of gallbladder
  Can occur in biliary tract with signs of cholecystitis
  Tx: cholecystectomy
Cholesterolosis – speckled cholesterol deposits on the gallbladder wall
Gallbladder polyps – >1 cm, worry about malignancy
  Polyps in patients >60 years more likely malignant
  Tx: cholecystectomy
Delta bilirubin – bound to albumin covalently, half-life of 18 days; may take awhile to clear after long-standing jaundice
Mirizzi syndrome – compression of the common hepatic duct by a stone in the infundibulum of the gallbladder or inflammation arising from the gallbladder or cystic duct extending to the contiguous hepatic duct, causing stricture and hepatic duct obstruction
Ceftriaxone – can cause gallbladder sludging and cholestatic jaundice
Indications for asymptomatic cholecystectomy – in patients undergoing liver TXP or gastric bypass procedure

CHAPTER 33. PANCREAS

Anatomy and physiology

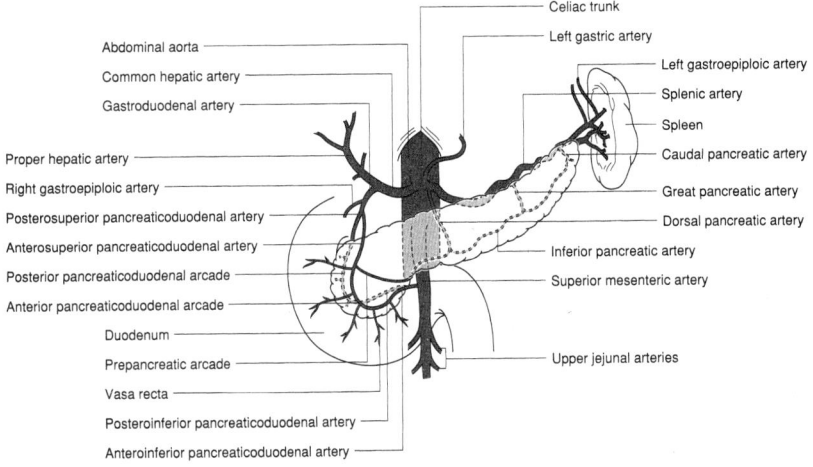

Arterial supply to the pancreas.

Head (including uncinate), **neck, body, and tail**
Uncinate process – rests on aorta, behind SMA
SMA and SMV – lay behind neck of pancreas
Portal vein – forms behind the neck (SMV and splenic vein)
Blood supply
    Head – superior (off GDA) and inferior (off SMA) pancreaticoduodenal arteries (anterior and posterior branches for each)
    Body – great, inferior, and caudal pancreatic artery (all off **splenic artery**)
    Tail – splenic, gastroepiploic, and dorsal pancreatic arteries
Venous drainage into the portal system
Lymphatics – celiac and SMA nodes

Ductal cells – have carbonic anhydrase and secrete HCO_3^- solution
    ↑ flow leads to ↑HCO_3^- and ↓ Cl^-
Acinar cells – secrete Cl^- and digestive enzymes

Exocrine function fo the pancreas – amylase, lipase, trypsinogen, chymotrypsinogen, carboxypeptidase; HCO_3^-
    Amylase – <u>only pancreatic enzyme secreted in active form</u>; hydrolyzes alpha 1-4 linkages of glucose chains

Endocrine function of the pancreas
    Alpha cells – glucagon
    Beta cells (at center of islets) – insulin
    Delta cells – somatostatin
    PP or F cells – pancreatic polypeptide
    Islet cells – also produce vasoactive intestinal peptide (VIP), serotonin, neuropeptide Y, gastrin-releasing peptide (GRP)

Islet cells receive majority of blood supply related to size.
After islets, blood goes to acinar cells.
Enterokinase – released by the duodenum, activates trypsinogen to trypsin
Trypsin activates other pancreatic enzymes including trypsinogen

Hormonal control of pancreatic excretion
- **Secretin** – ↑ HCO₃⁻ mostly
- **CCK** – ↑ enzymes mostly
- **Acetylcholine** – ↑ HCO⁻ and enzymes
- **Somatostatin and glucagons** – ↓ exocrine function
- **CCK and secretin** – most released by cells in the duodenum

Ventral pancreatic bud
Connected to duct of Wirsung; migrates posteriorly, to the right, and clockwise to fuse with dorsal bud
Forms uncinate and inferior portion of the head
Dorsal pancreatic bud – body, tail, and superior aspect of the pancreatic head; has duct of Santorini
Duct of Santorini – small accessory pancreatic duct that drains directly into duodenum
Duct of Wirsung – major pancreatic duct that merges with CBD before entering duodenum

Annular pancreas
2nd portion of duodenum trapped in pancreatic band; can see double bubble on abdominal x-ray
Associated with Down's syndrome; forms from the ventral pancreatic bud from failure of clockwise rotation
Tx: duodenojejunostomy or duodenoduodenostomy and sphincteroplasty
- Pancreas not resected

Pancreas divisum
Failed fusion of the pancreatic ducts; can result in pancreatitis from duct of Santorini (accessory duct) stenosis
Most are asymptomatic; some get pancreatitis
Dx: ERCP – **minor papilla** will show long and large duct of Santorini; **major papilla** will show short duct of Wirsung
Tx: sphincteroplasty and stent placement if symptomatic
- May need open sphincteroplasty of that fails
- If longstanding, sphincteroplasty, may not work → then need longitudinal pancreaticojejunostomy

Heterotopic pancreas
Most commonly found in duodenum
Usually asymptomatic
Surgical resection if symptomatic

Acute pancreatitis
Stones and ETOH most common causes in US
Other causes – ERCP, trauma, hyperlipidemia, hypercalcemia, viral infection, medications (azathioprine, furosemide, steroids, cimetidine), *Ascaris lumbricoides* and *C. sinesis*
Symptoms: abdominal pain radiating to the back, nausea, vomiting, anorexia
- Jaundice can occur in 40%; can also get left pleural effusion and sentinel loop (dilated small bowel near the pancreas as a result of the inflammation)

Caused by impaired extrusion of zymogen granules and activation of degradation enzymes → leads to autodigestion
Mortality rate 10%; hemorrhagic pancreatitis mortality 50%
Pancreatitis without obvious cause → need to worry about malignancy

Ranson's criteria
On admission → age >55, WBC >16, glucose >200, AST >250, LDH >350
After 48 hours: Hct ↓ 10%, BUN ↑ of 5, Ca <8, PaO2 <60, base deficit >4, fluid sequestration >6 L
- 8 Ranson criteria met → mortality rate near 100%

Labs: ↑ amylase, lipase, and WBCs
Tx: NPO, aggressive fluid resuscitation
- Antibiotics for those with stones, if severe, failure to improve or thought to have infection
- TPN may be necessary during recovery period

Chapter 33. Pancreas

ERCP may be needed in patients with gallstone pancreatitis and retained stone still in the CBD → perform sphincterotomy and stone extraction
Patients with gallstone pancreatitis should undergo cholecystectomy when recovered from pancreatitis.
Morphine should probably be avoided in patients with pancreatitis as it can contract the sphincter of Oddi and could worsen attack
Abdominal CT – needed only to check for complications (dead pancreas will not light up)
Ultrasound – needed to check for gallstones and possible CBD dilatation

Bleeding
- **Grey Turner sign** – flank ecchymosis
- **Cullen's sign** – periumbilical ecchymosis
- **Fox's sign** – inguinal ecchymosis

15% get necrosis – generally leave sterile necrosis alone
- 10% of those patients require surgery for infected necrosis → may need to sample this with CT-guided aspiration.
- CT-guided drainage of pancreatic abscesses is often ineffective

Infection – leading cause of death; usually GNRs
- Need to remove infected material – see gas in pancreas on abdominal CT
- May need ultrasound- or CT-guided aspiration to diagnose infection

Obesity – most important risk factor for necrotizing pancreatitis
ARDS – related to release of phospholipases
Coagulopathy – related to release of proteases
Pancreatic/fat necrosis – related to release of phospholipases

Mildly ↑ amylase and lipase can be seen with cholecystitis, perforated ulcer, sialoadenitis, SBO, and intestinal infarction.

Pancreatic pseudocysts

Most common in patients with chronic pancreatitis
Symptoms; pain, fever, weight loss, bowel obstruction from compression
Often occurs in the head of the pancreas; small cysts likely to resolve spontaneously (<5 cm)
Nonepithelialized sac
Expectant management up to 3 months – allows pseudocyst to mature
Only need to treat patients with **continued symptoms or pseudocysts that are growing**
May need to place these patients on TPN if unable to eat
Usually in head of pancreas
Can present with persistent **pain, fever, ↑ WBCs, palpable mass, jaundice**

Patients with symptomatic or growing pseudocyst need MRCP or ERCP to check for duct involvement.
- If <u>duct involved</u>, will need **cystogastrostomy (endoscopic or open)**
- If <u>duct not involved</u>, may get away with **percutaneous drainage of pseudocyst**

Complications of pancreatic pseudocyst – SBO, infection, portal or splenic vein thrombosis
Incidental cysts should be resected unless associated with pancreatitis or unless the cyst is purely serous.

Pancreatic fistulas

Most close spontaneously (especially if low output <200 cc/day)
Tx: allow drainage, TPN, octreotide
If failure to resolve with medical management, can try ERCP, sphincterotomy, and pancreatic stent placement
If that fails, for distal lesions perform **distal pancreatectomy**; for proximal lesions **may need Whipple**
Pancreatitis-associated recurrent pleural effusion or ascites – thoracentesis or paracentesis followed by ERCP and stent placement initially; may need resection if that fails
Amylase will be elevated in the fluid.

Chronic pancreatitis

Corresponds to irreversible parenchymal fibrosis
ETOH most common cause; idiopathic 2nd most common

Pain most common problem; anorexia, weight loss, malabsorption, steatorrhea, recurrent acute pancreatitis
Exocrine tissue gets calcified and fibrotic; **islet cells usually preserved**
Advanced disease – **chain of lakes** → alternating segments of dilation and stenosis in pancreatic duct
Can cause **malabsorption of fat-soluble vitamins**
    Stents – have a temporizing role
Dx: abdominal CT will show shrunken pancreas with calcifications
    Ultrasound – shows pancreatic ducts >4 mm, cysts, and atrophy
    ERCP – very sensitive at diagnosing chronic pancreatitis
Tx: supportive care, including pain control and nutritional support (tube feeds, TPN)

Surgical indications – pain that inteferes with quality of life, nutrition abnormalities, addiction to narcotics, failure to rule out malignancy, biliary obstruction

Surgical options
    Puestow procedure – pancreaticojejunostomy, for ducts >8 mm (most patients improve) → open along main pancreatic duct and drain into jejunum
    Distal pancreatic resection – for normal duct anatomy, failed Peustow procedures, or when only a small portion of the gland is affected
    Whipple – may be needed to patients with pancreatic head disease
    Splanchnicectomy or celiac ganglionectomy (ablation) may be used for postop pain control
Common bile duct stricture – proximal dilation that can occur with chronic pancreatitis
    Tx: hepaticojejunostomy or choledochojejunostomy for pain, jaundice, cholangitis

Splenic vein thrombosis – chronic pancreatitis most common cause of splenic vein thrombosis
Can get bleeding from gastric varicies that form as collaterals
Tx: splenectomy for bleeding gastric varicies

Pancreatic insufficiency
Usually the result of longstanding pancreatitis or occurs after total pancreatectomy (over 90% of the function must be lost)
Generally refers to exocrine function
Symptoms: malabsorption and steatorrhea
Dx: fecal fat testing
Tx: high-carbohydrate, high-protein, low-fat diet with pancreatic enzyme replacement
Steatorrhea – give pancrease (pancreatic enzymes)

Biliary stenosis (pancreatic etiologies)
Secondary to pseudocysts, fibrosis
Complications: biliary cirrhosis, cholangitis
Surgery indicated with persistent jaundice, cirrhosis, progressive dilatation of hepatic ducts, or cholangitis; also if cannot exclude pancreatic cancer
Tx: hepaticojejunostomy

Jaundice workup
Ultrasound 1st
    Positive stones, no mass → ERCP
    No stones, no mass → abdominal CT or MRI
    Positive mass → abdominal CT or MRI

Pancreatic adenocarcinoma
Male predominance; typically occurs in the 6th–7th decades of life
Symptoms: **weight loss, jaundice, pain**
20% 5-year survival rate with resection
Risk factors – **tobacco #1**
CA 19-9 – serum marker for pancreatic CA
Lymphatic spread 1st

70% in head
    50% invade portal vein, SMV, or retroperitoneum at time of diagnosis (unresectable disease)
    Metastases to peritoneum, omentum, and liver – indicate unresectable disease
    Metastases to celiac or SMA nodal system (nodal systems outside area of resection) – indicate unresectable disease
    Most cures in patients with pancreatic head disease
90% ductal adenocarcinoma
    Other tumors of the exocrine pancreas (have more favorable prognosis) – papillary cystic adenocarcinoma, serous cystadenomas (vast majority benign), mucinous cystadenomas (considered premalignant),

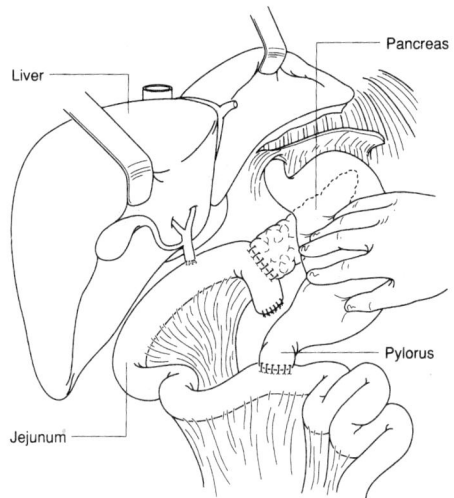

Reconstruction after pylorus-preserving pancreaticoduodenectomy.

Labs: typically show ↑ conjugated bilirubin and alkaline phosphatase
Patient with mass in pancreas does <u>not</u> need a biopsy because you are taking it out regardless.
ERCP good at differentiating dilated ducts secondary to chronic pancreatitis vs cancer
    Signs of CA on ERCP – duct with irregular narrowing, displacement, destruction
Abdominal CT – may show the lesion and double-duct sign for pancreatic head cancers (dilation of both the pancreatic duct and CBD)
    May want preop <u>MR angiogram or contrast angiogram</u> if worried about vessel involvement

Can consider stents, hepaticojejunostomy, or gastrojejunostomy **as palliation** for jaundice or obstruction
Chemotherapy **(gemcytibine) and XRT**

Complications from Whipple
    Delayed gastric emptying #1
        Tx – metoclopramide
    Anastomotic breakdown
    Marginal ulceration
    Abscess or infection
    Pancreatitis
    Fistulas

Pancreatic duct leak – Tx: drain and possible ERCP and stenting of pancreatic duct
Celiac plexus block – for painful unresectable disease
Prognosis related to vascular and nodal invasion and ability to get a clear margin

Nonfunctional endocrine tumors
Represent ⅓ of pancreatic endocrine neoplasms
90% of the nonfunctional tumors are malignant.
Symptoms: pain, weight loss, jaundice
Tend to have a more indolent and protracted course compared with pancreatic adenocarcinoma
Dx: abdominal CT or MRI
Resect these lesions: metastatic disease precludes resection
5FU and steptozosin may be effective
Liver metastases most common
    50% 5-year survival rate after resection

Functional endocrine pancreatic tumors
Represents ⅔ of pancreatic endocrine neoplasms
Octreotide – effective for insulinoma, glucagonoma, gastrinoma, VIPoma
Most common in pancreatic head – gastrinoma, somatostatinoma
All tumors can respond to debulking.
Liver spread – 1st for all
Streptozosin works well in all.

Insulinoma
Most common islet cell tumor of the pancreas
Symptoms: **Whipple's triad** → fasting hypoglycemia (<50), symptoms of hypoglycemia, (catecholamine surge → palpitations, ↑ HR, and diaphoresis), relief with glucose
85%–95% benign and evenly distributed throughout pancreas
Dx: Insulin to glucose ratio >0 .4 after fasting, ↑ C peptide and proinsulin → otherwise suspect **Munchausen's syndrome**
Tx: enucleate if <2 cm; formal resection if >2 cm
    For metastatic disease → streptozocin, octreotide, 5FU

Gastrinoma (Zollinger-Ellison syndrome; ZES)
Most common pancreatic islet cell tumor in MEN I patients
50% **malignant** and 50% **multiple**
75% spontaneous and 25% MEN I

Majority in gastrinoma triangle – common bile duct, neck of pancreas, third portion of the duodenum

Symptoms: refractory ulcer disease (abdominal pain) **and diarrhea** (improved with H2 blockers)

Serum gastrin usually >200; 1000s is diagnostic
Secretin stimulation test – ZES patients: ↑ gastrin (>200); normal patients: ↓ gastrin
Suspect ZES with refractory ulcer disease, ulcers occurring with diarrhea, bleeding, obstruction, perforation

Tx: enucleation if <2 cm; formal resection if >2 cm
    Malignant disease → excise suspicious nodes
    Can't find tumor → perform duodenostomy and look inside duodenum for tumor (15% of microgastrinomas there)
    Duodenal tumor – resection with primary closure; may need Whipple if extensive; be sure to check pancreas for primary
    Debulking – can improve symptoms
    Somatostatin receptor scintigraphy – single best study for localizing tumor
MRI and CT scan can also be effective.

Somatostatinoma
Very rare
Symptoms: diabetes, gallstones, steatorrhea, hypochlohydria
Diagnosis: fasting somatostatin level
Most **malignant**; most in **head of pancreas**
Perform cholecystectomy with resection.

Glucagonoma
- Symptoms: diabetes, stomatitis, dermatitis (necrolytic migratory erythema), weight loss
- Diagnosis: fasting glucagon level
- Most **malignant**; most in **distal pancreas**
- Zinc, amino acids, or fatty acids may treat skin rash.

VIPoma (Verner-Morrison syndrome)
- Symptoms: watery diarrhea, hypokalemia, and achlorhydria (WDHA)
- Hypokalemia from diarrhea
- Dx: exclude other causes of diarrhea; ↑ VIP levels
- Most **malignant**; most in **distal pancreas**, 10% extrapancreatic (retroperitoneal, thorax)
- Can measure VIP levels

CHAPTER 34. SPLEEN

Anatomy and physiology
Short gastrics and splenic artery are end arteries.
Splenic vein is posterior and inferior to the splenic artery.
Spleen serves as antigen-processing center for macrophages; **largest producer of IgM**
85% red pulp – acts as a filter for aged or damaged RBCs
  Pitting – removal of abnormalities in RBC membrane
    Howell-Jolly bodies – nuclear remnants
    Heinz bodies – hemoglobin
  Culling – removal of less deformable RBCs
15% white pulp – immunologic function; contains lymphocytes and macrophages
  Major site of **bacterial clearance that lacks preexisting antibodies**
  Site of removal of **poorly opsonized bacteria, particles, and cellular debris**
  Antigen processing occurs with interaction between macrophages and helper T cells

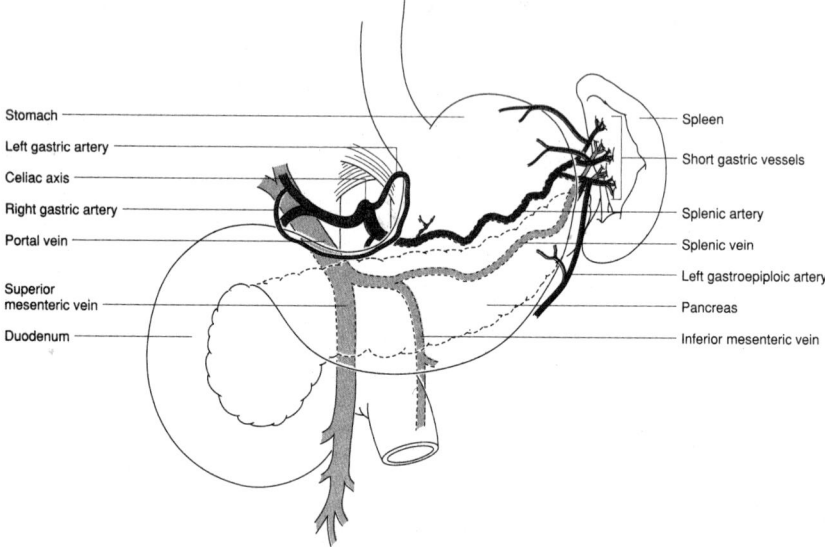

The arterial blood flow to the spleen is derived from the splenic artery, the left gastroepiploic artery, and the short gastric arteries (vasa brevia). The venous drainage into the portal vein is also shown.

  Tuftsin – an opsonin; facilitates phagocytosis → produced in the spleen
  Properdin – activates alternate complement pathway → produced in spleen
  Hematopoiesis – occurs in spleen before birth and in conditions like myeloid dysplasia
  Accessory spleen – most commonly found at splenic hilum (20%)
  Indication for splenectomy – ITP far greater than for TTP
  ITP most common nontraumatic condition requiring splenectomy

Idiopathic thrombocytopenic purpura (ITP)
  Antiplatelet antibodies (IgG) – bind platelets, cause ↓ platelets
  Petechiae, gingival bleeding, bruising, soft tissue ecchymosis
  Spleen is normal.
  In children <10 years, usually resolves spontaneously
  Tx: **steroids** (primary therapy), plasmapheresis, gammaglobulin for steroid-resistant disease
  Splenectomy indicated for those who fail steroids → removes IgG production and source of
    phagocytosis; 80% respond after splenectomy
  Give platelets 1 hour before surgery.

Chapter 34. Spleen

Thrombotic thrombocytopenic purpura (TTP)
    Loss of platelet inhibition – leads to thrombosis and infarction, profound thrombocytopenia
    Purpura, fever, mental status changes, renal dysfunction, hematuria, hemolytic anemia
    80% respond to medical therapy.
    Tx: **plasmapheresis** (primary), steroids, ASA
    Death most commonly due to intracerebral hemorrhage or acute renal failure
    Splenectomy rarely indicated

Postsplenectomy sepsis syndrome (PSSS)
    0.1% risk; ↑ risk in **children**
    S. pneumoniae (#1), H. influenzae, N. meningitidis – most common
    Secondary to specific lack of immunity (immunoglobulin, IgM) to capsulated bacteria
    Highest in patients with splenectomy for **hemolytic disorders or malignancy**
    Children also have ↑ risk of mortality after developing PSSS.
    Try to wait until at least 5 years old before performing splenectomy → allows antibody
        formation; child can get fully immunized
    Most episodes occur within 2 years of splenectomy.
    Children <10 years should be given prophylactic antibiotics for 6 months (controversial),
    Vaccines needed before splenectomy – Pneumococcus, Meningococcus, H. influenzae
        Try to give before splenectomy

    Postsplenectomy changes – ↑ RBCs, ↑ WBCs, ↑ platelets; if platelets $>1 \times 10^6$, need ASA
    Hemangioma – #1 splenic tumor overall; #1 benign splenic tumor
        Splenectomy if symptomatic
    Non-Hodgkin's lymphoma – #1 malignant splenic tumor
    Splenic cysts – surgery if symptomatic or >10 cm

Hypersplenism
    Results in ↓ platelets, RBCs, and WBCs; splenomegaly occurs as well
    Secondary hyperplenism (most common)
        Associated most commonly with ↑ venous pressure (portal hypertension, CHF),
            malignant disease (leukemia), chronic inflammatory disease (Felty's syndrome,
            SLE, sarcoidosis), myeloproliferative disease, infectious disease, amyloidosis,
            AIDS, hemolytic anemias, polycythemia vera
        Splenectomy may be indicated for **symptomatic hypersplenism** associated with CLL,
            CML, NHL, Hodgkin's, hairy cell leukemia, hemolytic anemias, sarcoidosis
    Primary hypersplenism (very rare) – need to rule out other causes
        Splenectomy indicated for primary hypersplenism
    Sarcoidosis of spleen – anemia, ↓ platelets
        Tx: splenectomy for symptomatic splenomegaly
    Felty's syndrome – rheumatoid arthritis, hepatomegaly, splenomegaly
        Tx: splenectomy for symptomatic splenomegaly
    Gaucher's disease – lipid metabolism disorder leading to splenomegaly
        Partial splenectomy may be effective.

Hemolytic anemias – membrane protein defects
    Spherocytosis
        Most common congenital hemolytic anemia requiring splenectomy
        Spectrin deficit (**membrane protein**) deforms RBCs and leads to splenic sequestration.
        Causes pigmented stones, anemia, reticulocytosis, jaundice, splenomegaly
        Try to perform splenectomy after age 5; give immunizations 1st
        Tx: splenectomy and cholecystectomy
        Splenectomy curative
    Elliptocytosis
        Symptoms and mechanism similar to spherocytosis; less common
        Spectrin and protein 4.1 deficit (**membrane protein**)

Hemolytic anemias – non–membrane protein defects
    Pyruvate kinase deficiency
        Results in congenital hemolytic anemia
        Causes altered glucose metabolism; RBC survival enhanced by splenectomy

Most common congenital hemolytic anemia **not** involving a membrane protein that requires splenectomy
G6PD deficiency
    Precipitated by infection, certain drugs, fava beans
    Splenectomy usually not required
Warm antibody–type acquired immune hemolytic anemia – indication for splenectomy
Sickle cell anemia – HgbA replaced with HgbS
    Spleen usually autoinfarcts and splenectomy not required
Beta thalassemia
    Most common thalassemia
    Major – both chains affected; minor – 1 chain, asymptomatic
    Symptoms: pallor, retarded body growth, head enlargement
    Persitent HgbF
    Splenectomy may ↓ hemolysis and symptoms.
    Most die in teens secondary to hemosiderosis.

Hodgkin's disease[1]
    A – asymptomatic
    B – symptomatic (night sweats, fever, weight loss) → unfavorable prognosis
    Stage I – 1 area or 2 contiguous areas on same side of diaphragm
    Stage II – 2 noncontiguous areas on same side of diaphragm
    Stage III – involved on each side of diaphragm
    Stage IV – liver, bone, lung, or any other nonlymphoid tissue except spleen

    See **Reed-Sternberg cells**
    Lymphocyte predominant – best prognosis
    Lymphocyte depleted – worst prognosis
    Nodular sclerosing – most common
    Tx: XRT and chemotherapy with vincristine, cyclophophamide, prednisone, procarbazine

Non-Hodgkin's lymphoma
    Worse prognosis than Hodgkin's
    Generally systemic disease by the time the diagnosis is made
    90% are B cell lymphomas.
    Tx: XRT and chemotherapy with vincristine, cyclophosphamide, prednisone, Adriamycin

Hairy cell leukemia – Tx: splenectomy, INF-gamma
Spontaneous splenic rupture – mononucleosis, malaria, sepsis, sarcoid, leukemia, polycythemia vera
Splenosis – splenic implants; usually related to trauma
Hyposplenism – see Howell-Jolly bodies
Pancreatitis – most common cause of splenic artery or splenic vein thrombosis
Splenic artery aneurysms – females; secondary to fibromuscular dysplasia, atherosclerosis (see Chap. 27, Vascular)

---

[1] Modified from AJCC. Cancer staging handbook. Ed 6. New York: Springer-Verlag, 2002:440–441.

CHAPTER 35. SMALL BOWEL

Anatomy and physiology
- **Small intestine** – nutrient and water absorption
- **Large intestine** – water absorption
- **Duodenum**
    - **Bulb (1st)** – 90% of ulcers here
    - **Descending (2nd)** – contains ampulla of Vater (duct of Wirsung) and duct of Santorini
    - **Transverse (3rd)**
    - **Ascending (4th)**
    - Descending and transverse portions are **retroperitoneal**.
    - 3rd and 4th portions – transition point at the acute angle between the aorta (posterior) and SMA (anterior)
    - Vascular supply is superior (off gastroduodenal artery) and inferior (off SMA) pancreaticoduodenal arteries.
        - Both have anterior and posterior branches.
        - Many communications between these arteries

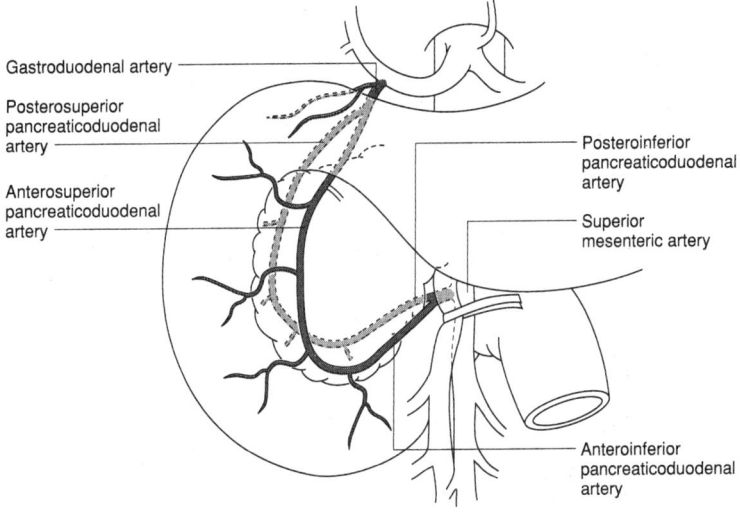

Arterial supply to the duodenum.

- **Jejunum**
    - 100 cm long; long vasa recta, circular muscle folds
    - **Maximum site of all absorption** except B_{12} (terminal ileum), bile acids (ileum – nonconjugated; terminal ileum – conjugated), iron (duodenum), and folate (terminal ileum)
    - 95% NaCl absorbed, 90% water absorbed in jejunum
    - Vascular supply – SMA
- **Ileum** – 150 cm long; short vasa recta, flat
    - Vascular supply – SMA
- **Intestinal brush border** – maltase, sucrase, limit dextrinase, lactase
- **Normal sizes** – small bowel/transverse colon/cecum → **3/6/9 cm**
- SMA eventually branches off **ileocolic artery**.

- **Cell types**
    - **Absorptive cells**
    - **Goblet cells** (mucin secretion)
    - **Paneath cells** (secretory granules, enzymes)
    - **Enterochromaffin cells** (APUD, 5-hydroxytryptamine release, carcinoid precursor)

175

Brunner's glands (alkaline solution)
Peyer's patches (lymphoid tissue); increased in the ileum
M cells – antigen-presenting cells in intestinal wall

IgA – released into gut; also in mother's milk
Fe – both heme and Fe transporters

Migrating motor complex (gut motility)
Phase I – rest
Phase II – acceleration and gallbladder contraction
Phase III – peristalsis
Phase IV – deceleration
Motilin is most important hormone in migrating motor complex.

Fat and cholesterol
Broken down by cholesterol esterase, phospholipase A_2, lipase, colipase in combination with bile salts
Converted to free fatty acids and monacylglycerides → form **micelles**
TAGs are re-formed in intestinal cells and released as chylomicrons into the lymphatics via terminal villous lacteals
Chylomicrons – 90% TAGs, 10% phopholipid, cholesterol, protein; released into lymphatics
Long-chain fatty acids – released into lymphatics
Short- and medium-chain fatty acids – released into portal vein

Carbohydrate and protein digestion – see Chap. 10, Nutrition

Bile salts
95% of bile salts are reabsorbed.
50% passive absorption – 45% ileum and 5% colon
50% active resorption in **terminal ileum** (Na/K ATPase)
Conjugated bile is absorbed only in the terminal ileum.
Bile is conjugated to **taurine and glycine**.
Can also be deconjugated in the colon by bacteria and absorbed there (small amount)
Primary bile acids – cholic and chenodeoxycholic
Secondary bile acids – deoxycholic and lithocholic (from bacterial action on primary bile acids in gut)
Gallstones can form after terminal ileum resection from malabsorption of bile acids

Short-gut syndrome
Diagnosis is made on symptoms, not length of bowel.
Symptoms: diarrhea, steatorrhea, weight loss, nutritional deficiency
Lose fat, B_{12}, electrolytes, water
Sudan red stain – checks for fecal fat
Schilling test – checks for B_{12} absorption (radiolabeled B_{12} in urine)
Probably need at least 75 cm to survive off TPN; 50 cm with competent ileocecal valve
Tx: try to restrict fat with diet resumption, H2 blockers to reduce acid, Lomotil

Causes of steatorrhea
Gastric hypersecretion of acid → ↓ pH → ↑ intestinal motility; intefers with fat absorption
Interruption of bile salt resorption intefers with micelle formation (terminal ileum resection).
Tx: control diarrhea (codeine, Lomotil); ↓ oral intake, especially fats; Pancrease, H2 blocker

Nonhealing fistula
"**FRIENDS**" – pneumonic for causes of nonhealing fistula: **f**oreign body, **r**adiation, **i**nflammatory bowel disease, **e**pithelialization, **n**eoplasm, **d**istal obstruction, **s**epsis/Infection
High output fistulas are more likely with proximal bowel (duodenum or proximal portion of jejunum) and are less likely to close with conservative management
Colonic fistulas are more likely to close than those in small bowel.

Patients with persistent fever – need to check for abscesses (fistulogram, abdominal CT, upper GI with small bowel follow-through series)
Most fistulas **iatrogenic** and treated conservatively 1st → TPN, skin protection, NG tube, stoma appliance, octreotide
40% close spontaneously.
Surgical options: resect bowel segment containing fistula and perform primary anastamosis

Obstruction
Without previous surgery (most common)
   Small bowel – hernia
   Large bowel – cancer
With previous surgery (most common)
   Small bowel – adhesions
   Large bowel – cancer

Symptoms: nausea and vomiting, crampy abdominal pain, failure to pass gas or stool
Adbominal x-ray: air-fluid level, distended loops of small bowel, distal decompression
Get bacterial overgwoth; 3rd spacing of fluid into bowel lumen
Air with bowel obstruction – from **swallowed nitrogen**
Tx: bowel rest, NG tube, IV fluids → cures 80% of partial SBO, 20%–40% of complete SBO
Surgical indications: **progressing pain, peritoneal signs, fever, increasing WBCs→ signs of strangulation or perforation**

Gallstone ileus
Small bowel obstruction from **gallstone in terminal ileum**
Classically see **air in the biliary tree** in a patient with small bowel obstruction
Caused by a **fistula between gallbladder and second portion of duodenum**
Tx: remove stone from terminal ileum
   Can leave gallbladder and fistula if patient too sick
   If not too sick, perform cholecystectomy and close duodenum

Meckel's diverticulum (a true diverticula)
2 ft from ileocecal valve; 2% of population; usually presents in 1st 2 years of life with bleeding
Caused by failure of closure of the omphalomesenteric duct
Accounts for 50% of all **painless lower GI bleeds in children <2 years**
Pancreas tissue – most common tissue found in Meckel's
Gastric mucosa – most likely to be symptomatic
Obstruction – most common presentation in adults
Incidental → usually not removed unless gastric mucosa suspected (diverticulum feels thick) or has a very narrow neck
Dx: can get a Meckel's scan (^{99}Tc) if having trouble localizing (mucosa lights up)
Tx: diverticulectomy for uncomplicated diverticulitis
   Need segmental resection for complicated diverticulitis or neck >⅓ the diameter of the normal bowel lumen

Duodenal diverticula
Need to rule out gallbladder disease (chronic cholecystitis) origin
Observe unless perforated, bleeding, causing obstruction, or highly symptomatic
Frequency of diverticula – duodenal > jejunal > ileal
Tx: segmental resection; may need temporary gastrojejunostomy for duodenal diverticula perforation

Crohn's disease
Intermittent abdominal pain, diarrhea, and weight loss
15–35 years old at 1st presentation
↑ in Askenazi Jews
Can have extraintestinal manifestations (arthritis, arthralgias, pyoderma gangrenosum, erythema nodosum, ocular diseases, growth failure, megaloblastic anemia from folate and vitamin B$_{12}$ malabsorption)
Can occur anywhere from mouth to anus

Terminal ileum – most commonly involved bowel segment
Anal/perianal disease – 1st presentation in 10%
Anal disease most common symptom – large skin tags
Most common sites for initial presentation
  Terminal ileum and cecum – 40%
  Colon only – 35%
  Small bowel only – 20%
  Perianal – 5%

Dx: colonoscopy with biopsies and enteroclysis can help make the diagnosis
Pathology – transmural involvement, segmental disease (skip lesions), cobblestoning, narrow deep ulcers, creeping fat, fistulas; small bowel may be involved, perianal disease common
Medical Tx: 5-ASA, sulfasalazine, steroids, azathioprine, methotrexate, Remicade (infliximab; TNF-alpha inhibitor, usually just used for abscess or fistula)
  <u>No</u> agents affect the natural course of disease.
TPN – may induce remission and fistula closure with small bowel Crohn's's disease
90% patients with Crohn's disease eventually need an operation.

Surgical indications
  Unlike ulcerative colitis, surgery is not curative.
  Obstruction – usually just partial and can be initially treated conservatively
  Abscess – can usually be treated with percutaneous drainage
  Megacolon – perforation occurs in 15%, usually contained
  Hemorrhage – unusual in Crohn's but can occur
  Blind loop obstruction
  Fissures – <u>no</u> lateral internal sphincteroplasty in patients with Crohn's disease
  Enterocutaneous fistula – can usually be treated conservatively
  Perineal fistula – unroof and rule out abscess; let heal on its own
  Anorectovaginal fistulas – may need rectal advancement flap; usually need colostomy
  Do not need clear margins; just get 2 cm away from gross disease.

Perirectal disease may respond to resection of small bowel.
Patients with diffuse disease of colon and rectum – proctocolectomy and ileostomy the procedures of choice
Incidental finding of inflammatory bowel disease in patient with presumed appendicitis who has normal appendix – remove **appendix if cecum not involved**

Stricturoplasty
  Consider if patient has multiple strictures to save small bowel length
  Probably not good for patient's 1st operation as it leaves disease behind
  10% leakage/abscess/fistula rate with stricturoplasty
  50% recurrence rate requiring surgery for Crohn's disease after resection

Complications from removal of terminal ileum
  ↓ B_{12} uptake can result in **megaloblastic anemia**.
  ↓ bile salt uptake causes osmotic **diarrhea and steatorrhea** in colon.
  ↓ oxalate binding secondary to ↑ intraluminal fat that binds calcium → oxalate then gets absorbed in colon → released in urine → **Ca oxalate kidney stones (hyperoxaluria)**
  Gallstones can form after terminal ileum resection from malabsorption of bile acids.

Carcinoid
  Serotonin is produced by **Kulchitsky cells** (enterochromaffin cell or argentaffin cell).
  Part of amine precursor uptake decarboxylase system **(APUD)**
  5-HIAA is a breakdown product of serotonin – can measure this in urine
  Tryptophan is the precursor to serotonin.
    Increased use of tryptophan can lead to **niacin deficiency and pellagra** (diarrhea, dermatitis, dementia).
  Bradykinin – also released by carcinoid tumors

  Carcinoid syndrome – caused by bulky liver metastases
    Intermittent **flushing and diarrhea** – hallmark symptoms
    Can also get **asthma-type symptoms and right heart valve lesions**

Chapter 35. Small Bowel

If patient has carcinoid syndrome with small bowel carcinoid primary, it **indicates metastasis to liver** (liver usually clears serotonin).
All patients with carcinoid syndrome need abdominal exploration unless unresectable.
If resection of liver metastases is performed, perform cholecystectomy in case of future embolization.
GI symptoms from **vasoconstriction and fibrosis (desmoplastic reaction)**
Octreotide scan – good for localizing tumor not seen on CT scan

Appendix carcinoid – most common site for carcinoid tumor (50% of carcinoids arise here; ileum and rectum next most common)
Small bowel carcinoid – patients at ↑ risk for **multiple primaries** and **second unrelated malignancies**
   Carcinoid in appendix – <2 cm → appendectomy; ≥2 cm or involving base → right hemicolectomy
   Carcinoid anywhere else in GI tract → treat like cancer (segmental resection with lymphadenectomy)
   Chemotherapy – **streptozocin and 5FU**; usually just for patients with **unresectable disease and carcinoid syndrome**
   Octreotide – useful for patients with carcinoid syndrome
   Bronchospasm – Tx: **Aprotinin**
   Flushing – Tx: **alpha-blockers** (phenothiazine).
   False 5-HIAA – fruits
   Pentagastrin – can exacerbate symptoms

Benign small bowel tumors
Rare
Benign small bowel tumors are more common than malignant.
Leiomyomas – most common benign small bowel tumor; usually extraluminal
Adenomas – most found in ileum; present with bleeding, obstruction
   Need resection when identified

Peutz-Jeghers syndrome (autosomal dominant) – jejunal and ileal hamartomas; mucocutaneous melanotic skin pigmentation; patients have ↑extraintestinal malignancies
   Slight ↑ risk of colon CA in patients who have these polyps
   Lipomas, neurogenic tumors, and hemangiomas can occur in these patients as well

Intussusception in adults
Can occur from small bowel or cecal tumors
Most common presentation is bleeding or obstruction
Worrisome in adults it often has a malignant lead point (i.e., cecal CA)
Tx: resection

Malignant small bowel tumors
Adenocarcinoma (rare) – most common malignant small bowel tumor
   High proportion are in the **duodenum**.
   Symptoms: obstruction, jaundice
   Tx: resection and adenectomy; Whipple if in duodenum
Duodenal CA – risk factors: FAP, Gardner's, polyps, adenomas, von Reckinghausen's
Leiomyosarcoma
   Usually in **jejunum and ileum**; most extraluminal
   Hard to differentiate compared with leimyoma (>5 mitoses/HPF, atypia, necrosis)
   Tx: resection; no adenectomy required
Lymphoma
   Usually in **ileum**; ↑ incidence in patients with Wegener's disease, SLE, AIDS, Crohn's disease, celiac sprue
   Posttransplantation – ↑ **risk of bleeding and perforation**
   Dx: abdominal CT, UGI, node sampling
   Tx: XRT, chemotherapy, wide en bloc resection may be needed; include nodes
   40% 5-year survival rate
   Usually NHL B cell type
   Mediterranean variant occurs in young males and they get **clubbing**.

Stomas

Loop ileostomies – 1%–2% obstruction rate
Parastomal hernias ↑ with loop colostomies – relocation best treatment
Candida – most common stomal infection
Diversion colitis (Hartmann's pouch) – secondary to ↓ short-chain fatty acids
    Tx: short-chain fatty acid enemas
Ischemia – most common cause of stenosis of stoma
    Tx: dilation if mild
Crohn's disease – most common cause of fistula near stoma site
Abscesses – underneath stoma site often caused by irrigation device
Gallstones and uric acid kidney stones – ↑ in patients with ileostomy

Appendix

Appendicitis – 1st: anorexia; 2nd: abdominal pain (periumbilical); 3rd: vomiting
Pain gradually migrates to the RLQ as peritonitis sets in.
Most commonly occurs in patients 20–35 years
Patients can have normal WBC count.
    CT scan – <u>diameter >7 mm or wall thickness >2 mm</u> (looks like a bull's eye), fat stranding, no contrast in appendiceal lumen; try to give rectal contrast
    Midpoint of antimesenteric border – most likely to perforate

Hyperplasia – most common cause in children; can follow a viral illness

Fecalith – most common cause in adults
Luminal obstruction is followed by distention of the appendix, venous congestion and thrombosis, ischemia, gangrene necrosis, and finally rupture.

Nonoperative situation – CT scan shows walled-off perforated appendix
    Tx: percutaneous drainage and interval appendectomy at later date as long as symptoms are improving
    Consider follow-up barium enema or colonoscopy to rule out perforated colon CA

Children and elderly have higher propensity to rupture secondary to <u>delayed diagnosis</u>.
    Children often have **higher fever and more vomiting and diarrhea**.
        Elderly – signs and symptoms can be minimal; may need right hemicolectomy if cancer suspected
Appendicitis is infrequent in infants.

Perforation – patient generally more ill; can have evidence of sepsis

Appendicitis during pregnancy
    Most common cause of acute abdominal pain in the 1st trimester
    More likely to occur in the 2nd trimester but is not the most common cause of abdominal pain
    More likely to perforate in the 3rd trimester – confused with contractions
    May have symptoms of RUQ pain in the 3rd trimester
    35% fetal mortality with rupture
    Women with suspected appendicitis need beta-HCG drawn +/– abdominal ultrasound to rule out OB/GYN causes of abdominal pain

Mucocele – can be benign or malignant mucous papillary adenocarcinoma; needs resection
    Need right hemicolectomy if malignant
    Can get pseudomyxoma peritonei with rupture

Regional ileitis – can mimic appendicitis; 10% go on to Crohn's disease

Gastroenteritis – nausea, vomiting, diarrhea

Presumed appendicitis but find ruptured ovarian cyst, or thrombosed ovarian vein, or regional enteritis not involving cecum → **still perform appendectomy**

Ileus
Causes include surgery (most common), electrolyte abnormalities (↓ K), peritonitis, ischemia, trauma, drugs
Ileus – dilatation is uniform throughout the stomach, small bowel, colon, and rectum without decompression
Obstruction – there is bowel decompression distal to the obstruction

Typhoid enteritis (salmonella)
Rare bleeding/perforation; fever, headaches, maculopapular rash, leukopenia, abdominal pain
Tx: Bactrim

CHAPTER 36. COLORECTAL

Anatomy and physiology
Colon secretes **K** and reabsorbs **Na and water** (mostly in right colon and cecum).
4 layers – mucosa (columnar epithelium) → submucosa → muscularis propria → serosa
Ascending, descending, and sigmoid colon are all **retroperitoneal**.
Peritoneum – covers anterior upper and middle ⅓ of the rectum

Muscularis mucosa – circular/longitudinal interwoven inner layer
Muscularis propria – circular layer of muscle
Plicae semilunaris – transverse bands that form haustra
Taenia coli – three bands that run longitudinally along colon. At rectosigmoid junction, the taeniae become broad and completely encircle the bowel as two discrete muscle bands.

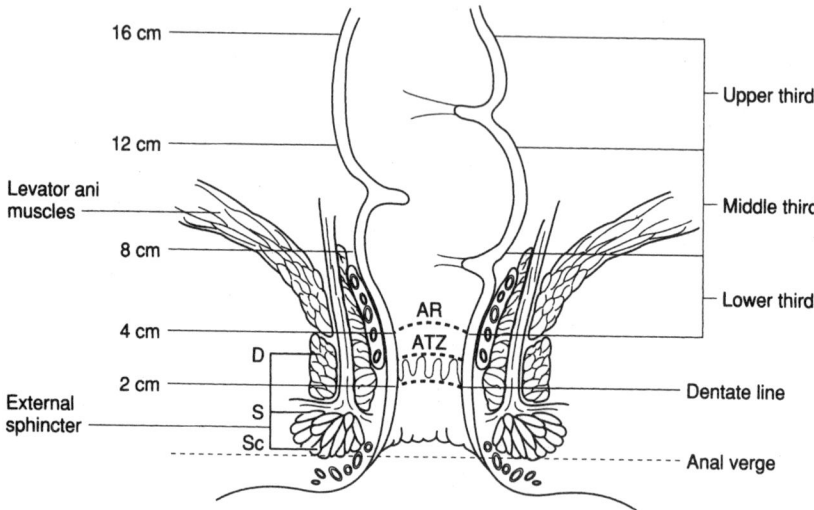

Anorectal anatomy with important landmarks. Approximate measurements are relative to the anal verge. D, deep; S, superficial; Sc, subcutaneous; AR, anorectal ring; ATZ, anal transition zone.

Vascular supply
Ascending and ⅔ of transverse colon supplied by SMA (ileocolic, right and middle colic arteries)
⅓ transverse, descending colon, sigmoid colon, and upper portion of the rectum supplied by IMA (left colic, sigmoid branches, superior rectal artery)
Marginal artery – runs along colon margin, connecting SMA to IMA (provides collateral flow)
Arc of Riolan – short direct connection between IMA and SMA
80% of blood flow goes to mucosa and submucosa.

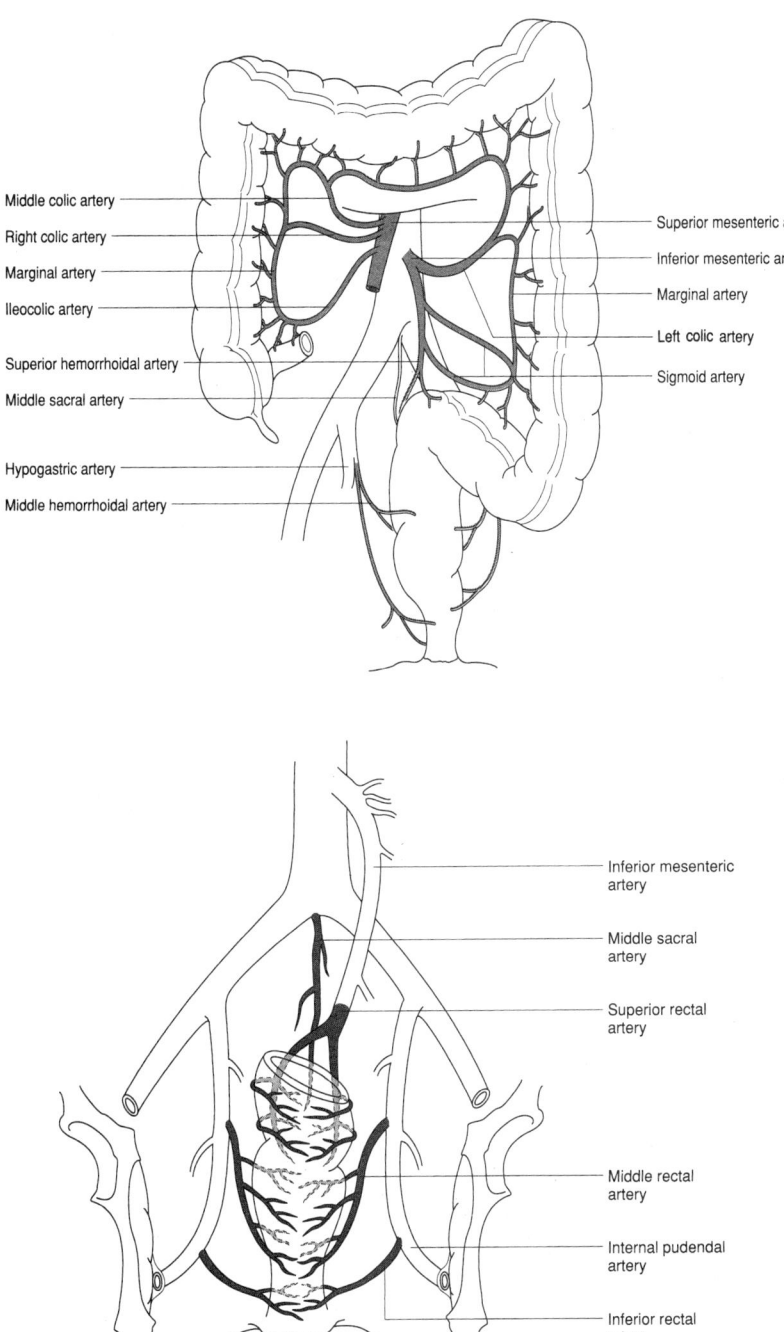

Arterial blood supply of the colon (*top*) and rectum and anal canal (*bottom*).

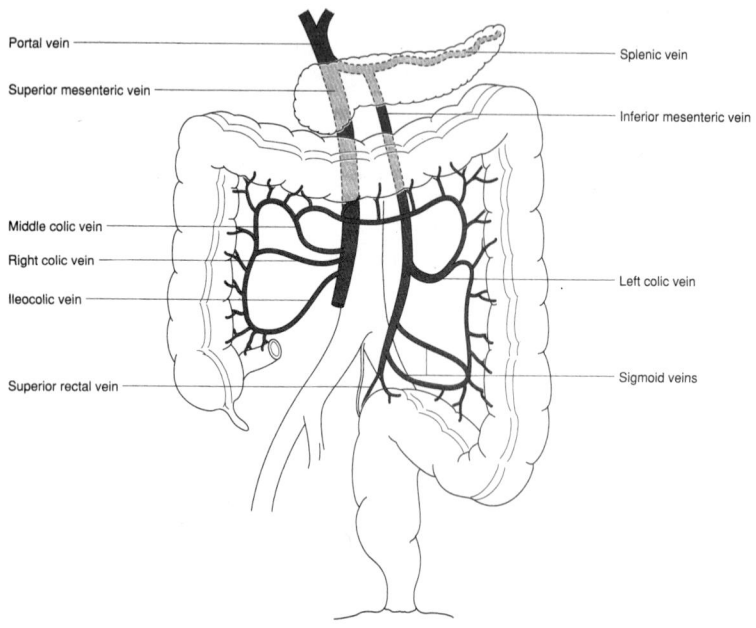

Venous drainage of the colon by the portal vein.

Venous drainage follows arterial except IMV, which goes to the splenic vein.
   Splenic vein joins the SMV to form the portal vein.
Superior rectal artery – branch of IMA
Middle rectal artery – branch of internal iliac
Inferior rectal artery – branch of internal pudendal (which is a branch of internal iliac)

Superior and middle rectal veins drain into the IMV and eventually the portal vein.
Inferior rectal veins drain into the internal iliac veins and eventually the caval system.

Superior and middle rectum – drain to IMA nodal lypmphatics
Lower rectum – primarily to IMA nodes, also to internal iliac nodes
Bowel wall contains submucosal and mucosal lymphatics.

Watershed areas
   Splenic flexure (Griffith's point) – SMA and IMA junction
   Rectum (Sudak's point) – superior rectal and middle rectal junction
   Colon more sensitive to ischemia than small bowel secondary to ↓ collaterals

External sphincter (puborectalis muscle) – under CNS (voluntary) control
   Inferior rectal branch of internal pudendal nerve and perineal branch of S4
   Is the continuation of the levator ani muscle (striated muscle)
Internal sphincter – involuntary control
   Is the continuation of the circular band of colon muscle (smooth muscle)
   Is normally contracted

Meissner's plexus – inner nerve plexus
Auerbach's plexus – outer nerve plexus
Pelvic nerves – parasympathetic
Lumbar, splanchnic, and hypogastric nerves – sympathetic

From anal verge – anal canal 0–5 cm, rectum 5–15 cm, rectosigmoid junction 15–18 cm
Levator ani – marks the transition between anal canal and rectum
Crypts of Lieberkuhn – mucus-secreting goblet cells

Dentate line – squamocolumnar junction at anal verge
Colonic inertia – slow transit time; patients may need subtotal colectomy
Short-chain fatty acids – main nutrient of colonocytes
Stump pouchitis (diversion or disuse proctitis) – Tx: short-chain fatty acids
Infectious pouchitis – Tx: Flagyl
Lymphocytic colitis – watery diarrhea and inflammatory bowel symptoms. Tx: sulfasalazine
Denonvillier's fascia (anterior) – rectovesicular fascia in men; rectovaginal fascia in women
Waldeyer's fascia (posterior) – rectosacral fascia

Polyps
Hyperplastic polyps – most common polyp; no cancer risk
Tubular adenoma – most common (75%) intestinal neoplastic polyp
    These are generally pedunculated.
Villous adenoma – most likely to produce symptoms
    These are generally sessile and larger than tubular adenomas.
    50% of villous adenomas have **cancer**.
>2 cm, sessile, and villous lesions have ↑ cancer risk.
Polyps have left side predominance.
Most **pedunculated polyps** can be removed endoscopically.
If not able to get all of the polyp (which usually occurs with **sessile polyps**) → need **segmental resection**
30% of patients >50 years with guaiac-positive stool have polyps.

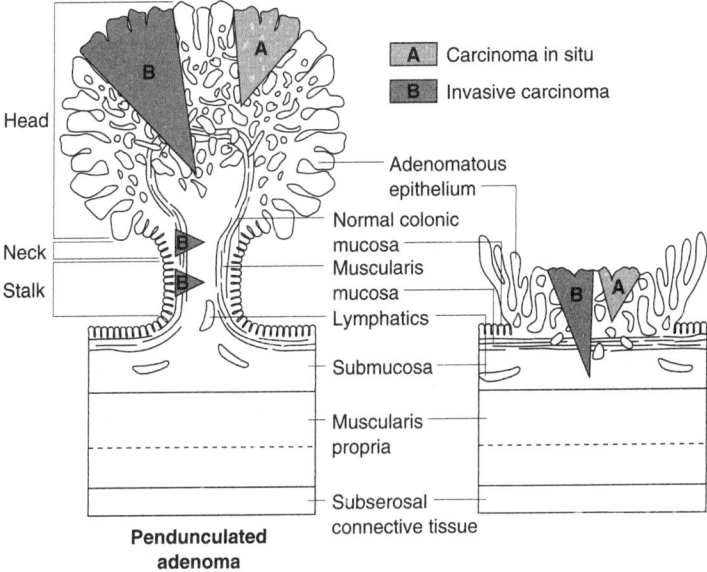

Diagrammatic representation of cancer-containing polyps. Pedunculated adenoma is described on the left and a sessile adenoma on the right. In carcinoma in situ, malignant cells are confined to the mucosa. These lesions are adequately treated by endoscopic polypectomy. Polypectomy is adequate treatment for invasive carcinoma only if there is a sufficient margin (perhaps 2 mm), if the carcinoma is not poorly differentiated, and if there is no evidence of venous or lymphatic invasion.

High-grade dysplasia – basement membrane is intact (carcinoma in situ)
Intramucosal cancer – into muscularis mucosa (carcinoma in situ → still has not gone through basement membrane)
Invasive cancer – into submucosa (T1)
Screening

Normal risk – flexible sigmoidoscopy (goes to 60 cm) every 3–5 years starting at age 50; stool guaiac (x3) and digital rectal exam every year starting at age 40
Positive stool guaiac requires colonoscopy.
Positive polyp on sigmoidoscopy requires colonoscopy.
If worried about getting all the polyp, repeat colonoscopy in 3 months.
High-risk – colonoscopy every 2–3 years starting at age 40; stool guaiac (x3) every year starting at 40
False-positive guaiac – beef, vitamin C, iron, antacids, cimetidine
No colonoscopy with recent MI, splenomegaly, pregnancy if fluoroscopy planned

Polypectomy shows T1 lesion – polypectomy adequate if margins clear (2 mm), is well differentiated, and no vascular/lymphatic invasion; otherwise need formal colon resection
Extensive low rectal villous adenomas with atypia – transanal excision (can try mucosectomy) as much of the polyp as possible
No APR unless cancer is present
Pathology shows T1 lesion after transanal excision of rectal polyp → transanal excision adequate if margins are clear (2 mm), is well differentiated, or has no vascular/lymphatic invasion
Pathology shows T2 lesion after transanal excision of rectal polyp → patient needs APR or LAR

Colorectal cancer
2nd leading cause of CA death
Symptoms: **anemia, constipation, and bleeding**
Fat → O_2 radicals thought to have a role
Colon CA has had an association with *Clostridium septicum* infection.
Colon CA – main gene mutations are **APC, DCC, p53, and k-ras**
Sigmoid colon – most common site of primary

Disease spread
Spreads to nodes 1st
Nodal status – most important prognostic factor
Liver – #1 site of metastases; **lung** – #2 site of metastases
Portal vein → **liver metastases**; iliac vein → **lung metastases**
Liver metastases – if resectable and leaves adequate liver function, patients have 25% 5-year survival rate
Lung metastases – 20% 5-year survival rate in selected patients
Isolated liver and lung metastases should be resected.

5% get drop metastases to **ovaries**.
Rectal CA – can metastasize to **spine directly via Batson's plexus (venous)**
Colon CA typically does not go to bone.
Colorectal CA growing into adjacent organs can be resected en bloc with a portion of the adjacent organ (i.e., partial bladder resection).

Lymphocytic penetration – patients have an improved prognosis
Mucoepidermoid – worst prognosis

Rectal ultrasound – good at assessing depth of invasion (sphincter involvement), recurrence, presence of enlarged nodes
Need **colonoscopy** to rule out **synchronous** lesions

Goals of resection
En bloc resection, adequate margins, regional adenectomy
Most right-sided colon CAs can be treated with primary anastamosis without ostomy.
Rectal pain with rectal CA – patient needs APR
Need 2-cm margins

Intraoperative ultrasound – best method of picking up intrahepatic metastases
Conventional ultrasound: 10 mm
Abdominal CT: 5–10 mm
Abdominal MRI: 5–10 mm (better resolution than CT)
Intraoperative ultrasound: 3–5 mm
Abdominoperineal resection (APR)

Permanent colostomy; anal canal is excised along with the rectum
Can have impotence and bladder dysfunction
Indicated for malignant lesions only (not benign tumors) that are not amenable to low anterior resection (LAR)
Need at least a 2-cm margin (2 cm from levator ani muscles) for LAR
High rate of impotence in men after rectal resection, especially with APR, due to disruption of nerve supply
Risk of local recurrence higher with rectal CA than with colon CA in general
Unresectable large liver metastases at time of APR → may not need APR
   If obstructed or nearly obstructed → place colostomy and mucous fistula
      Avoid morbidity of APR in patient with terminal CA.
   If bleeding was a significant symptom, probably best to proceed with APR
   If rectal pain was a significant symptom, probably best to proceed with APR
Unresectable large liver metastases during preop workup for colon or rectal CA → no resection unless obstructed or nearly obstructed, or unless bleeding is a significant symptom

Preoperative chemotherapy/XRT – produces complete response in some patients with rectal CA; preserves sphincter function in some

---

TNM Staging System for Colorectal Cancer

T1: into submucosa. **T2**: into muscularis propria. **T3**: into serosa or through muscularis propria if no serosa present. **T4**: through serosa or into adjacent organs/structures if no serosa present
N0: nodes negative. **N1**: 1–3 nodes positive, **N2**: ≥4 nodes positive
M1: distant metastases

Stage	TNM Status
I	T1–2, N0, M0
II	T3–4, N0, M0
III	Any N1 disease
IV	Any M1 disease

(Modified from AJCC. Cancer staging handbook. Ed 6. New York: Springer-Verlag, 2002:131–132)

Low rectal T1 (limited to submucosa) – can be excised transanally if <4 cm, has negative margins (need 1 cm), is well differentiated, and there's no neurologic or vascular invasion; otherwise patient needs APR or LAR
Low rectal T2 or higher – Tx: APR or LAR

Chemotherapy
   Stage III and IV colon CA (nodes positive or distant metastases) → **postop chemo**, no XRT
   Stage II and III rectal CA → preop or postop chemo and XRT
   Stage IV rectal CA → chemo and XRT +/– **surgery** (possibly just colostomy)

   Stage II (rectal) and III (colon or rectal) – 5FU and levamisole
   Stage IV (colon or rectal) – 5FU and leucovorin

XRT
   ↓ local recurrence and ↑ survival when combined with chemotherapy
   Postop XRT for rectal CA – needed for T3 tumors or positive nodes (stage II or higher)
   XRT damage – rectum most common site of injury → vasculitis, thrombosis, ulcers, strictures
   Preop XRT and chemotherapy may help shrink tumor, allowing downstaging of the tumor and possibly allowing LAR vs APR.

20% of patients have a recurrence
   50% have recurrence within 6 months.
   100% have recurrence by 3 years.
   5% have another primary – **main reason for surveillance colonoscopy**

Follow-up
History and physical exam, CEA, and stool guaiac – every 6 months for 3 years, then annually
Yearly LFTs, abdominal CT, colonoscopy, CXR
These vary and there is no consensus.
Colonoscopy mainly to check for new colon CAs (metachronous)

Familial adenomatous polyposis (FAP)
Autosomal dominant; all have cancer by age 40
APC gene – chromosome 5
20% of FAP syndromes are spontaneous.
Polyps not present at birth; are present in puberty
Do not need colonoscopy for surveillance in patients with suspected FAP → just need flexible sigmoidoscopy to check for polyps
Need **total colectomy prophylactically at age 20**
Also get duodenal polyps → need to check duodenum for cancer with esophagogastroduodenoscopy every 2 years

Surgery – **proctocolectomy, rectal mucosectomy, and ileoanal pouch** (J-pouch)
Need lifetime surveillance of residual rectal mucosa
Following colectomy, most common cause of death in FAP patients is **periampullary tumors of duodenum**.
Total proctocolectomy with end ileostomy also an option

Gardner's syndrome – patients get colon CA (associated with APC gene) and desmoid tumors/osteomas
Turcot's syndrome – patients get colon CA (associated with APC gene) and brain tumors

Lynch syndromes (hereditary nonpolyposis colon cancer)
5% of population, autosomal dominant
Associated **with DNA mismatch repair gene**
Predilection for right-sided and multiple cancers
Lynch I – just colon CA risk
Lynch II – patients also have ↑ risk of ovarian, endometrial, bladder, and stomach cancer
Amsterdam criteria – "3, 2, 1" → at least **3** 1st degree relatives, over **2** generations, **1** with cancer before age 50
Need surveillance colonoscopy starting at age 25 or 10 years before primary relative got cancer
50% get metachronous lesions within 10 years; often have multiple primaries
Women need **endometrial biopsy** every 3 years and annual pelvic exams; earlier mammograms
Consider **total abdominal hysterectomy and bilateral salpingoophorectomy** after child-bearing years
Consider subtotal colectomy with 1st cancer operation

Juvenile polyposis
Hamartomatous polyps – cancer is dependent on adenomatous change in these polyps
Symptoms: anemia, ↓ energy, failure to thrive, anergy
Colonic surveillance every 2 years; total colectomy probably best option if CA develops
Juvenile polyps do not have malignant potential, but **patients with juvenile polyposis do have ↑ CA risk**.

Peutz-Jeghers syndrome
GI hamartoma polyposis and dark pigmentation around mucous membranes
Now believed to ↑ risk of gastrointestinal CAs
These patients need polypectomy if possible (may be too many polyps to resect) – 2% colon/duodenal CA risk
↑ risk of other cancers – gonadal, breast, biliary

Cronkite-Canada syndrome
Hamartomatous polyps; get atrophy of nails and hair, hypopigmentation
Thought to have no malignant potential

Sigmoid volvulus
More common with high-fiber diets (Iran, Iraq)
Occurs in debilitated, psychiatric patients; neurologic dysfunction, laxative abuse
Symptoms: pain, distention, obstipation
Causes closed loop obstruction
Abdominal x-ray – bent inner tube sign; gastrograffin enema may show bird's beak sign (tapered colon)
Do not attempt decompression with gangrenous bowel or peritoneal signs → go to OR for sigmoidectomy
Tx: decompress with colonoscopy (80% reduce, 50% will recur), give bowel prep, and perform sigmoid colectomy during same admission

Cecal volvulus
Less common than sigmoid volvulus; occurs in 20–30s
Can appear as a SBO, with dilated cecum in the RLQ
Can try to decompress with colonoscopy but unlikely to succeed (only 20%);
Tx: OR → right hemicolectomy probably best treatment, can try cecopexy if colon is viable and patient is frail

Ulcerative colitis
Symptoms: **bloody diarrhea, abdominal pain, fever, and weight loss**
Involves the mucosa and submucosa
Strictures and fistulae unusual with ulcerative colitis

Pathologic features of Crohn's disease and ulcerative colitis

Pathology	Crohn's Disease	Ulcerative Colitis
Transmural inflammation	Yes	Uncommon
Granulomas	50%–75%	No
Fissures	Common	Rare
Submucosal thickening, fibrosis	Common	No
Submucosal inflammation	Common	Uncommon

Distinguishing characteristics of Crohn's colitis and ulcerative colitis

Characteristic	Crohn's Colitis	Ulcerative Colitis
Location	Small bowel involvement	Colon only (rare backwash ileitis) 10%
Anatomic distribution	Asymmetric distribution (skip lesions)	Contiguous involvement beginning distally
Rectal involvement	Rectal sparing common 50%	Involved 90%
Gross bleeding	Absent in 25%–30%	Universal
Perianal disease	≤75%	Rare, may be severe
Fistulization	Yes	No
Granulomas	50%–75%	No

Endoscopic features of Crohn's disease and ulcerative colitis

Endoscopic Feature	Crohn's Disease	Ulcerative Colitis
Mucosal involvement	Discontinuous	Contiguous
Discrete ulcers (aphthous ulcers)	Common	Rare
Surrounding mucosa	Relatively normal	Abnormal
Longitudinal ulcer	Common	Rare
Cobblestoning	In severe cases	No
Rectal involvement	Sparing common	Involved in 90%
Mucosal friability	Uncommon	Common
Vascular pattern	Normal	Distorted

Spares anus – unlike Crohn's disease
  Starts distally in **rectum**, is contiguous (no skip areas like Crohn's disease)
  Bleeding is universal and has mucosal friability with <u>pseudopolyps and collar button ulcers</u>.
  Always need to rule out infectious etiology
  Backwash ileitis can occur with proximal disease.
Barium enema – with chronic disease see loss of haustra, narrow caliber, short colon, loss of redundancy
Medical Tx: sulfasalazine, 5-ASA, steroids, methotrexate, Imuran, Remicade
  5-ASA and sulfasalazine have been shown to maintain remission in ulcerative colitis.

Toxic megacolon
  Clinical Dx: fever, ↑ HR, bloating, abdominal radiographs→ dilated colon
  Initial Tx: NGT, fluids, steroids, bowel rest, TPN, and antibiotics will treat 50% adequately; other 50% require surgery.
    Follow clinical response and abdominal radiographs.

Perforation with ulcerative colitis – <u>transverse colon</u> more common
Perforation with Crohn's – <u>distal ileum</u> most common

Surgical indications: hemorrhage, toxic megacolon, acute fulminant ulcerative colitis (occurs in 15%), obstruction, low-grade dysplasia, cancer, intractability, systemic complications, failure to thrive, longstanding disease (>10 years) as prophylaxis against colon CA
  Ileoanal anastamosis – rectal mucosectomy, ileaoanal anastamosis, and J-pouch; <u>not</u> used with Crohn's disease
    Protects bladder and sexual function
    Need lifetime surveillance of residual rectal area
    Many ileoanal anastamoses need resection secondary to cancer, dysplastic changes, or refractory proctitis
    Need temporary diverting ileostomy (6–8 weeks) while pouch heals
    Leak – most common major morbidity after surgery → can lead to sepsis
      Infectious pouchitis – Tx: Flagyl
  APR with ileostomy – can also be performed

Cancer risk is 1%–2% per year starting 10 years after initial diagnosis.
  Cancer more evenly distributed throughout colon
  Need yearly colonoscopy starting 8–10 years after diagnosis

Extraintestinal manifestations:
  Most common extraintestinal manifestation requiring total colectomy – **failure to thrive in children**
  Does <u>not</u> get better with colectomy → primary sclerosing cholangitis, ankylosing spondolytis
  Gets better with colectomy → most ocular problems, arthritis, anemia
  50% get better → pyoderma gangrenosum
  HLA B27 – sacroiliitis and ankylosing spondylitis
  Can get **thromboembolic disease**
  Pyoderma gangrenosum – Tx: steroids

Carcinoid of the colon and rectum
Represents 15% of all carcinoids; infrequent cause of carcinoid syndrome
Metastases related to size of tumor
⅔ of colon carcinoids have either local or systemic spread.
Low rectal carcinoids – <2 cm → wide local excision with negative margins; >2 cm or invasion of muscularis propria → APR
Colon or high rectal carcinoids – formal resection with adenectomy

Colonic obstruction
Colon perforation with obstruction – most likely to occur in cecum
  Law of LaPlace: tension = pressure x diameter
Closed-loop obstructions – can be worrisome; can have rapid progression and perforation with minimal distention
  Competent ileocecal valve can lead to closed-loop obstruction.

Colonic obstruction – #1 cancer; #2 diverticulitis
Pneumotosis intestinalis – air on the bowel wall, associated with ischemia and dissection of air through areas of bowel wall injury; most often an indication for surgery
Air in the portal system – usually indicates significant infection or necrosis of the large or small bowel; often an ominous sign

Ogilvie's syndrome
Pseudoobstruction of colon
Associated with opiate use, bedridden or older patients recent surgery, infections, trauma
Get a massively dilated colon
Check electrolytes; discontinue drugs that slow the gut, such as morphine
Tx: **colonoscopy with decompression and neostigmine**; cecostomy if that fails

Amoebic colitis
10% become carriers for ***Entamoeba histolytica***; from contaminated food and water with feces that contain cysts
Primary infection – occurs in colon; **secondary infection** – occurs in liver
Risk factors – travel to Mexico, ETOH; fecal-oral transmission
Symptoms: similar to ulcerative colitis (dysentery); chronic more common form (3–4 bowel movements/day, cramping and fever)
Dx: endoscopy → ulceration, trophozoites; 90% have antiamebic antibodies
Tx: Flagyl, diiodohydroxyquin

Actinomyces
Can present as a mass, abscess, fistula, or induration; suppurative and granulomatous
Cecum most common location
Tx: tetracycline or penicillin, drainage

Lymphogranuloma venereum
Chlamydia; homosexuals
Causes proctitis, tenesmus, bleeding; may produce fistulas
Tx: doxycycline, hydrocortisone

Diverticuli
Herniation of mucosa through the colon wall at sites where arteries enter the muscular wall
Thickening of circular muscle adjacent to diverticulum with luminal narrowing
Caused by **straining (↑ intraluminal pressure)**
More diverticuli occur on **left side** (80%) in the sigmoid colon.
  Bleeding is more likely with right-sided diverticuli (50% of bleeds occur on right).
  Diverticulitis is more likely to present on left side.
Present in 35% of the population

Lower GI bleeding
Stool guaiac can stay positive up to 3 weeks after bleed.
Hematemesis – pharynx to ligament of Treitz
Melena – passage of tarry stools; need as little as 50 cc
Azotemia after GI bleed – caused by production of urea from bacterial action on intraluminal blood (↑ BUN, total bilirubin)
Arteriography – bleeding must be ≥0.5 cc/min
Tagged RBC scan – bleeding must be ≥0.1 cc/min

Diverticulitis
Result of perforations in the mucosa in the diverticulum with adjacent fecal contamination
Denotes infection and inflammation of the colonic wall as well as surrounding tissue
LLQ pain, tenderness, fever, ↑ WBCs
Dx: CT scan needed only if worried about complications of disease
Need follow-up barium enema to rule out cancer

25% of patients will have a complication, **most likely abscess formation,** which can usually be percutaneously drained
- **Signs of complication** – obstruction symptoms, fluctuant mass, peritoneal signs, temperature >39, WBCs >20

Uncomplicated diverticulitis – Tx: Flagyl and Bactrim, bowel rest for 3–4 days

Surgery for recurrent disease (2nd attacks associated with 50% recurrence rate), **significant emergent complications** (obstruction, perforation, or abscess formation not amenable to percutaneous drainage), **inability to exclude cancer**
- Some say patients with any complicated diverticulitis (i.e., abscess formation) or if young should undergo sigmoidectomy with 1st time diverticulitis

Right-sided diverticulitis – 80% discovered at the time of incision for appendectomy
- Tx: right hemicolectomy

Colovesicular fistula – fecaluria, pneumonuria
- Occurs in men; women more likely to get **colovaginal fistula**
- **Cystoscopy** more likely to identify
- Tx: close bladder opening, resect involved segment of colon, perform reanastamosis, diverting ileostomy

Diverticulosis bleeding

Most common cause of lower GI bleed
Usually causes significant bleeding
75% stop spontaneously; recurs in 25%
Caused by disrupted vasa rectum; creates **arterial bleeding**
Dx: **colonoscopy 1st** or **angio 1st** if massive bleed → these can be therapeutic and will localize the bleeding should surgery be required
- **Go to operating room** if hypotensive and not responding to resuscitation → subtotal colectomy if bleeding source has not been localized
- **Tagged RBC scan** for intermittent bleeds that are hard to localize
- **NG tube to rule out upper GI source**

Tx: with colonoscopy can coagulate bleeder
- With arteriography can use vasopressin or highly selective coil embolization
  - Vasopressin can allow time for resuscitation.
- May need segmental colectomy or even subtotal colectomy when bleeding not localized and not controlled

Patients with recurrent diverticular bleeds should have resection of the area if it can be localized or they may need subtotal colectomy if the area cannot be localized

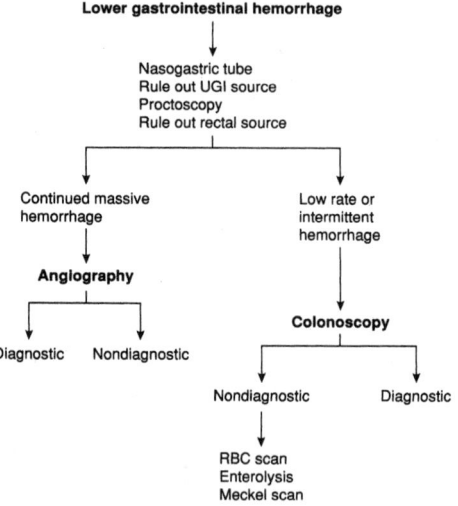

Diagnostic steps in the evaluation of acute lower gastrointestinal hemorrhage.

Angiodysplasia bleeding
↑ on right side of colon
Bleeds are usually less severe than diverticular bleeds but are more likely to recur (80%).
Causes **venous bleeding**
Soft signs of angiodysplasia on angiogram – tufts, slow emptying
20%–30% of patients with angiodysplasia have **aortic stenosis**.

Ischemic colitis
Symptoms: abdominal pain, bright red bleeding
Can be caused by a low-flow state, ligation of the IMA at surgery (i.e., AAA repair), embolus or thrombosis of the IMA
Splenic flexure and descending colon most vulnerable to low-flow state
Griffith's point – SMA and IMA junction
Sudack's point – superior rectal and middle rectal artery junction
Dx: made by endoscopy → cyanotic edematous mucosa covered with exudates
  Lower ⅔ of the rectum is spared → supplied by the middle (off the internal iliac) and inferior (off the internal pudendal) rectal artery
    If gangrenous colitis suspected (peritonitis), no colonoscopy and go to OR→ sigmoid or left hemicolectomy usual

Pseudomembranous colitis (*C. difficile* colitis)
Symptoms: watery, green, mucoid diarrhea; pain and cramping
Can occur up to 3 weeks after antibiotics; increased in postop, elderly, and ICU patients
Carrier state not eradicated; 15% recurrence
Key finding – **PMN inflammation of mucosa and submucosa**
  Pseudomembranes, plaques, ringlike lesions
Most common in the distal colon
Dx: fecal leukocytes, stool cultures for *C. difficile*, *C. difficile* toxin
  Only ⅓ patients with *C. difficile* colitis are positive for fecal leukocytes with each test
  If tests are negative at 1st, need to repeat if your suspicion is high or just treat empirically
Tx: oral – vancomycin or Flagyl. IV – Flagyl
  Lactobacillus can also help; stop other antibiotics or change them

Neutropenic typhlitis (enterocolitis)
Follows chemotherapy when WBCs are low
Can mimic surgical disease
Can often see pneumotosis on plane film
TX: antibiotics, patients will improve when WBCs ↑

Other colon diseases
Other causes of colitis – *Salmonella, Shigella, Campylobacter*, CMV, *Yersinia* (can mimic appendicitis in children), other viral infections, *Giardia*
TB enteritis – presents like Crohn's disease (stenoses)
  Tx: INH, rifampin; surgery with obstruction
Yersinia – can mimic appendicitis; comes from contaminated food (feces/urine)
  Tx: tetracycline or Bactrim
Megacolon – propensity for volvulus; enlargement is proximal to nonperistalsing bowel
  Hirschsprung's disease – rectosigmoid most common. Dx: rectal biopsy
    Trypanosoma cruzi – most common acquired cause, secondary to destruction of nerves

CHAPTER 37. ANAL AND RECTAL

Arterial supply to the anus – inferior rectal artery
Venous drainage – above the dentate is internal hemorrhoid plexus and below the dentate is external hemorrhoid plexus

Hemorrhoids
Left lateral, right anterior, and right posterior hemorrhoidal plexuses
External hemorrhoids cause pain when they thrombose
  Distal to the dentate line, covered by sensate squamous epithelium, can cause pain, swelling and itching
Internal hemorrhoids cause bleeding or prolapse
  Primary – slides below dentate with strain
  Secondary – prolapse that reduces spontaneously
  Tertiary – prolapse that has to be manually reduced
  Quaternary – not able to reduce
Tx: fiber and stool softeners
Thrombosed external hemorrhoid → lance open to relieve pain
Surgical indications: recurrent disease (bleeding), thrombosis multiple times, large external component
Can band primary, secondary, and tertiary internal hemorrhoids
Surgery needed for some tertiary and quaternary internal hemorrhoids
Do not band external hemorrhoids (painful)

Rectal prolapse
Starts 6–7 cm from anal verge
Secondary to pudendal neuropathy and laxity of the anal sphincters
↑ with female gender, straining, chronic diarrhea, previous pregnancy, redundant sigmoid colons
Prolapse involves all layers of the rectum
Primary – occult
Secondary – to anal verge
Tertiary – through anal verge
Tx: high-fiber diet
  Rectosigmoid resection (Altmier) transanally if patient older and frail
    LAR; in the absence of a large redundant colon or constipation symptoms may perform just rectopexy

Condylomata acuminata
Cauliflower mass; papillomavirus (HPV)
Tx: laser surgery

Anal fissure
Caused by a split in the anoderm
90% in posterior midline
Cause pain and bleeding after defecation;; chronic ones will see a **sentinel pile**
Medical Tx: **Sitz baths, bulk, lidocaine jelly, stool softners** (90% heal).
Surgical Tx: **lateral subcutaneous internal sphincterotomy**
Fecal incontinence is the most serious complication of surgery.
Do <u>not</u> perform sugery if secondary to Crohn's disease or ulcerative colitis.
Lateral or recurrent fissures – worry about inflammatory bowel disease

Anorectal abscess
Can cause severe pain
Perianal, intersphincteric, and ischiorectal abscesses can be drained through the skin (all are below the levator muscles).
  Intersphincteric and ischiorectal abscesses can form horseshoe abscess.
Supralevator abscesses need to be drained transrectally.
Antibiotics are needed for cellulitis, patient with DM, immunosuppressed, or artificial valve.

Pilonidal cysts
Sinus or abscess formation over the sacrococcygeal junction; ↑ in men
Tx: drainage and packing; follow-up surgical resection of cyst

Fistula-in-ano
Unroof fistula and eliminate the primary opening with rectal advancement flap.
Do **not** need to excise the tract
Often occur after anorectal abscess formation
Goodsall's rule – anterior fistulas connect with rectum in a straight line
Posterior fistulas go toward a midline internal opening in the rectum

Rectovaginal fistulas
Simple – secondary to infection or obstetrical trauma, low to mid vagina, and <2.5 cm
Tx: transanally unroof and place rectal advancement flap
Many obstetrical fistulas heal spontaneously.
Complex – secondary to inflammatory bowel disease, XRT, neoplasm or high in vagina or >2.5 cm
Tx: abdominal or combined approach usual; resection and reanastomosis with placement of colostomy; need good tissue for anastomosis

Anal incontinence
Neurogenic (gaping hole) – no good treatment
Abdominoperineal descent – damage to levator ani muscle and anus falls below levators, also stretches the pudendal nerves
Tx: high-fiber diet, limit to 1 bowel movement a day; sphincteroplasty if related to trauma (childbirth)

AIDS anorectal problems
Kaposi's sarcoma – see nodule with ulceration; most common cancer in patients with AIDS
CMV – see shallow ulcers; similar presentation as appendicitis. Tx: ganciclovir
HSV – #1 rectal ulcer
B cell lymphoma – can look like abscess or ulcer
Need biopsies of ulcers to rule out cancer

Anal cancer
Association with **HPV** and **XRT**
Anal canal – above dentate line
Anal verge – below dentate line

Anal canal lesions (above dentate line)
Squamous cell CA (type of epidermal CA)
Symptoms: pruritus, bleeding, palpable mass
Tx: **chemotherapy 1st line** (Nigro protocol, chemo – 5FU and mitomycin, and XRT), **not** surgery
Cures 80%
APR for persistent or recurrent cancer
Basaloid (cloacogenic) CA, mucoepidermoid CA
Tx: same as squamous cell CA
Adenocarcinoma
Tx: APR usual; WLE if <3 cm, <⅓ circumference, limited to submucosa (T1), well differentiated, and no vascular/lymphatic invasion; need about 1-cm margin
Postoperative chemo/XRT same as rectal CA
Melanoma
3rd most common site for melanoma (skin and eyes #1 and #2)
⅓ have spread to mesenteric lymph nodes.
Hematogenous spread to the liver and lung is early and accounts for most deaths.
Symptomatic disease is often associated with significant metastatic disease.
Most common symptom – rectal bleeding
Most tumors are lightly pigmented or not pigmented at all.
Tx: APR usual; margin dictated by depth of lesion standard for melanoma

Anal margin lesions (below dentate line) – have better prognosis than anal canal lesions
  Squamous cell CA
    Ulcerating, slow growing; men with better prognosis
    Metastases – go to inguinal nodes
    Tx: WLE for lesions <3 cm and can get 0.5-cm margin
      May need APR for larger lesions or if sphincter is involved
      Need inguinal node dissection if clinically positive
  Basal cell CA – central ulcer, raised edges, rare metastases
    Tx: WLE usually sufficient, only need 3 mm margins; rare need for APR unless sphincter involved
  Bowen's disease (malignant)
    Intraepidermal squamous cell CA
    Many of these patients have or will develop 1 or more primary internal malignancies or will develop a primary cancer of the skin with internal metastases.
    Tx: WLE with clear margins; check for other internal malignancies
  Paget's disease (rare)
    Intraepidermal apocrine gland CA
    Slow growing; has positive PAS stain
    Many of these patients have intractable itching.
    Many of these patients have or will develop a rectal or colon CA.
    Tx: WLE with clear margins; groin dissection for positive nodes; check for other internal malignancies

Nodal metastases
  Superior and middle rectum – IMA nodes
  Lower rectum – primarily IMA nodes, also to internal iliac nodes
  Upper ⅔ of anal canal – internal iliac and pelvic nodes
  Lower ⅓ of anal canal – inguinal nodes

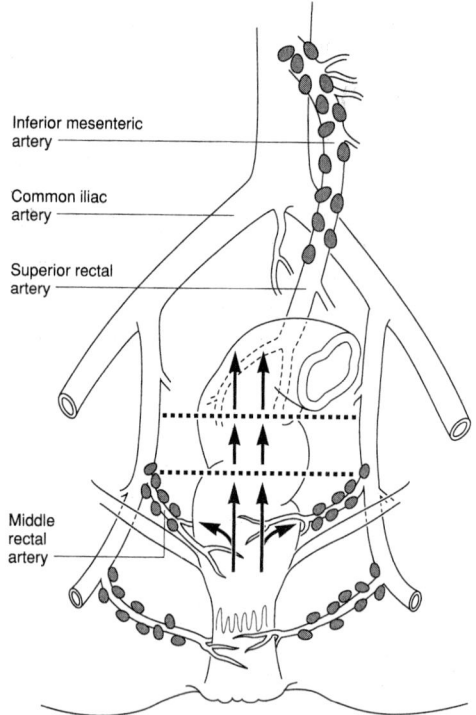

Lymphatic drainage of the rectum.

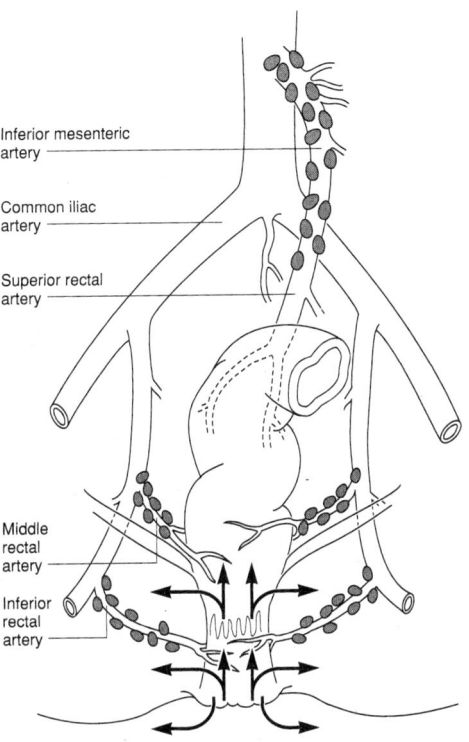

Lymphatic drainage of the anal canal.

CHAPTER 38. HERNIAS, ABDOMEN, AND SURGICAL TECHNOLOGY

Inguinal hernias
  External abdominal oblique – forms external abdominal oblique fascia and shelving edge
  Internal abdominal oblique – forms cremasteric muscles
  Transversalis muscle – forms inguinal canal floor
  Inguinal ligament (Poupart's ligament) – from external abdominal oblique, runs from anterior superior iliac spine to the pubis
    Lacunar ligament – where the inguinal ligament splays out to insert in the pubis
  Ileopubic tract – from transversalis, runs from anterior, superior, iliac spine to pubis
    Is below the inguinal ligament
  Cooper's ligament – pectineal ligament
  Conjoined tendon – composed of the aponeurosis of the internal abdominal oblique and transversus abdominus muscles
  Vas deferens – runs medial to cord structures

  Hesselbach's triangle – rectus muscle, inferior inguinal ligament, inferior epigastrics
    Direct hernias are inferior/medial to the epigastric vessels.
    Indirect hernias are superior/lateral to the epigastric vessels.

  Risk factors for inguinal hernia in adults: age, obesity, heavy lifting, COPD (coughing), chronic constipation, straining (BPH), ascites, pregnancy, peritoneal dialysis

  Indirect hernias – most common; from persistently patent processus vaginalis
  Direct hernias – lower risk of incarceration; rare in females, higher recurrence than indirect
  Pantaloon hernia – direct and indirect components
  Incarcerated hernia – can lead to bowel strangulation; should be repaired emergently

  Sliding hernias
    Females – ovaries or fallopian tubes most common
    Males – cecum or sigmoid most common
    Bladder can also be involved.

  Females with ovary in canal
    Ligate the round ligament.
    Return ovary to peritoneum.
    Perform biopsy if looks abnormal.

  Hernias in infants and children
    Just perform high ligation (nearly always indirect).
    Open sac prior to ligation.

  Lichtenstein repair = mesh; recurrence ↓ with use of **mesh** (↓ tension)
  Bassini repair – approximation of the conjoined tendon and transversalis fascia (superior) to the free edge of the inguinal ligament (inferior)
  McVay (Cooper's ligament) repair – approximation of the conjoined tendon and transversalis fascia (superior) to Cooper's ligament (pectineal ligament, inferior)
    Need a relaxing incision in the external abdominal oblique fascia
  Laparoscopic hernia repair – indicated for bilateral or recurrent inguinal hernia

  Urinary retention – most common early complication following hernia repair
  Wound infection – 2%
  Recurrence rate – 2%
  Testicular atrophy – usually secondary to dissection of the distal component of the hernia sac causing vessel disruption
    Thrombosis of **spermatic cord veins**
    Usually occurs with indirect hernias
  Pain after hernia – usually compression of ileoinguinal nerve
    Tx: local infiltration can be diagnostic and therapeutic
  Ileoinguinal nerve injury – loss of cremasteric reflex; numbness on ipsilateral penis, scrotum, thigh
    Nerve is usually injured at the external ring; nerve runs on top of cord.

Genitofemoral nerve injury – usually injured with laparoscopic hernia repair
    Genital branch – cremaster (motor) and scrotum (sensory)
    Femoral branch – upper lateral thigh (sensory)
Cord lipomas – should be removed
Trapezoid of doom
    Laparoscopic hernia repairs – femoral branch of genitofemoral nerve, lateral cutaneous nerve, femoral artery
    Need to dissect lateral to vessels; stay along inguinal ligament

Femoral hernia
Most common in males; more common than inguinal hernias in females
Femoral canal boundries – Cooper's ligament, inguinal ligament, femoral vein (Poupart's ligament is medial)
Femoral hernia is medial to the femoral vein and lateral to the lymphatics (in empty space).
High risk of incarceration → **may need to divide the inguinal ligament to reduce the bowel**
Hernia passes under the inguinal ligament
Characteristic bulge on the anterior-medial thigh below the ligament
Hernia is usually repaired through an inguinal approach with McVay or Bassini repair.

Other hernias
Umbilical hernia
    ↑ incidence in African-Americans
    Delay repair until age 5
    Risk of incarceration in adults, not children
Spigelian hernia
    Lateral border of rectus muscle, **through linea semilunaris**
    Almost always inferior to the semicircularis
    Occurs between the muscle fibers of the internal abdominal oblique muscle and line of insertion of the external abdominal oblique aponeurosis into the rectus sheath
Richter's hernia – noncircumferential incarceration of the nonmesenteric bowel wall
Littre's hernia – incarcerated Meckel's
Petit's hernia – inferior lumbar hernia
    External abdominal oblique
    Latissimus dorsi (or lumbodorsal aponeurosis)
    Iliac crest
Grynfelt's hernia – superior lumbar hernia
    Internal abdominal oblique
    Lumbodorsal aponeurosis
    12th rib (or posterior lumbocostal ligament)
Sciatic hernia (posterior pelvis)
    Herniation through the greater sciatic foramen; high rate of strangulation
Obturator hernia (anterior pelvis)
    Howship-Romberg sign – inner thigh pain with internal rotation
    Elderly women, previous pregnancy, bowel gas below superior pubic ramus
    Tx: operative reduction, may need mesh; check other side for similar defect
    Diagnosis usually made at time of surgery for small bowel obstruction
Incisional hernia – most likely to recur; inadequate closure most common cause
Peristomal hernia
    True hernias – need to remove and place in rectus muscle (missed the rectus)
    Prolapse – keep stoma at same site, fix mesentery (is in rectus but prolapsing through)
    Pseudohernia – secondary to being in the oblique muscle; need to move to rectus

Rectus sheath
Anterior – complete
Posterior – absent below semicircularis (below umbilicus)
The posterior aponeurosis of the internal abdominal oblique and transversalis aponeurosis move anterior.
Rectus sheath hematomas
    Most common after trauma; epigastric vessel injury
    Painful abdominal wall mass
    Mass more prominent and painful with flexion of the rectus muscle (Fothergill's sign)
    Tx: nonoperative usual, surgery if expanding

Desmoid tumors
   Women, benign but locally invasive; ↑ recurrences
   Gardner's syndrome
   Painless mass
   Tx: wide local excision; if involving small bowel, excision may not be indicated → often not completely resectable and can cause worsening fibrosis
   NSAIDs and antiestrogens may help.

Retroperitoneal fibrosis
   Can occur with hypersensitivity to methlysergide
   IVP most sensitive test
   Symptoms usually related to **trapped ureters and lymphatic obstruction**.
   Tx: steroids, nephrostomy if infection present, surgery if renal function becomes compromised (free up ureters and wrap in omentum)

Mesenteric tumors
   Of the primary tumors, most are cystic.
   Malignant tumors – closer to the **root** of the mesentery
   Benign tumors – more **peripheral**
   Malignant – **liposarcoma**, leiomyosarcoma
   Most solid tumors of the mesentery are benign.
   Dx: abdominal CT
   Tx: resection

Retroperitoneal tumors
   15% in children, others in 5–6th decade
   Malignant > benign
   Most common malignant retroperitoneal tumor – #1 **lymphoma**, #2 liposarcoma
   Symptoms: vague abdominal and back pain
   Retroperitoneal sarcomas
      <25% resectable; local recurrence in 40%; 10% 5-year survival rate
      Have pseudocapsule but cannot shell out → leaves residual tumor
      Metastases go to lung.

Omental tumors
   Most common omental solid tumor is metastatic disease.
   Omentectomy for metastatic cancer has a role for some cancers (e.g., ovarian CA)
   Omental cysts usually asymptomatic, can undergo torsion
   Primary solid omental tumors rare; ⅓ malignant
   No biopsy → can bleed
   Tx: resection

Peritoneal membrane
   Saline absorbed at 35 cc/hr
   Blood absorbed through fenestrated lymphatic channels
   Most drugs are not removed with peritoneal dialysis; NH_3, Ca, Fe, and lead are removed.
   Movement into the peritoneal cavity with hypertonic intraperitoneal saline load → 300–500 cc/hr; can cause hypotension

CO_2 pneumoperitoneum
   Cardiopulmonary dysfunction can occur with intra-abdominal pressure >20.
   ↑ pulmonary artery pressure, HR, systemic vascular resistance, central venous pressure, mean airway pressure, peak inspiratory pressure, CO_2
   ↓ pH, venous return (IVC compression), renal flow secondary to renal vein compression, cardiac output
   Hypovolemia lowers pressure necessary to cause compromise.
   PEEP has additive effect → pressure causes ↓ renal blood flow and can ↑ renin production
   CO_2 can cause some ↓ in myocardial contractility.
   CO_2 embolus – head down, turn patient to the left (sudden rise in $ETCO_2$ hypotension)

Chapter 38. Hernias, Abdomen, and Surgical Technology

Physiologic effects of pneumoperitoneum

Parameter	Effect
Mean arterial pressure	↑
Systemic vascular resistance	↑
Pulmonary vascular resistance	↑
Heart rate	↑
Central venous pressure	↑
Venous return	↓
Cardiac output	↓
Cardiac index	↓

Surgical technology
Harmonic scalpel
  Cost-effective for medium vessels (short gastrics)
  Disrupts protein H-bonds, causes coagulation
Ultrasound
  B-mode used most common (B = brightness; assesses relative density of structures)
  Shadowing – dark area posterior to object indicates mass
  Enhancement – brighter area posterior to object, indicates fluid-filled cyst
  Duplex
    Lower frequencies – deep structures
    Higher frequencies – superficial structures
Argon beam – energy transferred across argon gas
  Depth of necrosis related to power setting (2 mm); pretty superficial coagulation
  Noncontact – good for hemostasis of the liver and spleen; smokeless
Laser – return of electrons to ground state releases energy as heat → coagulates and vaporizes
  Used for condylomata accuminata (wear mask)
Nd:YAG laser – good for deep tissue penetration; good for bronchial lesions
  1–2 mm cuts, 3–10 mm vaporizes, 1–2 cm coagulates
Gortex (PTFE) – cannot get fibroblast ingrowth
Dacron (polypropylene) – allows fibroblast ingrowth
Incidence of vascular or bowel injury with Veress needle or trocar – 0.1%

CHAPTER 39. UROLOGY

Anatomy and physiology
Gerota's fascia – around kidney
Anterior to posterior – renal vein, renal artery, renal pelvis
  Right renal artery crosses posterior to the IVC.
Ureters cross over iliac vessels.
Left renal vein – can be ligated from IVC secondary to increased collaterals (left adrenal vein, left gonadal vein, left ascending lumbar vein)
Epididymis – connects to vas deferens
Hypotension – most common cause of acute renal insufficiency following surgery

Kidney stones
Symptoms: severe colicky pain, restlessness
Urinalysis – blood or stones
Abdominal CT – can demonstrate stones and associated hydronephrosis
Calcium oxalate (phosphate) stones – most common (75%); radiopaque
Mg ammonium phosphate (struvite) stones – 15%; radiopaque
Uric acid stones – 7%; radiolucent
Cysteine stones – 2%; radiolucent to radiopaque

Calcium oxalate stones – ↑ in patients with terminal ileum resection due to ↑ oxalate absorption in colon
Struvite stones – occur with infections (*Proteus mirabilis*) that are urease producing
  Can cause staghorn calculi (fill the renal pelvis)
Uric acid stones – ↑ in patients with ileostomies, gout, myeloproliferative disorders
Cysteine stones – associated with congenital disorders in the reabsorption of cysteine

Surgery for kidney stones
Intractable pain or infection
Progressive obstruction
Progressive renal damage
Solitary kidney
90% of kidney stones opaque; >6 mm not likely to pass
  Tx: ESWL, ureteroscopy with stone extraction or placement of stent past the stone obstruction, percutaneous nephrostomy tube, open nephrolithotomy, or urethrotomy

Testicular cancer
#1 cancer killer in men 25–35
Symptom: painless hard mass
Testicular mass – patient needs an **orchiectomy** through an **inguinal incision** (not a transscrotal incision → do not want to disrupt lymphatics)
  The testicle and attached mass constitute the biopsy specimen.
Most testicular masses are **malignant**.
Ultrasound can help with diagnosis.
Chest x-ray – to check for pulmonary metastases
Chest and abdominal CT – to check for retroperitoneal and mediastinal burden
LDH correlates with tumor bulk
90% of tumors are germ cell – seminoma or nonseminoma

Undescended testicles (cryptorchidism) – ↑ risk of testicular CA
  Most likely to get seminoma (see also Chap. 32, Pediatric Surgery)

Seminoma
#1 testicular tumor
10% of seminomatous tumors have beta-HCG elevation
Should not have AFP elevation (if elevated, need to treat like nonseminomatous)
Spreads to retroperitoneum
Seminoma is extremely sensitive to XRT.

Tx: all stages get **orchiectomy and retroperitoneal XRT** – some patients have occult retroperitoneal metastases
Positive nodes, metastatic disease, or bulky retroperitoneal disease → chemo (cisplatin, bleomycin, VP-16)

Nonseminomatous testicular CA
- **Types** – embryonal, teratoma, choriocarcinoma, yolk sac
- **Alpha fetoprotein and beta-HCG** – 90% have these markers
- Spreads hematogenously to **lungs**
- Also spreads to **retroperitoneum**
- Classically, tumors with ↑ teratoma components more likely to metastasize to the retroperitoneum
- Surgical Tx
    - **Stage I – orchiectomy**, prophylactic **retroperitoneal node dissection**
    - **Stage II or greater – orchiectomy, XRT, and chemo (cisplatin, bleomycin, VP-16); surgical resection of residual metastases**

Prostate cancer
- **Posterior lobe** – most common site
- **Bone** – most common site of metastases
    - **Osteoblastic; x-ray demonstrates hyperdense areas**
- Many patients impotent after resection; can get incontinence
- Can also get urethral strictures
- **Intracapsular tumors and no metastases (T1 and T2)** → XRT, radical prostatectomy (if life span >10 years), or nothing depending on age and health
- **Extracapsular invasion or metastatic disease**
    - **Hormonal Tx**: leuprolide (LH-RH blocker), flutamide (testosterone blocker), bilateral orchiectomy, ketoconazole, XRT for bone pain
    - **Chemotherapy**: reserved for metastatic disease not responding to hormonal therapy
- **Stage IA disease found with TURP** – Tx: nothing
- **With prostatectomy, PSA should go to 0 after 3 weeks** → if not, get bone scan to check for metastases
- **Normal PSA <4 in a patient that has a prostate gland**
    - PSA can be ↑ with prostatitis, BPH, and chronic catheterization
- ↑ alkaline phosphatase in patient with prostate CA → metastases or extracapsular disease

Renal cell carcinoma (hypernephroma)
- #1 primary tumor of kidney (15% calcified)
- Risk factor: smoking
- **Abdominal pain, mass, and hematuria**
- ⅓ have metastatic disease at time of diagnosis → can perform **wedge resection of isolated lung and colon metastases**
- **Lung** – most common location for RCC metastases
- **Erythrocytosis** can occur secondary to ↑ erythropoietin (HTN).
- Tx: radical nephrectomy with regional nodes; XRT, chemotherapy
    - Radical nephrectomy takes kidney, adrenal, fat, Gerota's fascia, and regional nodes.
    - Predilection for growth in the IVC; can still resect even if going up IVC → can pull the tumor thrombus out of the IVC
    - Partial nephrectomies should be considered only for patients who would require dialysis after nephrectomy.
    - Embolization can be used to palliate large tumors or as preop for large tumors to facilitate removal.

Most common tumor in kidney – **metastasis from the breast**
Paraneoplastic syndromes associated with RCC – erythropoietin, PTHrp, ACTH, insulin
Transitional cell CA of renal pelvis – Tx: radical nephroureterectomy
Oncocytomas – treat like RCC
Angiomyolipomas – hamartomas; can occur with tuberous sclerosis; large tumors (>4 cm) may be symptomatic and require excision or embolization
Von Hippel–Lindau syndrome – multifocal and recurrent RCC, renal cysts, CNS tumors, pheochromocytomas

Bladder cancer
Usually transitional cell CA
Painless hematuria
Males; prognosis based on stage and grade
Risk factors: smoking, aniline dyes, cyclophosphamide
Dx: cystoscopy, IVP
Tx: **intravesical BCG or transurethral resection if muscle not involved (T1)**
    If muscle wall invaded (T2 or greater) → cystectomy with ileal conduit, chemotherapy (MVAC: methotrexate, vinblastine, Adriamycin [doxorubicin], cisplatin) and XRT
    Metastatic disease – chemotherapy
Ileal conduit standard – avoid stasis as this predisposes to infection, stones (calcium resorption), ureteral reflux
Squamous cell CA of bladder – schistosomiasis infection

Testicular torsion
Peaks in 15-year-olds
Involved testis almost never viable
Usually have intravaginal torsion of the spermatic cord if viable
Torsion is usually toward the midline.
Tx: **bilateral orchiopexy**
    If not, resection and orchiopexy of contralateral testis

Ureteral trauma
If going to repair end to end:
    Spatulate ends.
    Use **absorbable suture** to avoid stone formation.
    Stent the ureter to avoid stenosis.
    Place drains to identify and potentially help treat leaks.
Avoid stripping the soft tissue on the ureter, as it will compromise blood supply.

Urethral and bladder trauma – see Chap. 15, Trauma

Benign prostatic hypertrophy (BPH)
Arises in **transitional zone**
Symptoms: nocturia, frequency, dysuria, weak stream, urinary retention
Initial therapy
    Alpha blockers – terazosin, doxazosin
    5-alpha-reductase inhibitors – finasteride → inhibits the conversion of testosterone to dihydrotestosterone
Surgery (TURP): for recurrent UTIs, gross hematuria, stones, renal insufficiency, failure of medical therapy
    Post-TURP syndrome – hyponatremia secondary to irrigation with water; can precipitate **seizures** from cerebral edema
    Tx: careful correction of Na with diuresis
Most patients with TURP have retrograde ejaculation.

Neurogenic bladder
Most commonly secondary to spinal compression
Patient urinates all the time.
Injury above T-12
Tx: surgery to improve bladder resistance

Neurogenic obstructive uropathy
Incomplete emptying.
Injury below T-12; can occur with APR
Tx: intermittent catheterization.

Chapter 39. Urology

Incontinence

Stress incontinence (cough, sneeze)
Due to hypermobile urethra or loss of sphincter mechanism
Tx: Kegel exercises, alpha-adrenergic agents, surgery for urethral suspension or pubovaginal sling

Urge incontinence
Sense of urgency or frequency
Due to involuntary detrusor contraction without neurologic disorder
Tx: anticholinergics, behavior modification, cystoplasty, urinary diversion (last resort)

Neuropathic incontinence
Urgency or frequency
↓ bladder capacity; associated with neurologic conditions → spinal cord dysfunction, stroke, multiple sclerosis, stroke
Tx: underlying neurologic disorder, behavior modification; surgical options cystoplasty or urinary diversion

Overflow incontinence
Incomplete emptying and enlarged bladder
Obstruction (BPH) leads to the distention and leakage.
Tx: TURP

Congenital incontinence
Continuous leakage and nocturnal emuresis; sphincter mechanism is bypassed
Tx: surgical correction (bladder exstrophy, ureteral diversion)

Other urologic diseases

Ureteropelvic obstruction – Tx: pyeloplasty
Vesicoureteral reflux – Tx: reimplantation with long bladder portion
Ureteral duplication – most common urinary tract abnormality. Tx: reimplantation
Ureterocele – Tx: resect and reimplant
Hypospadias – ventral. Tx: repair at 6 months with penile skin
Epispadias – dorsal. Tx: surgery
Horseshoe kidney – usually joined at lower poles
  Complications: UTI, urolithiasis, hydronephrosis
  Tx: may need pyeloplasty
Polycystic kidney disease – resection only if symptomatic
Failure of closure of urachus – connection between umbilicus and bladder; occurs in patients with bladder outlet obstructive disease (wet umbilicus)
  Tx: resection of sinus/cyst and closure of the bladder; relieve obstruction
Epididymitis – sterile epididymitis can occur from ↑ abdominal straining
Varicocele – worrisome for renal cell CA (left gonadal vein inserts into left renal vein, obstruction by renal tumor causes varicocele)
Hydrocele in adult – if acute, suspect tumor elsewhere; translucent
Pneumaturia – most common cause is diverticulitis and subsequent formation of colovesical fistula
WBC casts – pyelonephritis, glomerulonephritis
RBC casts – glomerulonephritis
Interstitial nephritis – fever, rash, arthralgias, eosinophils
Vasectomy – 50% pregnancy rate after repair of vasectomy
Priapism – Tx: aspiration of the corpus cavernosum with dilute epinephrine or phenylephrine.
  May need to create a communication through the glans with scalpel
  Risk factors: sickle cell anemia, hypercoagulable states, trauma, intracorporeal injections for impotence
SCC of penis – penectomy with 2-cm margin
Indigo carmine or methylene blue – used to check for urine leak
Phimosis found at time of laparotomy – Tx: dorsal slit
Erythropoietin – ↓ production in patients with renal failure

CHAPTER 40. GYNECOLOGY

Ligaments
Round ligament – allows anteversion of the uterus
Broad ligament – contains uterine vessels
Infundibular ligament – contains ovarian artery, nerve, and vein
Cardinal ligament – holds cervix and vagina

Ultrasound
Very good at diagnosing disorders of the female genital tract

Pregnancy
Can see most pregnancies on ultrasound at 6 weeks
Fetal pole usually is seen with beta-HCG of 6000.
Gestational sac is seen with beta-HCG of 1500.

Abortions
Missed – 1st trimester bleeding, closed os, positive sac on ultrasound, no heartbeat
Threatened –1st trimester bleeding, positive heartbeat
Incomplete – tissue protrudes through os
Ectopic – acute abdominal pain; positive beta-HCG, negative ultrasound for sac (life-threatening); missed period, vaginal bleeding, hypotension
  Risk factors for ectopic pregnancy: previous tubal manipulation, PID, previous ectopic pregnancy
Significant shock and hemorrhage can occur from an ectopic pregnancy.

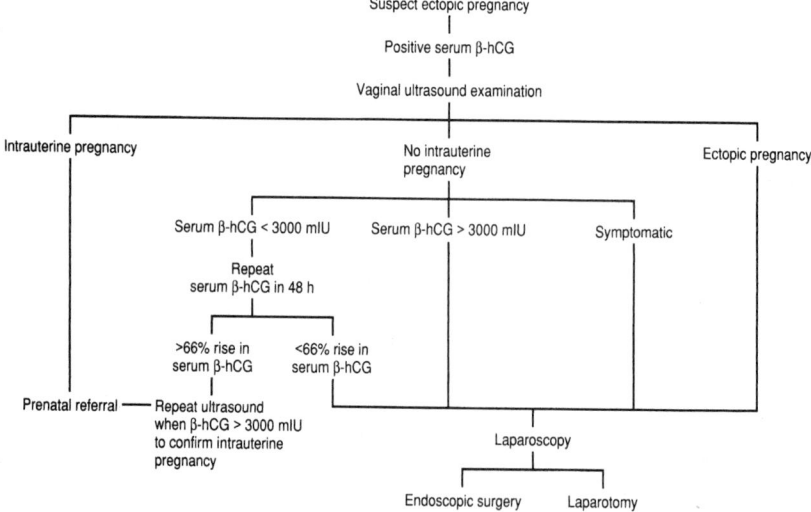

Management of suspected ectopic pregnancy. The level of serum beta-hCG at which intrauterine pregnancy is detected by vaginal ultrasound examination can vary according to institution.

Endometriosis
Symptoms: dysmenorrhea, infertility, dyspareunia
Can involve the rectum and cause bleeding during menses → endoscopy shows **blue mass**
Ovaries – most common site
Tx: OCPs

Pelvic inflammatory disease
Have ↑ risk of infertility and ectopic pregnancy
Symptoms: pain, nausea, vomiting, fever, vaginal discharge
  Most commonly occurs in the first ½ of the menstrual cycle
Risk factors: multiple sexual partners
Dx: cervical motion tenderness, cervical cultures, Gram stain
Tx: ceftriaxone, doxycycline
Gonococcus – diplococci
Chlamydia – granuloma lymphadenopathy
Complications: persistent pain, infertility, ectopic pregnancy

HSV – condylomata, vesicles
Syphilis – positive darkfield microscopy, chancre

Mittelschmirtz
Rupture of graafian follicle
Causes pain that can be confused with appendicitis
Occurs 14 days after the 1st day of menses

Vaginal cancer
#1 primary – squamous cell CA
DES – can cause clear cell CA of vagina
Botryoides – rhabdosarcoma that occurs in young girls
XRT – used for most cancers of vagina

Vulvar cancer
Elderly, nulliparous, obese
Usually unilateral
Tx: <2 cm – WLE and ipsilateral inguinal node dissection; >2 cm – vulvectomy with bilateral inguinal dissection, **postop XRT if close margins** (<1 cm)
  Paget's VIN III or higher – **premalignant**

Ovarian cancer
Leading cause of gynecologic death
↓ **risk** with OCPs and bilateral tubal ligation
↑ **risk** with nulliparity, late menopause, early menarche
Types – teratoma, granulosa-theca (estrogen secreting, precocious puberty); Sertoli-Leydig (androgens, masculinization); struma ovarii (thyroid tissues); choriocarcinoma (beta-HCG); mucinous; serous; papillary
Clear cell type – worst prognosis

Staging of ovarian cancer

Stage	Location
I	One or both ovaries only
II	Limited to pelvis
III	Spread throughout abdomen
IV	Distant metastases

(Modified from AJCC. Cancer staging handbook. Ed 6. New York: Springer-Verlag, 2002:309–310)

Bilateral ovary involvement still stage I
Initial site of regional spread – other ovary
Debulking tumor – can be effective; including omentectomy (helps chemo and XRT)
Tx: **total abdominal hysterectomy and bilateral oophorectomy for all stages**
  Chemotherapy: cisplatin and Taxol
Krukenberg tumor – stomach CA that has metastasized to ovary
  Pathology classically shows **signet ring cells**.
Meige's syndrome – pelvic ovarian fibroma that causes ascites and hydrothorax
  Excision of tumor cures syndrome.

Endometrial cancer
Most common malignant tumor in female genital tract
Risk factors – nulliparity, late 1st pregnancy, obesity, tamoxifen, unopposed estrogen, tamoxifen
Vaginal bleeding in postpartum patient is endometrial CA until proved otherwise.
Uterine polyps have very low chance of malignancy (0.1%)
Serous and papillary subtypes – worst prognosis

Staging and treatment

Stage	Location	Treatment
I	Endometrium	Total abdominal hysterectomy or XRT
II	Cervix	Total abdominal hysterectomy or XRT
III	Vagina, peritoneum, ovary	Total abdominal hysterectomy and XRT
IV	Bladder, rectum	Total abdominal hysterectomy and XRT

(Modified from AJCC. Cancer staging handbook. Ed 6. New York: Springer-Verlag, 2002:301–302)

Cervical cancer
Goes to **obturator nodes 1st**
Associated with **HPV 16 and 18**
Squamous cell CA – most common

Staging of cervical cancer

Stage	Location
I	Cervix
II	Upper ⅔ of vagina
III	Pelvis, side wall, lower ⅓ of vagina; hydronephrosis
IV	Bladder, rectum

(Modified from AJCC. Cancer staging handbook. Ed 6. New York: Springer-Verlag, 2002:294–296)

Tx: microscopic disease without basement membrane invasion – cone biopsy (conization)
    Stages I and IIa – total abdominal hysterectomy (TAH)
    Stages IIb to IV – XRT

Ovarian cysts
Postmenopausal patient
    If septated, has ↑ vascular flow on Doppler, has solid components, or has papillary projections → oophorectomy with intraoperative frozen sections; TAH if ovarian CA
    If none of the above are present, follow with ultrasound for 1 year → if persists or gets larger → oophorectomy with intraoperative frozen sections; TAH if ovarian CA

Premenopausal patient
    If septated, has ↑ vascular flow on Doppler, has solids components, or has papillary projections → oophorectomy with intraoperative frozen sections
    Algorithm becomes very complicated after this, weighing how aggressive the cancer is (based on histology and stage at time of operation) compared with whether the patient desires future pregnancy
    If none of the above are present → can follow with ultrasound; surgery if suspicious findings appear

Incidental ovarian mass at time of laparotomy for another procedure
Postmenopausal patient
    Oophorectomy, frozen section, TAH if ovarian CA at time of initial surgery
Premenopausal patient
    Much more complicated; likely will need partial oophorectomy and frozen section
    If cancer → removal of the tube and ovary (need to have gynecologist look at this)
    Then determine whether patient wants children → if not, go with TAH (usually at 2nd procedure)

Abnormal uterine bleeding
<40 years old – **anovulation**. Tx: medroxyprogesterone; if leiomyomas → GnRH
>40 years old – **cancer or menopause** → need biopsy

Other gynecologic considerations
Contraindications to estrogen therapy – endometrial CA, active thromboembolic disease, undiagnosed vaginal bleeding, breast CA
Uterine endometrial polyp – can present as progressively heavier menses
Uterine fibroids (leiomyomas) – under hormonal influence; recurrent abortions, infertility, bleeding
Most common vaginal tumor – invasion from surrounding or distant structure
Appendicitis with pregnancy – ↑ risk of premature labor and fetal mortality
Hydatidiform mole – malignancy risk with partial mole; complete mole is of paternal origin
    Tx: chemo (methotrexate)
Toxic shock syndrome – fever, erythema, diffuse desquamation, nausea, vomiting; associated with highly absorbent tampons
Ovarian torsion – Tx: remove torsion and check for viability
Adnexal torsion with vascular necrosis – Tx: adnexectomy
Ruptured tuboovarian abscess – Tx: drainage
Ovarian vein thrombosis – Dx: CT scan. Tx: heparin
Postpartum pelvic thrombophlebitis – Tx: heparin and antibiotics

CHAPTER 41. NEUROSURGERY

See also Chap. 15, Trauma

Circle of Willis
Vertebral arteries – come together to form a single **basilar artery**, which branches into two **posterior cerebral arteries**
Posterior communicating arteries – connect **middle cerebral arteries** to **posterior cerebral arteries**
Anterior cerebral arteries – branches off **middle cerebral arteries** and are connected to each other through the one **anterior communicating artery**

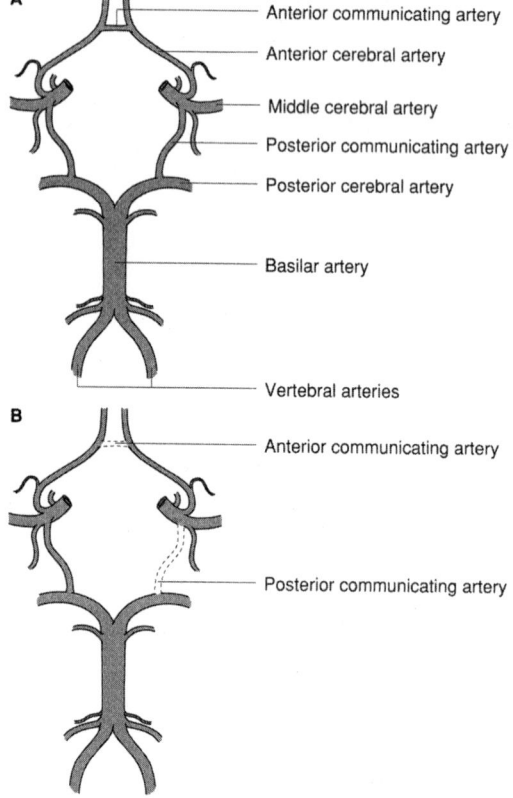

Circle of Willis. (*A*) The normal circle of Willis provides an efficient collateral circulation in the event of internal carotid artery occlusion or clamping. (*B*) An isolated hemisphere with inadequate anterior and posterior communicating arteries places the brain at risk when internal carotid artery occlusion or clamping occurs.

Nerve injury
Neurapraxia – no axonal injury (temporary loss of function, foot falls asleep)
Axonotmesis – disruption of **axon** with preservation of axon sheath, will improve
Neurotmesis – disruption of **axon and axon sheath (whole nerve is disrupted)**, may need surgery for recovery
Regeneration of nerves occurs at rate of **1 mm/day**.
Nodes of Ranvier – bare sections; allow salutatory conduction

Antidiuretic hormone (ADH)
Release controlled by **supraoptic nucleus of hypothalamus**, which descends into the posterior pituitary gland
Released in response to high plasma osmolarity; ↑ water absorption in collecting ducts
Diabetes insipidus (↓ ADH) – ↑ urine output, ↓ urine specific gravity, ↑ serum Na, and ↑ serum osmolarity
  Can occur with ETOH, head injury
  Tx: DDAVP, free water
SIADH (↑ ADH) – ↓ urine output, concentrated urine, ↓ serum Na, ↓ serum osmolarity
  Can occur with head injury
  Tx: fluid restriction, then diuresis; can give hypertonic saline if initial treatment fails

Hemorrhage
Arteriovenous malformations – 50% present with hemorrhage
  Usually in patients <30; sudden headache and loss of consciousness; are congenital
  Tx: resection if possible for both symptomatic and asymptomatic AVMs
  Can coil embolize these prior to resection

Cerebral aneurysms – usually occur in patients >40
  Can present with bleeding, mass effect, seizures, or infarcts.
  Occur at branch points in artery, most in carotid or anterior circulation; most congenital
  Often place coils before clipping and resecting the aneurysm if elective resection

Subdural hematoma – caused by **torn bridging veins**
  Has crescent shape on head CT and conforms to brain
  Higher mortality than epidural hematoma

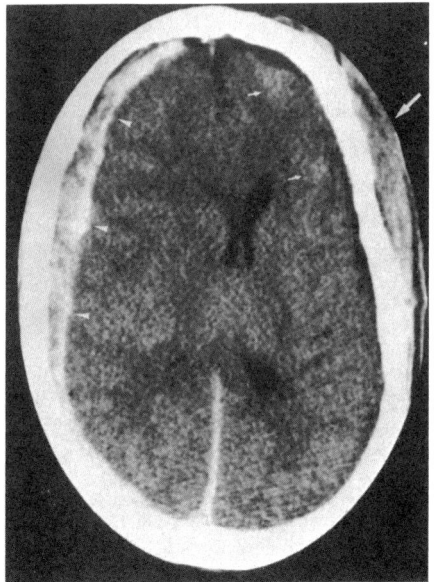

Acute subdural hematoma imaged by noncontrast CT.

Epidural hematoma – caused by injury to **middle meningeal artery**
  Has lens shape on head CT and pushes brain away
  Patients classically lose consciousness, have a lucid interval, and then lose consciousness again

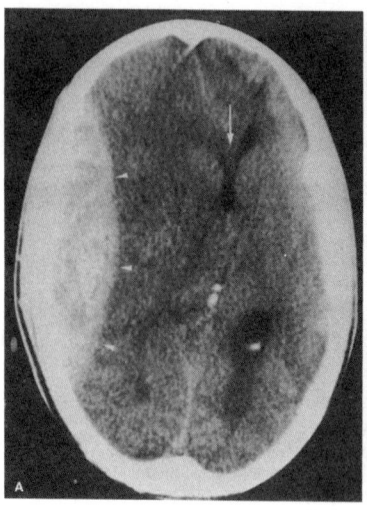 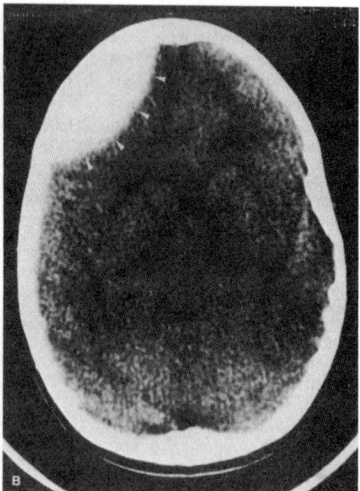

Two examples of acute epidural hematoma imaged by noncontrast CT.

Subarachnoid hemorrhage (nontraumatic)
 Caused by cerebral aneurysms (50% middle cerebral artery) and AVMs
 Symptoms: stiff neck (nuchal rigidity), severe headache, photophobia, neurologic defects
 Goal is to isolate the aneurysm from systemic circulation (clipping vascular supply),
  maximize cerebral perfusion to overcome vasospasm, and prevent rebleeding.
 Tx: hypervolemia, calcium channel blockers.
 Go to **OR only if neurologically intact**
 Can get subarachnoid hemorrhages with trauma as well

Intracerebral hematomas – temporal lobe most often affected
 Those that are large and cause focal deficits should be drained.

Cerebral perfusion pressure
 Cerebral perfusion pressure (CPP) = mean arterial pressure *minus* intracranial pressure
 Keep >60–70
 Head trauma and ↓ CPP
  Elevate head of bed
  Sedate and paralyze
  Moderate hyperventilation (pCO$_2$ 30–35)
  Mannitol to ↓ brain edema
  May need craniectomy if these measures fail
 Maximum brain swelling occurs 48–72 hours after trauma.
 Symptoms of ↑ ICP – stupor, headache, nausea and vomiting, stiff neck
 Signs of ↑ ICP – hypertension, HR lability, slow respirations
  Intermittent bradycardia is a sign of severely elevated ICP and impending herniation.
  Cushing's triad – hypertension, bradycardia, and slow respiratory rate
 Dilated pupil after trauma – ipsilateral temporal herniation onto 3rd cranial nerve

Spinal cord injury
 Cord injury with deficit → give **high-dose steroids (↓ swelling)**
 Complete cord transection – areflexia, flaccidity, anesthesia, and autonomic paralysis below
  the level of the lesion
 Spinal shock – hypotension, normal or slow heart rate, and warm extremities
  (vasodilated)
  Occurs with spinal cord injuries above T5 (loss of sympathetic tone)
  Tx: fluids initially, may need phenylephrine drip (alpha agonist)

Anterior spinal artery syndrome – most commonly occurs with acutely ruptured cervical disc
Bilateral loss of motor, pain, and temperature sensation below level of lesion
Preservation of position-vibratory sensation and light touch
About 10% recover to ambulation

Brown-Sequard syndrome – incomplete cord transection (hemisection of cord); most commonly due to penetrating injury
Loss of ipsilateral motor, contralateral pain, and temperature below level of lesion
About 90% recover to ambulation

Central cord syndrome – most commonly occurs with hyperflexion of the cervical spine
Bilateral loss motor, pain, and temperature sensation in upper extremities; lower extremities spared

Cauda equina syndrome – pain and weakness in lower extremities due to compression of lumbar nerve roots

Spinothalamic tract – carries pain and temp sensory neurons
Corticospinal tract – carries motor neurons
Rubrospinal tract – carries motor neurons
Doral nerve roots – are generally afferent; carry sensory fibers
Ventral nerve roots – are generally efferent; carry motor neuron fibers

Brain tumors
Symptoms: headache, seizures, progressive neurologic deficit, persistent vomiting
Adults – ⅔ supratentorial
Children – ⅔ infratentorial

Gliomas – most common primary brain tumor
Glioma multiforme – most common subtype, uniformly fatal
Lung – #1 metastasis to brain

Most common brain tumor in children – medulloblastoma
Most common metastatic brain tumor in children – neuroblastoma

Spine tumors
Overall most are benign, #1 tumor overall **neurofibroma**
Intradural tumors more likely benign and **extradural tumors** are more likely malignant
Paraganglionoma – check for metanephrine in urine; MIBG for extramedullary chromatin tissue

Pediatric neurosurgery
Intraventricular hemorrhage (subependymal hemorrhage)
Seen in premature infants secondary to rupture of the fragile vessels in germinal matrix
Patients go on to get intraventricular hemorrhage
Risk factors: ECMO, cyanotic congenital heart disease
Symptoms: bulging fontanelle, neurologic deficits, ↓ BP, ↓ Hct
Tx: ventricular catheter for drainage and prevention of hydrocephalus

Myelomeningocele
Neural cord defect – herniation of spinal cord and nerve roots through defect in vertebra
If sac ruptured – surgery needed to prevent infection of spinal cord
Most commonly occurs in the lumbar region

Wernicke's area – speech comprehension, temporal lobe
Broca's area – speech motor, posterior part of anterior lobe
Pituitary adenoma, undergoing XRT, patient now in shock
Dx: pituitary apoplexy
Tx: steroids
Cervical nerves roots 3–5 innervate diaphragm
Microglial cells – act as brain macrophages

Cranial nerves

Nerve	Name	Function	Muscle
I	Olfactory	Smell	
II	Optic	Sight	
III	Oculomotor		Motor to eye
IV	Trochlear		Superior oblique (eye)
V	Trigeminal: ophthalmic, maxillary, mandibular branches	Sensory to face	Muscles of mastication
VI	Abducens		Lateral rectus (eye)
VII	Facial	Taste to anterior ⅔ of tongue	Motor to face
VIII	Vestibulocochlear	Hearing	
IX	Glossopharyngeal	Taste to posterior ⅓ of tongue	Swallowing muscles
X	Vagus	Many functions	
XI	Accessory		Trapezius Sternocleidomastoid
XII	Hypoglossal		Tongue

CHAPTER 42. ORTHOPAEDICS

See also Chap. 15, Trauma

Background
- **Osteoblasts** – synthesize nonmineralized bone cortex
- **Osteoclasts** – reabsorb bone
    - Stages of bone healing – inflammation, soft callus formation, mineralization of the callus, removal of the callus
- Cartilage receives nutrients from synovial fluid.

Salter-Harris fractures III, IV, and V – cross the epiphyseal plate and can affect the growth plate of the bone; need open reduction and internal fixation (ORIF)
Salter Harris type I and I – closed reduction

Fractures associated with AVN – scaphoid, femoral neck, talus
Fractures associated with nonunion – <u>clavicle, 5th metatarsal fracture (Jones' fracture)</u>
Fractures associated with compartment syndrome – <u>supracondylar humerus and tibia</u>
Biggest risk factor for nonunion – smoking

Lower extremity nerves
- **Obturator nerve** – hip adduction
- **Superior gluteal nerve** – hip abduction
- **Inferior gluteal nerve** – hip extension
- **Femoral nerve** – knee extension

Lumbar disc herniation
Presents with back pain, sciatica
Herniated **nucleus pulposus**
Nerve root compression affects one nerve root below disc.
- **L3 nerve** compression (L2–3 disc) – weak hip flexion
- **L4 nerve** compression (L3 – 4 disc) – weak knee extension (quadriceps), weak patellar reflex
- **L5 nerve** compression (L4–5 disc) – weak dorsiflexion (foot drop)
    - ↓ sensation in big toe web space
- **S1 nerve** compression (L5–S1 disc) – weak plantarflexion, weak Achilles reflex
    - ↓ sensation in lateral foot

Dx: patients with neurologic findings need MRI
Tx: NSAIDs, heat, rest; surgery for substantial/progressive neurologic deficit, refractory cases, severe sciatica, disc fragments that have herniated into the cord

Terminal branches of brachial plexus
- **Ulnar nerve**
    - Motor – <u>intrinsic musculature of hand</u> (palmar interossei, palmaris brevis, adductor pollicis, hypothenar eminence); finger abduction (spread fingers); wrist flexion
    - Sensory – all of 5th and ½ 4th fingers, back of hand
    - Injury results in **claw hand**.
- **Median nerve**
    - Motor – thumb apposition (anterior interosseous muscle, OK sign); thumb abduction; finger flexors
    - Sensory – most of palm and 1st 3½ fingers on palmar side
    - Nerve is involved in **carpal tunnel syndrome**.
- **Radial nerve**
    - Motor – wrist extension, finger extension, thumb extension, triceps; <u>no</u> hand muscles
    - Sensory – 1st 3½ fingers on dorsal side
- **Musculocutaneous nerve** – motor to biceps, brachialis, and coracobrachialis
- **Axillary nerve** – motor to deltoid (abduction)

Cervical radiculopathy
C1, C2, C3, and C4 nerve compression (C1–2, C2–3, C3–4 discs) – neck and scalp pain
C5 nerve compression (C4–5 disc) – weak deltoid and biceps
  Weak biceps reflex
C6 nerve compression (C5–6 disc) – weak deltoid and biceps, weak wrist extensors
  Weak biceps reflex and brachioradialis reflex
C7 nerve compression (most common, C6–7 disc) – weak triceps
  Weak triceps reflex
C8 nerve compression (C7–T1 disc) – weak triceps, weak intrinsic muscles of hand and wrist flexion
  Weak triceps reflex

Radial nerve – C5–C8
Median nerve – C6–T1
Ulnar nerve – C8-T1
Musculocutaneous nerve – C5–C7
Axillary nerve – C5–C6

Radial nerve roots – on the superior portion of the brachial plexus
Ulnar nerve roots – on inferior portion of the brachial plexus

Upper extremity
Clavicle fracture – usually just treated with sling (risk of vascular impingement)
Shoulder dislocation
  Anterior (85%–95%) risk of **axillary nerve injury**. Tx: closed reduction
  Posterior (seizures, electrocution) risk of **axillary artery injury**. Tx: closed reduction
Acromioclavicular separation – Tx: sling (risk of brachial plexus and subclavian vessel injury)
Scapula fracture – sling unless glenoid fossa involved, then need internal fixation
Midshaft humeral fracture – often treated just with sling
Supracondylar humeral fracture – adults → internal fixation; children → closed reduction
Monteggia fracture – proximal ulnar fracture and radial head dislocation.
  Tx: open reduction and internal fixation
Colles fracture – fall on outstretched hand, distal radius. Tx: closed reduction
Scaphoid fracture – snuffbox tenderness; can have negative x-ray.
  Tx: all patients require cast to elbow, may need fixation; risk of **avascular necrosis**
Volkmann's contracture – supracondylar humerus fracture → occluded **anterior interosseous artery** → closed reduction of humerus → artery opens up → reperfusion injury, edema, and **forearm compartment syndrome (flexor compartment)**
  Patients have pain in forearm with passive extension, weakness, tense forearm, hypesthesia.
  Median nerve affected by swelling
  Tx: **fasciotomy**
Dupuytren's contracture – associated with diabetes, ETOH
  Progressive proliferation of the **palmar fascia of hand** results in contractures that usually affect the **4th and 5th digits** (can't extend fingers).
  Tx: NSAIDs, steroid injections; excision of involved fascia for significant contraction
Carpal tunnel syndrome – median nerve compression by transverse carpal ligament
  Tx: splint, NSAIDs, steroid injections; transverse carpal ligament release if that fails
Trigger finger – tenosynovitis of the flexor tendon that catches at the MCP joint when trying to extend finger
  Tx: splint, tendon sheath steroid injections (not the tendon itself); if that fails can release the pulley system at the MCP joint
Suppurative tenosynovitis
  Infections that spread along the flexor tendon sheaths
  4 classic signs: tendon sheath tenderness, pain with passive motion, swelling along sheath, semiflexed posture of the involved digit
  Tx; elevation, splinting, and antibiotics
    If improvement not prompt → midaxial longitudinal incision and drainage
Rotator cuff tears – supraspinatus, infraspinatus, teres minor, and subscapularis
  Acutely → sling and conservative treatment
  Surgical repair if the patient needs to retain a high level of activity or if ADL affected
Forearm fasciotomies – need to open volar and dorsal compartments

Paronychia – infection under nail bed; painful. Tx: antibiotics; remove nail if purulent
Felon – infection in the terminal joint space of the finger
  Tx: incision over the tip of the finger and along the medial and lateral aspects to prevent necrosis of tip of finger

Lower extremity
Hip dislocation
  Posterior (85%–95%) – patients have internal rotation and adduction of leg; risk of **sciatic nerve injury**. Tx: closed reduction
  Anterior – patients have external rotation and abduction of leg; risk of injury to **femoral artery**. Tx: closed reduction
Hip fracture (isolated anterior ring with minimal ischial displacement) – Tx: weight bearing as tolerated
Femoral shaft fracture – open reduction and internal fixation (ORIF) with intramedullary rod
Femoral neck fracture – ORIF → risk of avascular necrosis if open reduction delayed
Lateral knee trauma – can result in injury to **anterior cruciate ligament, posterior cruciate ligament, and medial meniscus**
Anterior cruciate ligament injury – positive anterior drawer test
  Present with knee effusion and pain with pivoting action; MRI confirms diagnosis
  Tx: surgery with knee instability (reconstruction with patellar tendon or hamstring tendon); otherwise physical therapy with leg-strengthening exercise
Posterior cruciate ligament injury – positive posterior drawer test
  Much less common than ACL injury; present with knee pain and joint effusion
  Tx: conservative therapy initially; surgery for failure of medical management
Medial collateral ligament injury – lateral blow to knee
Lateral collateral ligament injury – medial blow to knee
  Tx: **small tear** – brace; **large tear** – surgery
  These injuries are associated with injuries to the corresponding **meniscus** (medial and lateral meniscus, respectively.
    Meniscus tears – joint line tenderness; can treat with arthroscopic repair or debridement
Posterior knee dislocation – all patients need angiogram to rule out popliteal artery injury
Patellar fracture – long leg cast unless comminuted, then need internal fixation
Tibial plateau fracture and tibia-fibula fracture – ORIF fixation unless open, then need external fixator until tissue heals
Plantaris muscle rupture – pain and mass below popliteal fossa (contracted plantaris) and ankle ecchymosis.
Ankle fracture – most treated with cast and immobilization; bimalleolar or trimalleolar fractures need ORIF
Metatarsal fracture – cast immobilization or brace for 6 weeks
Calcaneus fracture – cast and immobilization if nondisplaced; ORIF for displacement
Talus fracture – closed reduction for most; ORIF for severe displacement
Nerve most commonly injured with lower extremity fasciotomy – superficial peroneal nerve (foot eversion); can also injure the common peroneal
Footdrop after lithotomy position or after crossing legs for long periods or fibula head fracture – common peroneal nerve

Leg compartments
Anterior – anterior tibial artery, deep peroneal nerve
  Muscles – anterior tibialis, extensor hallucis longus, extensor digitorum longus, communis
Lateral – superficial peroneal nerve
  Muscles – peroneal muscles
Deep posterior – posterior tibial artery, peroneal artery, tibial nerve
  Muscles – flexor hallucis longus, flexor digitorum longus, posterior tibialis
Superficial posterior – sural nerve
  Muscles – gastrocnemius, soleus, plantaris

Compartment syndrome
Most likely to occur in the **anterior compartment of leg (get footdrop)** after vascular compromise
Can also occur from crush injuries

Distal pulses can be present with compartment syndrome → last thing to go
Pressure >20–30 mmHg abnormal → consider fasciotomies; leave open 5–10 days
Dx: based on clinical suspicion

Pediatric orthopaedics

Osteomyelitis – can occur in metaphysis of long bones in children; most commonly staph
  Symptoms: pain, ↓ used of extremity
  Dx: MRI, bone biopsy
  Tx: antibiotics, incision and drainage

Idiopathic adolescent scoliosis – prepubertal females, right thoracic curve most common, usually asymptomatic
  Curves >20°–45° need bracing to slow progression, which can occur with growth spurt
  Curves >45° or those likely to progress → spinal fusion

Osgood-Schlatter disease – tibial tubercle apophysitis; caused by traction injury from the quadriceps in adolescents aged 13–15; most commonly have pain in front of knee
  X-ray: irregular shape or fragmenting of the tibial tubercle
  Tx: mild symptoms → activity limitation; severe symptoms → cast 6 weeks followed by activity limitation

Legg-Calvé-Perthes disease – AVN of the femoral head; children 2 years and older
  Can result from a hypercoagulable state; bilateral in 10%
  Symptoms: painful gait limp
  X-ray: flattening of the femoral head
  Tx: maintain range of motion with limited exercise; **femoral head will remodel without sequelae**
  Surgery if femoral head not covered by the acetabulum

Slipped capital femoral epiphysis
  Males aged 10–13; ↑ risk of AVN of the femoral head; painful gait
  X-ray: widening and irregularity of the epiphyseal plate
  Tx: surgical pinning

Congenital dislocation of the hip
  More common in females
  Tx: Pavlik harness, which keeps the legs abducted and the femoral head reduced in the acetabulum

Clubfoot – Tx: serial casting

Bone tumors

Most common is metastatic disease (#1 breast, #2 prostate)
  Tx: internal fixation with impending fracture (> 50% cortical involvement); followed by XRT

Multiple myeloma – most common primary malignant tumor of bone
  Tx: chemotherapy for systemic disease; internal fixation for impending fractures

Pathologic fractures – treat with internal fixation
  XRT can be used for pain relief in patients with painful bony metastases

Osteogenic sarcoma – most common primary bone sarcoma, usually around the knee
  80% in patients <20 years
  X-ray: Codman's triangle → periosteal reaction
  Tx: limb-sparing resection; XRT and doxorubicin-based chemotherapy can be used preoperatively to increase chance of limb-sparing resection; also often given postoperatively

Benign bone tumors treated with curettage +/− bone graft – osteoid osteoma, endochondroma (may be able to observe), osteochondroma (resection only if cosmetic defect or causing symptoms), chondroblastoma, nonossifying fibroma (may be observed), fibrodysplasia

Giant cell tumor of bone – total resection +/− XRT (benign but 30% risk of recurrence; also has malignant degeneration risk)

Other orthopaedic conditions

Spondylolisthesis – formed by subluxation or slip if one vertebral body over another
  Most commonly occurs in lumbar region
  Most common cause of lumbar pain in adolescents (gymnasts)

Tx: depends on degree of subluxation and symptoms – ranges from conservative treatment to surgical fusion

Cervical stenosis – surgical decompression is significant myelopathy present
Lumbar stenosis – surgical decompression for cases refractory to medical treatment
Torus fracture – buckling of the metaphyseal cortex seen in children (i.e., distal radius)
Open fractures – need incision and drainage, antibiotics, fracture stabilization, soft tissue coverage

CHAPTER 43. PEDIATRIC SURGERY

Foregut – lungs, esophagus, stomach, pancreas, liver, gallbladder, bile duct, duodenum proximal to ampulla
Midgut – duodenum distal to ampulla, small bowel, large bowel to distal ⅓ of transverse colon
Hindgut – distal ⅓ of transverse colon to anal canal
Midgut rotates 270 degrees counterclockwise normally.

Low birthweight <2500 g; premature <37 weeks

Immunity at birth – **IgA** from mother's milk; **IgM** synthesized in child

#1 cause of childhood death – trauma
Trauma bolus – 20 cc/kg x 2, then give blood 10 cc/kg
Tachycardia – best indicator of shock (neonate >150; <1 year >120; rest >100)
Urine output 2–4 cc/kg/hr
Children (<6 months) have **25% GFR capacity of adults** – poor concentrating ability

↑ alkaline phosphatase in children compared to adults → **bone growth**
Umbilical vessels – 2 arteries and 1 vein

Maintenance intravenous fluids
4 cc/kg/hr for 1st 10 kg
2 cc/kg/hr for 2nd 10 kg
1 cc/kg/hr for everything after that

Caloric need

Age (yr)	Calories (kcal/day)
0–1	90–120
1–12	70–90
12–18	30–60

Congenital cystic disease of the lung
Pulmonary sequestration
Lung tissue has systemic arterial supply (aorta) and either systemic venous or pulmonary vein drainage
Can be **intralobar** (more likely pulmonary venous drainage) or **extralobar** (more likely systemic venous drainage)
Neither communicate with tracheobronchial tree
Most commonly present with infection; can also have respiratory compromise or an abnormal CXR
Tx: lobectomy
Congenital lobar overinflation (emphysema)
Cartilage fails to develop in bronchus, leading to air trapping with expiration.
Vascular supply and other lobes are normal (except compressed by hyperinflated lobe).
Can develop hemodynamic instability (same mechanism as tension PTX) or respiratory compromise
LUL or RML most commonly affected
Tx: lobectomy
Congenital cystic adenoid malformation
Communicates with airway
Alveolar structure is not well developed although lung tissue present.
Symptoms: respiratory compromise or recurrent infection
Tx: lobectomy
Bronchiogenic cyst
Extrapulmonary cysts formed from bronchial tissue and cartilage wall
Usually present with a mediastinal mass filled with milky liquid
Can compress adjacent structures or become infected
Occasionally are intrapulmonary
Tx: resect cyst

Mediastinal masses in children
Neurogenic tumors (neurofibroma, neuroganglionoma, neuroblastoma) – most common mediastinal tumor in children; usually located posteriorly
Respiratory symptoms, dysphagia – common to all mediastinal masses regardless of location
Anterior – T cell lymphoma, teratoma and other germ cell tumors (most common type of anterior mediastinal mass in children), thymoma, thyroid CA
Middle – T cell lymphoma, teratoma, cyst (cardiogenic or bronchiogenic)
Posterior – T cell lymphoma, neuroblastoma, neurogenic tumor

Choledochal cyst
Need to resect – risk of cholangiocarcinoma, pancreatitis, cholangitis, obstructive jaundice
Thought to be caused by **reflux of pancreatic enzymes** into the biliary system

Type	%	Description	Treatment
I	85%	Fusiform dilation of entire common bile duct, mildly dilated common hepatic duct, normal intrahepatic ducts	Resection, hepaticojejunostomy
II	3%	A true diverticulum that hangs off the common bile duct	Resection off common bile duct; may be able to preserve common bile duct and avoid hepaticojejunostomy
III	1%	Dilation of distal intramural common bile duct; involves sphincter of Oddi	Resection, choledochojejunostomy
IV	10%	Multiple cysts, both intrahepatic and extrahepatic	Resection; may need liver lobectomy
V	1%	Caroli's disease: intrahepatic cysts; get hepatic fibrosis; may be associated with congenital hepatic fibrosis and medullary sponge kidney	Resection; may need lobectomy

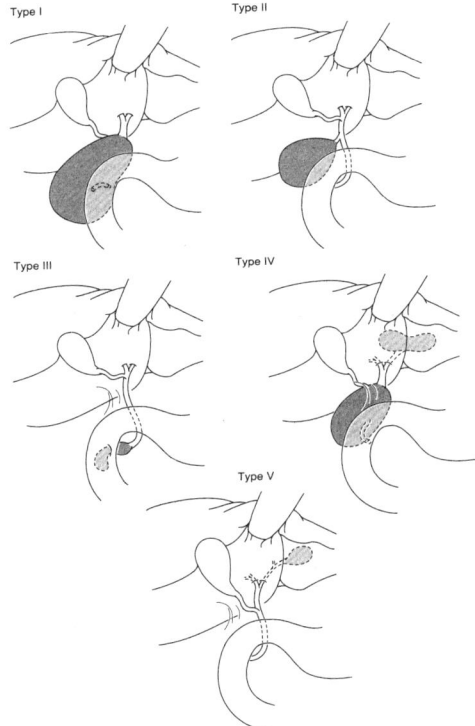

Choledochal cyst classification.

Lymphadenopathy
Usually acute suppurative adenitis associated with URI or pharyngitis
If fluctuant → FNA, culture and sensitivity, antibiotics; may need incision and drainage if it fails to resolve
- **Chronic causes** – cat scratch fever, atypical mycoplasma
- **Asymptomatic** – antibiotics for 10 days → excisional biopsy if no improvement
  - This is lymphoma until proved otherwise.
- **Cystic hygroma** (lymphangioma) – found in lateral cervical and submandibular regions in neck; get infected
  - Tx: resection

Diaphragmatic hernias
Overall survival 50%
Increased on **left side (80%)**; abdominal approach; can have severe **pulmonary HTN**
80% have associated anomalies (cardiac and neural tube defects mostly; malrotation)
Diagnosis can be made with prenatal ultrasound
Symptoms: respiratory distress
CXR – bowel in chest
Tx: high-frequency ventilation, may need ECMO, prostacyclin (pulmonary vasodilator).
- Stabilize these patients before operating on them
  - Need to reduce bowel and repair defect +/− mesh
Bochdalek's hernia – most common, located posteriorly
Morgagni's hernia – rare, located anteriorly
Eventration – failure of diaphragm to fuse

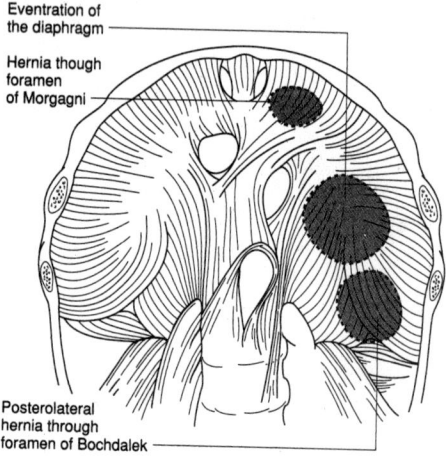

Locations of congenital diaphragmatic defects.

Pectus excavatum (sinks in) – sternal osteotomy, need strut; performed if causing respiratory symptoms or emotional stress
Pectus carinatum (pigeon chest) – strut not necessary; repair for emotional stress

Branchial cleft cyst
Lead to cysts, sinuses, and fistulas
- **1st branchial cleft cyst** – angle of mandible; may connect with external auditory canal
  - Often associated with facial nerve
- **2nd branchial cleft cyst (most common)** – on anterior border of SCM muscle
  - Goes through carotid bifurcation into tonsillar pillar
- **3rd branchial cleft cyst** – lateral neck
Tx for all cysts: resection

Chapter 43. Pediatric Surgery 223

Thyroglossal duct cyst
From the descent of the thyroid gland from the **foramen cecum**
May be only thyroid tissue patient has
Presents as a midline cervical mass
Tx: excision of **cyst, tract, and hyoid bone**

Hemangioma
Appears at birth or shortly after
Rapid growth during first 6–12 months of life, then begin to involute
Tx: **observation** – most resolve by age 7–8
If lesion has **uncontrollable growth, impairs function** (eyelid or ear canal), or is **persistent after age 8** → can treat with **steroids** → laser or resection if steroids not successful

Neuroblastoma
#1 solid abdominal malignancy in children
Usually presents as asymptomatic mass
Can have secretory diarrhea, raccoon eyes (orbital metastases), **HTN**, opsomyoclonus syndrome (unsteady gait)
Most often on **adrenals**; can occur anywhere along the sympathetic chain
Most common in **1st 2 years of life**
  Children <1 year have best prognosis.
Most have ↑ **catecholamines, VMA, HVA, and metanephrines**
Derived from **neural crest cells**
Encases vasculature rather than invades
Rare metastases – go to lung and bone

Abdominal x-ray: may show stippled calcifications in the tumor
NSE, LDH, HVA, diploid tumors, and N-myc – have worse prognosis
NSE ↑ in all patients with metastases
Tx: resection (30%–40% cured)
Initially unresectable tumors may be resectable after chemotherapy.

Staging of neuroblastoma

Stage	Description
I	Localized, complete
II	Incomplete excision but does not cross midline
III	Crosses midline +/– regional nodes
IV	Distant metastases (nodes or solid organ)
IV-S	Localized tumor with distant metastases

Wilms tumor (nephroblastoma)
Usually presents as asymptomatic mass; can have hematuria or HTN; 10% bilateral
Mean age at diagnosis – **3 years**
Prognosis based on tumor grade (anaplastic and sarcomatous variations have worse prognosis).
Frequent metastases to bone and lung
Can resect pulmonary metastases if resectable
May be associated with Beckwith-Wiedemann syndrome (hemihypertrophy, cryptorchidism, Drash syndrome, aniridia)
Abdominal CT – replacement of renal parenchyma and <u>not</u> displacement (as seen with neuroblastoma)

Tx: nephrectomy (80%–90% cured)
  If venous extension occurs in the renal vein, the tumor can be extracted from the vein.
  Need to examine the contralateral kidney and look for peritoneal implants
  Avoid rupture of tumor with resection, which will ↑ stage.
  All patients except stage I tumor weighing <500 g get **actinomycin and vincristine**.
  Patients with stage II tumor or greater or tumors >500 g get **actinomycin and vincristine plus doxorubicin**.
  Patients with stage III tumor or greater get **actinomycin, vincristine, and doxorubicin plus abdominal XRT**

Staging of Wilms tumor

Stage	Description
I	Limited to kidney, completely excised
II	Beyond kidney but completely excised
III	Residual nonhematogenous tumor
IV	Hematogenous metastases
V	Bilateral renal involvement

Hepatoblastoma
Most common malignant liver tumor in children; ↑ AFP in 90%
Fractures, precocious puberty (from beta-HCG release)
Better prognosis than hepatocellular CA
Associated with Beckwith-Wiedemann syndrome
Can be pedunculated; vascular invasion common; may develop areas of extramedullary hematopoiesis
Tx: resection optimal; otherwise doxorubicin- and cisplatin-based chemotherapy → may downstage tumors and make them resectable
Survival is primarily related to resectability.
Prefetal histology has best prognosis.

#1 children's malignancy overall – **leukemia (ALL)**
#1 solid tumor class – **CNS tumors**
#1 general surgery tumor – **neuroblastoma**
　#1 in child <2 years → **neuroblastoma**
　#1 in child >2 years → **Wilms tumor**
#1 cause of duodenal obstruction in newborns (<1 week) – **duodenal atresia**
#1 cause of duodenal obstruction after newborn period (>1 week) and overall – **malrotation**
#1 cause of colon obstruction – **Hirschsprung's disease**; some say constipation
#1 liver tumor in children – **hepatoblastoma**; ⅔ of liver tumors in children are malignant
#1 lung tumor in children – **carcinoid**
Painful lower GI bleeding – **#1 benign anorectal lesions** (fissures, etc)
Painless lower GI bleeding – **#1 Meckel's diverticulum**
Upper GI bleeding – 0–1 year → **gastritis, esophagitis**;
　1 year to adult → **esophageal varices, esophagitis**

Meckel's diverticulum
Found on **antimesenteric border** of small bowel
Embryology – **persistent vitelline duct**
Rule of 2s – 2 feet from ileocecal valve, 2% population, 2% symptomatic, 2 tissue types (pancreatic – most common; gastric – most likely to be symptomatic), 2 presentations (diverticulitis and bleeding)
#1 cause of painless lower GI bleeding in children
Can get Meckel's scan with pertechnetate if suspicious of Meckel's and having trouble locating
Tx: resection with symptoms, suspicion of gastric mucosa, or narrow neck

Pyloric stenosis
3–12 weeks, firstborn males
Projectile vomiting
Can feel olive mass in stomach
Get hypochloremic, hypokalemic metabolic alkalosis
Ultrasound – pylorus ≥4 mm thick, ≥14 mm long
Resuscitate with 10% dextrose before OR
Tx: pyloromyotomy

Intussusception
Usually 3 months to 3 years
Currant jelly stools (from vascular congestion, not an indication for resection), sausage mass, abdominal distention, RUQ pain, vomiting

Chapter 43. Pediatric Surgery

Invagination of one loop of intestine into another
Lead points in children – enlarged Peyer's patches (#1), lymphoma, Meckel's diverticulum
15% recurrence after reduction
Tx: reduce with air-contrast enema → 80% successful; no surgery required if reduced
    Max pressure with air-contrast enema – **120 mmHg**
    Max column height with barium enema – **1 meter (3 feet)**
    High perforation risk beyond these values → need to proceed to OR if you have reached these values
    Need to go to OR with peritonitis or free air, or if unable to reduce
        When reducing in OR, do not place traction on proximal limb of bowel; apply pressure to the distal limb
        Usually don't require resection unless associated with lead point (Meckel's, etc)
Adults presenting with intussusception – patient most likely has **malignant lead point** (i.e., colon CA in cecum) → OR

Intestinal atresias
Develop as a result of **intrauterine vascular accidents**
Symptoms: bilious emesis, distention; most do not pass meconium
More common in jejunum; can be multiple
    Tx: resection

Duodenal atresia
#1 cause of duodenal obstruction in newborns (<1 week)
Usually distal to ampulla of Vater and cause **bilious vomiting,** feeding intolerance
Associated with polyhydramnios in mother
Associated with cardiac, renal, and other GI anomalies
20% of these patients have **Down's syndrome**
Abdominal x-ray – shows **double-bubble sign**
Tx: resuscitation; duodenoduodenostomy or duodenojejunostomy

Tracheoesophageal (TE) fistulas
Type C – most common type (80%–90%)
    Proximal esophageal atresia (blind pouch) and distal TE fistula
        Symptoms: newborn spits up feeds, has excessive drooling, respiratory symptoms with feeding; can't place NG tube in stomach
Type A – second most common type (5%–10%)
    Esophageal atresia and no fistula
    Symptoms: similar to type C
    Abdominal x-ray – patients have gasless abdomen
Type E – most likely to present in adulthood (H configuration of esophagus and trachea), not associated with atresia
VACTERL = **v**ertebral, **a**norectal (imperforate anus), **c**ardiac, **T**E fistula, **r**adius/renal, and **l**imb anomalies
Tx: **right extrapleural thoracotomy** for most; perform primary repair
    Azygos vein often needs to be divided.
Infants that are premature, <2500 g, or sick → Replogle tube, treat respiratory symptoms; delay repair
Complications of repair – GERD, leak, empyema, stricture, fistula
Survival related to birthweight and associated anomalies.

Malrotation
Sudden onset of bilious vomiting (Ladd's bands cause duodenal obstruction, coming out from the right retroperitoneum)
Volvulus associated with compromise of the SMA, leading to infarction of the intestine
Failure of normal counterclockwise rotation (270°)
90% present by 1 year of age, 75% in the 1st month.
Any child with bilious vomiting needs an UGI to rule out malrotation.
Dx: UGI duodenum does not cross midline
Tx: resect Ladd's bands, counterclockwise rotation (may require multiple turns), cecum in LLQ (cecopexy), duodenum in RUQ, appendectomy

Meconium ileus
- Causes **distal ileal obstruction**, abdominal distention, bilious vomiting, and distended loops of bowel
- Need sweat chloride test or PCR for Cl channel defect
- Occurs in 10% of children with cystic fibrosis
- Abdominal x-ray: dilated loops of small bowel without air-fluid levels (because the meconium is too thick to separate from the bowel wall); can have ground-glass or soap suds appearance
- Can cause perforation, leading to meconium pseudocyst or free perforation → require laparotomy
- Tx: **Gastrografin enema** (effective in 80%); can also make the diagnosis and potentially treat the patient
- Can also use N-acetylcysteine enema
    - If surgery required, manual decompression and create a vent for **N-acetylcysteine antegrade enemas**

Necrotizing enterocolitis (NEC)
- Classically presents with bloody stools after 1st feeding in **premature infant (occurs in neonates)**
- Risk factors: prematurity, hypoxia, hypotension, anemia, polycythemia, sepsis
- Symptoms: lethargy, respiratory decompensation, abdominal distention, vomiting, blood per rectum
- Abdominal x-ray: may show pneumatosis intestinalis, free air, or portal vein air
- Initial Tx: resuscitation, NPO, antibiotics, TPN, orogastric tube
- Indications for operation: free air, peritonitis, clinical deterioration → resect dead bowel and bring up ostomies
- Need barium contrast enema before taking down ostomies to rule out distal obstruction from stenosis
- Mortality 10%

Congenital vascular malformation
- Surgery for hemorrhage, ischemia, CHF, nonbleeding ulcers, functional impairment, limb-length discrepancy
- Tx: embolization (may be sufficient on its own) and resection

Imperforate anus
- More common in males
- Need to check for associated anomalies such as renal, cardiac, and vertebral (VACTERL)
- **High (above levators)** – meconium in **urine or vagina** (fistula to bladder/vagina/prostatic urethra)
    - Tx: colostomy, later anal reconstruction with posterior sagittal anoplasty
- **Low (below levators)** – perform **posterior sagittal anoplasty** (pull anus down into sphincter mechanism); **no colostomy needed**
- Need postop anal dilatation to avoid stricture; these patients are prone to constipation

Gastroschisis
- **Intrauterine rupture of umbilical vein; does not have a peritoneal sac**
- ↓ congenital anomalies (only 10%) except malrotation
- To the right of midline, no peritoneal sac, stiff bowel from exposure to amniotic fluid
- Tx: initially place saline-soaked gauzes and resuscitate the patient; can lose a lot of fluid from the exposed bowel
    - Repair when patient is stable.
    - At operation, try place bowel back in abdomen, may need Vicryl mesh silo.
    - Primary closure at a later date if mesh used

Omphalocele
- **Failure of embryonal development**; midline defect
- ↑ congenital anomalies (50%); has peritoneal sac with cord attached
- Sac can contain intra-abdominal structures other than bowel (liver, spleen, etc)

Cantrell pentalogy
Cardiac defects
Pericardium defects (usually at diaphragmatic pericardium)
Sternal cleft or absence of lower sternum
Diaphragmatic septum transversum absence
Omphalocele

Tx: initially place saline soaked gauzes and resuscitate the patient; can lose a lot of fluid from the exposed bowel
  Repair when patient is stable.
    At operation, try place bowel back in abdomen; may need Vicryl mesh silo.
    Primary closure at a later date of mesh used
Worse overall prognosis compared with gastroschisis secondary to congenital anomalies
Malrotation can occur with both gastroschisis and omphalocele.

Hirschsprung's disease
1 cause of colonic obstruction in infants; more common in males
Most common sign → infants fail to pass meconium in 1st 24 hours
  Can also present in older age groups as chronic constipation (age 2–3)
Get distention, some get colitis
Can get explosive release of watery stool with anorectal exam
Barium enema can be normal, although often shows a spastic distal segment and dilated proximal segment
Rectal biopsy diagnostic (**absence of ganglion cells in myenteric plexus**)
Is due to failure of the neural crest cells (ganglion cells) to progress in craniocaudal direction
Need to resect colon until proximal to where ganglion cells appear
Tx: may need to bring up a colostomy initially, eventually connect the colon to the anus (Soave or Duhamel procedure)

Hirschsprung's colitis – may be rapidly progressive; manifested by abdominal distension and foul smelling diarrhea
  Lethargy and signs of sepsis may be present.
Tx: rectal irrigation; may need emergency colectomy

Hydrocele
Most disappear by 1 year; noncommunicating will resolve; should transilluminate
Tx: surgery at 1 year if not resolved or if thought to be communicating (waxing and waning size)

Umbilical hernia
Failure of closure of linea alba; most close by age 3
Increased in African-Americans and premature infants
Tx: surgery if not closed by age 5 or incarceration or if patient has a VP shunt

Inguinal hernia
Due to persistent processus vaginalis; 3% of infants, M > F
Right in 60%, left in 30%, bilateral in 10%
Extension of the hernia into the internal ring differentiates hernia from hydrocele
Tx: emergent operation if not able to reduce; otherwise elective repair with high ligation
Explore the contralateral side if left sided, female, or child <1 year

Cystic duplication
Most common in ileum; often on mesenteric border
Tx: resect cyst

Biliary atresia
Most common cause of neonatal jaundice requiring surgery
Jaundice persisting >2 weeks after birth suggests atresia
Can involve either the extrahepatic or intrahepatic biliary tree or both

Progressive jaundice
Dx: liver biopsy → periportal fibrosis, bile plugging, eventual cirrhosis
    Ultrasound and cholangiography can reveal atretic biliary tree
Get cholangitis, continued cirrhosis, eventual hepatic failure
Try Kasai procedure (hepaticoportojejunostomy) – ⅓ get better, ⅓ go on to liver transplant, ⅓ die
Need to perform Kasai procedure **before age 3 months**, o/w get irreversible liver damage

Osteosarcoma
Can get pulmonary metastases
Tx: resection of primary and pulmonary metastases if isolated

Teratoma
↑ AFP and beta-HCG
Neonates – sacrococcygeal; adolescents – ovarian
Tx: excision
Sacrococcygeal teratomas
    90% benign at birth (almost all have exophytic component)
    Great potential for malignancy
    AFP – good marker
    2-month mark is a huge transition – <2 months → 90% benign; >2 months → 90% malignant
Tx: coccygectomy and long-term follow-up

Undescended testicles
Wait until 2 years old to treat.
Higher risk of testicular CA in these children
Cancer risk stays the same even if testicles brought into scrotum.
Get **seminoma**
If undescended bilaterally, get chromosomal studies
Tx: orchiopexy through inguinal incision; if not able to get testicles down → close and wait 6 months and try again; if won't come down, perform division of spermatic vessels

Prune belly syndrome (rare) – hypoplasia of the abdominal wall, urinary tract abnormalities with dilated urinary system, and bilateral cryptorchidism

Laryngomalacia
Most common cause of airway obstruction in infants
Symptoms: intermittent respiratory distress and stridor exacerbation in the supine position
Caused by immature epiglottis cartilage with intermittent collapse of the epiglottis airway
Most children outgrow this by 12 months
Surgical tracheostomy reserved for a small number of patients

Choanal atresia
Obstruction of choanal opening by either bone or mucus membrane, usually unilateral
Symptoms: intermittent respiratory distress, poor suckling
Tx: surgical correction

Laryngeal papillomatosis
Most common tumor of the pediatric larynx
Frequently involutes after puberty
Can treat with endoscopic removal or laser but frequently come back
Thought to be caused from HPV in the mother during passage through the birth canal

Cerebral palsy
Many develop GERD

CHAPTER 44. STATISTICS

Type I error – rejects null hypothesis incorrectly → falsely assumed there was a difference when no difference exists
Type II error – accepts null hypothesis incorrectly because of **small sample size** → the treatments are interpreted as equal when there is actually a difference
Null hypothesis – hypothesis that no difference exists between groups
    $p < 0.05$ rejects the null hypothesis
$p < 0.05$ = >95% likelihood that the difference between the populations is true
    <5% likelihood that the difference is not true and occurred by chance alone
95% confidence interval – if it includes the value 1, it is <u>not</u> statistically significant
    The farther away from 1, the stronger the correlation (i.e., CI of 9–10 or 0.1–0.2 has stronger correlation than CI of 2–3 or 0.8–0.9)

Variance – spread of data around a mean
Parameter – population
Numeric terms – example: 2, 7, 7, 8, 9, 11, 15
    Mode – most frequently occurring value = 7
    Mean – average = 9
    Median – middle value of a set of data (50th percentile) = 8

Trials and studies
    Randomized controlled trial – prospective study with random assignment to treatment and nontreatment groups
        Avoids treatment biases
    Double-blind controlled trial – prospective study in which patient and doctor are blind to the treatment
        Avoids observational biases
    Cohort study – prospective study → compares disease rate between exposed and unexposed groups (nonrandom assignment)
    Case–control study – retrospective study in which those who have the disease are compared with a similar population who do not have the disease; the frequency of the suspected risk factor is then compared between the two groups
    Meta-analysis – combining data from <u>different studies</u>

Quantitative variables
    Student's t test – two independent groups and variable is **quantitative** → compares means (mean weight between two groups)
    Paired t tests – variable is **quantitative**; before and after studies (e.g., weight before and after, drug vs placebo)
    ANOVA – compares **quantitative** variables (means) for more than 2 groups

Qualitative variables
    Nonparametric statistics – compare categorical (qualitative) variables **(race, sex, medical problems and diseases, medications)**
    Chi-squared test – compares two groups with **categorical (qualitative) variables** (number of obese patients with and without diabetes vs number of nonobese patients with and without diabetes)
    Kaplan-Meyer – small groups → estimates survival

Relative risk = incidence in exposed/incidence in unexposed
Power of test = probability of making the correct conclusion = 1 – probability of type I error.
    Likelihood that the conclusion of the test is true
    Larger sample size increases power of a test

Prevalence – number of people with disease in a population (e.g., number of patients in US with colon CA)
    Longstanding diseases increases prevalence.
Incidence – number of new cases diagnosed over a certain time frame in a population (e.g., number of patients in US newly diagnosed with colon CA in 2003)

	Positive Test	Negative Test
Have disease	True-positive (TP)	False-negative (FN)
No disease	False-positive (FP)	True-negative (TN)

Sensitivity – ability to detect disease = true-positives/(true-positives + false-negatives)
    Indicates the number of people who have the disease who test positive
    With high sensitivity, a <u>negative test result means patient is very unlikely to have disease</u>.
Specificity – ability to state no disease is present = true-negatives/(true-negatives + false-positives)
    Indicates the number of people who do not have the disease who test negative
    With high specificity, a <u>positive test result means patient is very likely to have disease</u>.

Positive predictive value = true-positives/(true-positives + false-positives)
    Likelihood that with a positive result, the patient actually has the disease
Negative predictive value = true-negatives/(true-negatives + false-negatives)
    Likelihood that with a negative result the patient does not have the disease

Accuracy = true-positives + true-negatives/true-positives + true-negatives + false-positives + false-negatives

Predictive value – depends on disease prevalence
Sensitivity and specificity – independent of prevalence

Appendix. COMMON ABBREVIATIONS AND EPONYMS

↑	increased or high
↓	decreased or low
2,3-DPG	2,3-diphosphoglycerate
5FU	5-fluorouracil
AAA	abdominal aortic aneurysm
Ab	antibody
Abd	abdominal
abx	antibiotic
AC	doxorubicin (Adriamycin) and cyclophosphamide (Cytoxan)
ACE	angiotensin converting enzyme
Ach	acetylcholine
ACT	activated clotting time
ACTH	adrenocorticotropic hormone
AD	autosomal dominant
ADH	antidiuretic hormone
ADL	activities of daily living
AFP	alpha-fetoprotein
Ag	antigen
AIDS	acquired immunodeficiency syndrome
AKA	above knee amputation
ALL	acute lymphoblastic leukemia
ALND	axillary lymph node dissection
ALT	alanine aminotransferase
angio	angiography
ANOVA	analysis of variance
AP	aortopulmonary
APACHE	acute physiology and chronic health evaluation
APR	abdominoperineal resection
APUD	amine precursor uptake and decarboxylation
ARDS	acute/adult respiratory distress syndrome
ASA	acetylsalicylic acid
ASD	atrial septal defect
AST	aspartate aminotransferase
ATGAM	antithymocyte gamma globulin
AT-III	antithrombin III
ATN	acute tubular necrosis
ATP	adenosine triphosphate
ATPase	adenosine triphosphatase
A-V	arteriovenous
AV	atrioventricular
AVM	arteriovenous malformation
AVN	avascular necrosis
AXR	abdominal radiograph
BCG	bacille Calmette-Guérin
BKA	below-knee amputation
BM	bowel movement
BPH	benign prostatic hyperplasia
BSA	body surface area
BT shunt	Blalock-Taussig shunt
BUN	blood urea nitrogen
Bx	biopsy
Ca	calcium
CA	cancer, carcinoma
CABG	coronary artery bypass graft
cAMP	cyclic adenosine monophosphate
CaO_2	arterial oxygen content
CBD	common bile duct
CCK	cholecystokinin
cCMP	3',5'-cyclic monophosphate (cytidine)
CD	cluster of differentiation (e.g., CD4, CD8)
CEA	carcinoembryonic antigen
CEA	carotid endarterectomy
cGMP	cyclic guanosine 3,5'-monophosphate
chemo	chemotherapy
CHF	chronic heart failure
CI	cardiac index
CLL	chronic lymphocytic leukemia
CMF	cyclophosphamide (Cytoxan), methotrexate, and 5-fluorouracil
CML	chronic myelogenous leukemia
CMV	cytomegalovirus
CN	cranial nerve
CNS	central nervous system
CO	cardiac output
COPD	chronic obstructive pulmonary disease
CPAP	continuous positive airway pressure
CPP	cerebral perfusion pressure
CPR	cardiopulmonary resuscitation
Cr	creatinine
CRH	corticotropin (ACTH)-releasing hormone
CSA	cyclosporin A
CSF	cerebrospinal fluid
CT	computed tomography
CVA	cerebrovascular accident (stroke)
CVHD	continuous venovenous hemodialysis
CvO_2	venous oxygen content
CVP	central venous pressure
Cx	complication
CXR	chest radiograph
D/C	discontinue
DAG	diacylglycerol
DBP	diastolic blood pressure
DCIS	ductal carcinoma in situ
DDAVP	desmopressin acetate, 1-desamino-8-d-arginine-vasopressin
DES	diethylstilbestrol
DIC	disseminated intravascular coagulation
DIT	diiodotyrosine
DKA	diabetic ketoacidosis
DLCO	diffusing capacity of the lung for carbon monoxide
DM	diabetes mellitus
DPL	diagnostic peritoneal lavage
DVT	deep venous thrombosis
Dx	diagnosis
DZ	disease
EBV	Epstein-Barr virus

ECA	external carotid artery	GSH	glutathione
ECHO	echocardiogram	GU	genitourinary
ECMO	extracorporeal membrane oxygenation	H and P	history and physical
		HA	headache
EDRF	endothelium-derived relaxing factor	HBIG	hepatitis B immunoglobulin
		HBV	hepatitis B virus
EDV	end diastolic volume	HCG	human chorionic gonadotropin
EEG	electroencephalogram	HCl	hydrochloric acid; hydrochloride
EF	ejection fraction		
EGD	esophagogastroduodenoscopy	Hct	hematocrit
EGF	epidermal growth factor	HCT	hematocrit
EKG	electrocardiogram	HCV	hepatitis C virus
ELAM	endothelial leukocyte adhesion molecule	HETE	hydroxyeicosatetraenoic acid
		HGB/Hgb	hemoglobin
EPI	epinephrine	HIDA	hepatic iminodiacetic acid
ER	emergency room or endoplasmic reticulum	HIT	heparin-induced thrombocytopenia
ERCP	endoscopic retrograde cholangiopancreatography	HIV	human immunodeficiency virus
		HLA	human leukocyte antigen
ERV	expiratory reserve volume	HMG-CoA	β-hydroxy-β-methylglutaryl-CoA
ESR	erythrocyte sedimentation rate		
ESWL	extracorporeal shock wave lithotripsy	HMW	high molecular weight
		HPETE	hydroperoxyeicosatetraenoic acid
ET	endotracheal		
$ETCO_2$	end tidal CO_2	HPF	high-power field
ETOH	ethanol, alcohol	HPV	human papillomavirus
F/U	follow-up	HR	heart rate
FAP	familial adenomatous polyposis	HSV	herpes simplex virus
		HTLV-1	human T-cell leukemia virus 1
FAST	focused abdominal sonography for trauma	HTN	hypertension
		HUS	hemolytic uremic syndrome
Fc	antibody fragment, crystallizable	HVA	homovanillic acid
		IABP	intra-aortic balloon pump
FEV_1	forced expiratory volume in 1 second	IBW	ideal body weight
		ICA	internal corotid artery
FFP	fresh frozen plasma	ICAM	intracellular adhesion molecule
FGF	fibroblastic growth factor	ICP	intracranial pressure
FiO_2	fraction of inspired oxygen	ICU	intensive care unit
FNA	fine needle aspiration	Ig	immunoglobulin
FRC	functional residual capacity	IJ	internal jugular vein
FSH	follicle stimulating hormone	IL	interleukin
FTSG	full-thickness skin graft	IMA	inferior mesenteric artery or internal mammary artery
FTT	failure to thrive		
Fx	fracture	IMF	intermaxillary fixation
G6PD	glucose-6-phosphate dehydrogenase	IMV	inferior mesenteric vein
		INF	interferon
GCS	Glasgow Coma Scale	INH	isoniazid
GCSF	granulocyte colony–stimulating factor	INR	International Normalized Ratio
		ITP	idiopathic thrombocytopenic purpura
GDA	gastroduodenal artery		
GERD	gastroesophageal reflux disease	IV	intravenous
		IVC	inferior vena cava
GFR	glomerular filtration rate	IVF	intravenous fluid
GH	growth hormone	IVP	intravenous pyelogram
GHRH	growth hormone-releasing hormone	L	liter
		LA	left atrium
GI	gastrointestinal	LAD	left anterior descending (coronary artery)
GIP	gastric inhibitory peptide		
GIST	gastrointestinal stromal tumors	LAK	lymphokine-activated killer
GNR	gram-negative rods	LATS	long acting thyroid stimulator
GnRH	gonadotropin-releasing hormone	LAR	low anterior resection
		LCIS	lobular carcinoma in situ
GPC	gram-positive cocci	LD_{50}	dose that will kill 50% of test subjects
GPR	gram-positive rod		
GRP	gastrin-releasing peptide	LDH	lactate dehydrogenase

Appendix. Common Abbreviations and Eponyms

LES	lower esophageal sphincter	OCP	oral contraceptive pills
LFT	liver function test	OKT3	murine monoclonal anti-CD3 antibody therapy
LH	luteotropic hormone		
LHRH	luteinizing hormone–releasing hormone	Op-DDD	2,4′-dichlorodiphenyl-dichloroethane (mitotane)
LLQ	left lower quadrant	OR	operating room
LR	lactated ringers	ORIF	open reduction and internal fixation
LS ratio	lecithin:sphingomyelin ratio		
LTA_4	leukotriene A4	PA	pulmonary artery
LTB_4	leukotriene B4	PABA	p-aminobenzoic acid
LTC_4	leukotriene C4	PADP	pulmonary artery diastolic pressure
LTD_4	leukotriene D4		
LTE_4	leukotriene E4	PAF	platelet activating factor
LV	left ventricle or left ventricular	PAS	periodic acid–Schiff stain
LVEDV	left ventricular end-diastolic volume	PCN	penicillin
		PCR	polymerase chain
LVEF	left ventricular ejection fraction	PDA	patent ductus arteriosum
LVESV	left ventricular end-systolic volume	PDGF	platelet-derived growth factor
		PE	pulmonary embolism
LVOT	left ventricular outflow tract	PECAM	platelet/endothelial cell adhesion molecule
MAC	minimum alveolar concentration	PEEP	positive end-expiratory pressure
MALT	mucosal-associated lympho-proliferative tissue	PEG	percutaneous endoscopic gastrostomy
MAO	monoamine oxidase		
MAOI	monoamine oxidase inhibitor	PGD_2	prostaglandin D_2
MAP	mean arterial pressure	PGE_1	prostaglandin E_1
MEN	multiple endocrine neoplasia	PGE_2	prostaglandin E_2
MHC	major histocompatibility complex	PGF_2	prostaglandin F_2
		PGG_2	prostaglandin G_2
MI	myocardial infarction	PGH_2	prostaglandin H_2
MIBG	radioactive iodine meta-idobenzoguanidine	PGI_2	prostaglandin I_2 (prostacyclin)
		PMHx	past medical history
MIT	monoiodotyrosine	PMN	polymorphonuclear leukocytes
MRA	magnetic resonance angiogram	PNMT	phenylethanolamine-N-methyl-transferase
MRCP	magnetic resonance cholangiopancreatography	POD	postoperative day
		PNA	pneumonia
MRM	modified radical mastectomy	PPN	peripheral line parenteral nutrition
MRND	modified radical neck dissection		
		PRBC	packed red blood cells
MRSA	methicillin-resistant S. aureus	PSA	prostate-specific antigen
MS	mental status	PSSS	postsplenectomy sepsis syndrome
MSH	melanocyte-stimulating hormone		
		PT	prothrombin time
MTP	metatarsophalangeal	PTA	percutaneous transluminal angioplasty
MTX	methotrexate		
N/V	nausea and vomiting	PTC	percutaneous transhepatic cholangiography
NADH	nicotinamide adenine dinucleotide		
		PTCA	percutaneous transluminal coronary angioplasty
NADPH	nicotinamide adenine dinucleotide phosphate		
		PTFE	polytetrafluoroethylene
NAPA	n-acetylprocainamide	PTH	parathyroid hormone
NE	norepinephrine	PTHrP	parathyroid hormone-related peptide
NEC	necrotizing enterocolitis		
NGT	nasogastric tube	PTT	partial thromboplastin time
NHL	non-Hodgkin's lymphoma	PTU	propylthiouracil
NIF	negative inspiratory force	PTX	pneumothorax
NO	nitric oxide	PUD	peptic ulcer disease
NPO	nil per os (nothing by mouth)	PVC	premature ventricular contraction
NS	normal saline (solution)		
NSAID	nonsteroidal anti-inflammatory drug	PVR	pulmonary vascular resistance
		Qp/Qs	pulmonary-to-systemic flow ratio
NSE	neuron-specific enolase		
NTG	nitroglycerine	R/O	rule out

RA	right atrium	TMJ	temporomandibular joint
RBC	red blood cell	TNF	tumor necrosis factor
RLL	right lower lobe	TOS	thoracic outlet syndrome
RLN	recurrent laryngeal nerve	tPA	tissue plasminogen activator
RND	radical neck dissection	TPN	total parenteral nutrition
ROM	range of motion	TRALI	transfusion-related acute lung injury
RPR	rapid plasma reagin		
RQ	respiratory quotient	TRAM	transverse rectus abdominis myocutaneous
RR	respiratory rate		
RUG	retrograde urethrogram	TRH	thyrotropin-releasing hormone
RUL	right upper lobe	TSH	thyroid-stimulating hormone
RUQ	right upper quadrant	TSI	thyroid-stimulating immunoglobulin
RV	residual volume		
RV	right ventricle	TTP	thrombotic thrombocytopenic purpura
S/E	side effect		
S-B	Sengstaken-Blakemore (tube)	TURP	transurethral resection of the prostate; transurethral prostatectomy
SBFT	small bowel follow-through		
SBO	small bowel obstruction		
SBP	spontaneous bacterial peritonitis	TV	tidal volume
		Tx	treatment
SBP	systolic blood pressure	TXA_2	thromboxane A_2
SCC	squamous cell carcinoma	TXP	transplant
SCD	sequential compression device	U/S	ultrasound
SCM	sternocleidomastoid	UC	ulcerative colitis
SCV	subclavian	UDCA	ursodeoxycholic acid
SFA	superficial femoral artery	UES	upper esophageal sphincter
SIRS	systemic inflammatory response syndrome	UGI	upper gastrointestinal
		URI	upper respiratory tract infection
SLE	systemic lupus erythematosus	UTI	urinary tract infection
SMA	superior mesenteric artery	UV	ultraviolet
SMV	superior mesenteric vein	V/Q	ventilation/perfusion
SOB	shortness of breath	VC	vital capacity
STSG	split-thickness skin graft	VCAM	vascular cell adhesion molecule
SVC	superior vena cava		
SvO_2	mixed venous oxygen saturation	V-fib	ventricular fibrillation
		VIP	vasoactive intestinal peptide
SVR	systemic vascular resistance	VIPoma	vasoactive intestinal peptide–producing tumor
SVRI	systemic vascular resistance index		
		VLDL	very-low-density lipids
SVT	supraventricular tachycardia	VMA	vanillylmandelic acid
Sx	symptom	VO_2	oxygen consumption
T bili	total bilirubin	VP-16	etoposide
TAG	triacylglyceride	VRE	vancomycin-resistant *Enterococcus*
TAH	total abdominal hysterectomy		
TB	tuberculosis	VSD	ventricular septal defect
TBG	thyroid-binding globulin	V-tach	ventricular tachycardia
TCOM	transcutaneous oxygen measurement	vWD	von Willebrand's disease
		vWF	von Willebrand factor
TCR	T-cell receptor	W/U	work-up
TE	tracheoesophageal	WBC	white blood cell
TEN	toxic epidermal necrolysis	WDHA	watery diarrhea, hypokalemia, achlorhydria
TFT	thyroid function test		
TGF-beta	transforming growth factor-beta	wedge	pulmonary artery wedge pressure
TIA	transient ischemic attack		
TIPS	transjugular intrahepatic portosystemic shunt	WLE	wide local excision
		XRT	radiation therapy
TLC	total lung capacity	Z-E/ZES	Zollinger-Ellison syndrome

INDEX

Abdominal abscess, 13
Abdominal aortic disease, 120–122
Abdominal compartment syndrome, 49
Abdominal surgery, fluid loss, 26
Abdominoperineal resection, colorectal cancer, 187
ABO incompatibility, 9
Abortion, 206
Abscess
    abdominal, 13
    amebic, 156
    anorectal, 194
    breast, 97
    echinococcal, 157
    head and neck, 80
    hepatic, 156–157
    lung, 108
    pyogenic, 157
Acalculous cholecystitis, 161
Access grafts, 130
Accessory spleen, 172
Accuracy, 230
Acetylsalicylic acid (ASA), 6
    poisoning, 21
Achalasia, 138
Acid–base balance, 28t
Acid burn, 69
Acoustic neuroma, 79
Acquired hypercoagulability, 7
Acquired thrombocytopenia, 6
Acral lentigos melanoma, 73
Acromegaly, 2
Acromioclavicular separation, 216
ACTH, ectopic, 85
Actinic keratosis, 76
Actinomyces, 14
    large bowel, 191
Activated clotting time (ACT), 5
Acute phase response proteins, 43
Acyclovir, 19
Addison's disease, 84
Adenocarcinoma
    anal, 195
    esophageal, 140
    gallbladder, 162–163
    metaplastic, breast, 102
    pancreatic, 168–169
    small bowel, 179
Adenohypophysis, 82
Adenoid cystic carcinoma
    breast, 102
    salivary gland, 79
Adenoma
    adrenocortical, 83, 85
    bronchial, 107
    hepatic, 157
    parathyroid, 94
    pituitary, 82, 84, 213
    salivary gland, 79
    small bowel, 179
    thyroid, 91
    tubular, 185
    villous, 185
Adenomyomatosis, 164
Adenosine, 21
Adnexal torsion, 209
Adrenal disorders, 83–86
    adrenal cortex, 83–85
    adrenal medulla, 85–86
    mass lesions, 83
Adrenalectomy, 85
Adrenal insufficiency, 84
    shock, 63
Adrenocortical carcinoma, 85
Adson's test, 126
Adventitial cystic disease, lower extremity, 124
Afferent-loop obstruction, 150
Air emboli, 64
Albumin
    half-life, 29
    normal level, 29
Alcohol withdrawal, 67
Alkali burn, 69
Alkaline reflux gastritis, 149
Alkylating agents, 35
Alpha-2 antiplasmin, 5
Amaurosis fugax, 117
Ameloblastoma, 80
Amino acids, 33
Aminocaproic acid, 8
Aminoglutethimide, 21
Aminoglycosides, 18
    renal toxicity, 67
Amebic abscess, 156
Amebic colitis, 191
Amphotericin, 19
Amputation, lower extremity, 124
Amsterdam criteria, 188
Anaerobes, 13
Anal canal, lymphatic drainage, 197f
Anal fissure, 194
Anal incontinence, 195
Anaphylatoxins, 44
Anaphylaxis, transfusion-related, 9
Anaplastic thyroid cancer, 92
Ancrod, 8
Anesthesia
    complications, 24–25
    epidural, 24
    spinal, 24
Anesthetics, 22–25
    benzodiazepines, 24
    complications, 24–25
    induction agents, 22
    inhalational agents, 22
    local anesthetics, 23
    muscle relaxants, 22–23
    narcotics, 23–24
Aneurysms
    aortic, 118–119, 120
    cerebral, 211

Aneurysms (*contd.*)
    femoral, 128
    iliac, 128
    left ventricle, 113
    popliteal, 128
    renal, 128
    splenic artery, 128, 174
    visceral, 128
Angina, chronic mesenteric, 128
Angiodysplasia, colonic, 193
Angiofibroma, nasopharyngeal, 78
Angiogenesis factors, 42
Angiomyolipoma, renal, 203
Angiotensin-converting enzyme (ACE), 21
Angiotensin II, 66
Anion gap, 27
Anion gap acidosis, 27
Ankle-brachial index, 123
Ankle fracture, 217
Annular pancreas, 166
Anomalous pulmonary venous return, 113
Anorectum, 194–197
    abscess, 194
    anatomy, 182f
    arterial blood supply, 183f
    cancer, 195–196
    condylomata acuminata, 194
    fistula in ano, 195
    imperforate anus, 226
Anorexia, 134
ANOVA, 229
Anterior cruciate ligament injury, 217
Anterior spinal artery syndrome, 213
Antibiotics, 17–19. *See also specific drugs*
    mechanism of action, 17
    resistance to, 17
    for specific organisms, 19
Antibodies, 12
Anticoagulant agents, 8
Anticoagulation, 5
Antidiuretic hormone, 66, 211
Antifibrinolytic agents, 8
Antifungal agents, 19
Antigens
    processing and presentation, 11f
    T- and B-cell activation, 10f
Antioxidants, cellular defenses, 45t
Antiplatelet antibodies, 9
Antiseptics, 17
Antithrombin III, 5
Antithrombin III deficiency, 7
Antituberculosis agents, 19
Antiviral agents, 19
Aorta
    abdominal, 120–122
    coarctation, 113
    thoracic, 118–120
Aortic aneurysm
    abdominal, 120–121
    inflammatory, 121
    mycotic, 121
    thoracic, 118
    thoracoabdominal, 119
Aortic arch aneurysm, 119
Aortic dissection, 119–120

Aortic graft
    infections, 121
    stented tube grafts, 122
Aortic insufficiency, 115, 120
Aortic stenosis, 114–115, 193
Aortic transection, thoracic, 54, 118
Aortoenteric fistula, 121
Aortoiliac occlusive disease, 123
Apnea test, 67
Appendicitis, 180
Appendix, 180
    carcinoid, 179
Aprotinin, 8
ARDS (acute respiratory distress syndrome), 65
Argon beam, 201
Arsenical keratosis, 76
Arteriovenous fistula, acquired, 130
Arteriovenous malformation, 211
Arteriovenous malformations, 110
Arteritis, immune, 129
Arthritis, septic, 16
Asbestos exposure, 107
Ascites, 154
Aspiration, 54, 66
    fine-needle, 88
Atelectasis, 66
ATGAM, 37
Atheroma embolism, 125
Atherosclerosis, 116
Atrial natriuretic peptide, 66
Atrial septal defect, 112
Atropine, 21
    in anesthesia, 23
Auerbach's plexus, 184
Augmentin, 17
Autografts, burn wound, 69
Axillary lymph nodes
    anatomic classification, 100
    dissection, 103
Axillary nerve, 215
Axonotmesis, 210
Azathioprine, 37

Bacterial infection, immunology, 11
Bacterial peritonitis, 15
    spontaneous, 155
Bacterial thyroiditis, 90
Bacterial translocation, 30
Bacteroides fragilis, surgical wound infection, 13
Bactrim, 18
Barrett's esophagus, 139
Basal cell carcinoma
    anal, 196
    skin, 74
Basophils, 12, 42
Bassini repair, 198
Batson's plexus, 97
Battle's sign, 51
B cell lymphoma, anorectum, 195
B cells, 10
Benign prostatic hypertrophy, 204
Benzodiazepines, 24
Bernard-Soulier disease, 6

Beta-blockers, 21
Beta-HCG, 206
Beta-2 integrins, 43
Beta thalassemia, 174
Bile, 153
    composition, 159t
    excretion, 159
    functions, 159
Bile acids, 153, 176
    synthesis, 160
Bile salts, 176
Biliary atresia, 228
Biliary tract, 159–164
    anatomy and physiology, 159
    cholangiocarcinoma, 163
    cholesterol and bile acid synthesis, 160
    common bile duct injury, 57, 162
    cysts, 163
    disorders, 160–164
    gallstones, 160
    primary biliary cirrhosis, 164
    primary sclerosing cholangitis, 163–164
    stenosis, 168
    strictures, 162, 168
Bilirubin, 153
    delta, 164
Billroth I, 143
Billroth II, 143
Bioavailability, 20
Biopsy
    sentinel lymph node, 36, 103
    soft tissue sarcoma, 75
Bird's beak sign, 189
Bite wounds, 16
Bladder
    neurogenic, 204
    trauma, 60
Bladder cancer, 204
Bleeding disorders, 5–7
Blind-loop syndrome, 150
Blood products, 9
Blowout fracture, orbit, 52
Blue toe syndrome, 125
Blunt injury, 49
Bochdalek's hernia, 222
Body water, total, 26
Body weight, ideal, 29
Boerhaave's syndrome, 141
Bombesin, 134
Bone healing, 215
Bone tumors, 218
    sarcoma, 75
Bowditch effect, 62
Bowen's disease, 76
    anal, 196
Brachial cleft cyst, pediatric, 222
Brachial plexus
    irritation, 126–127
    terminal branches, 215
Bradykinin, 42
Brain, arterial blood supply, 117f
Brain death, 67
Brain tumors, 213

Breast
    anatomy and physiology, 97
    benign disease, 97–99
    mass lesion, in pregnancy, 104
    nipple discharge, 98–99
Breast cancer, 99–104
    benign conditions mimicking, 104
    bone metastases, 96
    chemotherapy, 103–104
    ductal, 102
    ductal carcinoma in situ, 99
    inflammatory, 102
    lobular, 102
    lobular carcinoma in situ, 99
    male, 102
    radiotherapy, 103
    risk factors, 101
    screening, 100
    staging, 101
    surgical management, 102–103
Broca's area, 213
Bronchial adenoma, 107
Bronchiectasis, 110
Bronchioalveolar carcinoma, 107
Bronchiogenic cyst, 220
Bronchogenic cysts, 109
Brown recluse spider, 16
Brown-Sequard syndrome, 213
Brunner's glands, 143, 176
Budd-Chiari syndrome, 156
Buerger's disease, 129
Burns, 68–71
    admission criteria, 68
    caloric needs, 29
    caustic esophageal injury, 140–141
    in children, 69
    classification, 68
    complications, 70–71
    lung injury, 69
    rule of 9s, 68
    treatment, 69–70
    wound infection, 70

CA 19-9, 168
Cachexia, 31
Calcitonin, 93
Calcium, normal value, 27
Calcium oxalate stones, 202
Caloric needs, 29
    burn patient, 69
    pediatric surgery, 220
Cancer, 34–36
    carcinogens, 36
    chemotherapy, 35
    genetics, 35–36
    metastasis, 36
    oncogenesis, 34
    post-transplantation malignancies, 37
    proto-oncogenes, 35
    radiation therapy, 34–35
    resection, 35
    therapy, 36
    tumor markers, 34
    tumor suppressor genes, 35
Candida, 15

Cantrell pentalogy, 227
Carbohydrate digestion, 33
Carbon monoxide poisoning, 67
Carbuncle, 16
Carcinogens, 36
Carcinoid
    colon and rectum, 190
    lung, 107
    small bowel, 178–179
Carcinoid syndrome, 178–179
Cardiac index, 62t
Cardiac output, 62t
Cardiac tamponade, 63
    echocardiography, 115
Cardiogenic shock, traumatic, 54
Cardiology workup, indications, 24
Cardiopulmonary bypass, 7
Cardiovascular drugs, 64–65
Cardiovascular system
    heart disease. See Heart disease
    normal parameters, 62t
    vascular disorders, 116–132
Carotid artery(ies), 117
    external, 77
    traumatic injury, 53, 117
Carotid body tumors, 118
Carotid endarterectomy, 118
Carpal tunnel syndrome, 216
Case-control study, 229
Catamenial pneumothorax, 110
Catecholamines, 45, 85
Catheter infection, peritoneal dialysis, 16
Cauda equina syndrome, 213
Cauliflower ear, 79
Caustic ingestion, 140–141
Cecum, volvulus, 189
Cell adhesion molecules, 43
Cell biology, 1–3
Cell cycle, 1
Cell-mediated immunity, 10
Cell membrane, 1
Cellular catabolism, 26
Cellular metabolism, 3
Central cord syndrome, 213
Central line, venous thrombosis, 132
Central venous pressure (CVP), 62t
Cephalosporins, 18
    platelet disorders, 6
Cerebral aneurysms, 211
Cerebral artery(ies), 117
Cerebral ischemia, 117
Cerebral palsy, 228
Cerebral perfusion pressure, 50, 212
Cerebrospinal fluid, rhinorrhea, 79
Cerebrovascular disease, 117–118
    vertebral disease, 118
Cervical cancer, 208
Cervical radiculopathy, 216
Cervical spine, 51
Cervical stenosis, 219
Cesarean section, in traumatic injury, 61
Chagas' disease, 9
Charcot's triad, 164
Chemodectoma, ear, 79
Chemokines, 45

Chemotactic factors, 42
Chemotherapy, 35
    breast cancer, 103
    colorectal cancer, 187
    lung cancer, 105
Chest trauma, 53
Chest tube, 53
Chest wall tumors, 110
Chest x-ray, whiteout, 110
Chief cells, 142
Child abuse, burn injury, 69
Chi-squared test, 229
Chloramphenicol, 19
Choanal atresia, 228
Cholangiocarcinoma, 163
Cholangiohepatitis, Oriental, 164
Cholangiosarcoma, 158
Cholangitis, 164
Cholecystectomy
    asymptomatic, 164
    laparoscopic, 162
Cholecystitis, 160–161
Cholecystokinin (CCK), 133
Choledochal cyst, 163
    classification, 221f, 221t
Cholesteatoma, 79
Cholesterol, synthesis, 160
Cholesterolosis, 164
Cholestyramine, 20
Chromium deficiency, 33t
Chronic granulomatous disease, 45
Chylomicrons, 32, 176
Chylothorax, 109
Cimetidine, 21
Circle of Willis, 210, 210f
Circumcision, bleeding disorders, 6
Cirrhosis, 154
    primary biliary, 164
Cis-atracurium, 23
Clark's levels, melanoma, 73t
Claudication, 122
Clavicle fracture, 216
Cleft lip, 81
Cleft palate, 81
Clindamycin, 19
Clopidogrel, platelet disorders, 6
Clostridium difficile colitis, 13, 193
Clostridium perfringens infection, 14
Clubfoot, 218
Coagulation, 4
    measurements, 5
Coagulation factors, 4
Coarctation of aorta, 113
Cobalamin deficiency, 33t
Coccidioidomycosis, 15
Cohort study, 229
Coin lesion, lung, 107
Colitis, 193
    amebic, 191
    Hirschsprung's, 227
    ischemic, 193
    pseudomembranous, 193
    ulcerative, 189–190
Collagen, in wound healing, 47
Collateral circulation, lower extremity, 123

Index 239

Collateral ligaments, injury, 217
Colles fracture, 216
Colon
   anatomy and physiology, 182–185
   angiodysplasia, 193
   arterial blood supply, 182, 183f
   carcinoid, 190
   diverticula, 191
   diverticulosis, 193
   familial adenomatous polyposis, 188
   juvenile polyposis, 188
   obstruction, 190–191
   Ogilvie's syndrome, 191
   polyps, 185–186
   sigmoid volvulus, 189
   toxic megacolon, 190
   venous drainage, 184f
Colon cancer, 186–188
   familial adenomatous polyposis, 188
   genetics, 36
   hepatic metastases, 158
   hereditary nonpolyposis, 188
Colonic inertia, 185
Colonoscopy, 186
Colon trauma, 56
Colorectal cancer, 186–188
Common bile duct
   injury, 57, 162
   strictures, 162, 168
Compartment syndrome, 58–59, 124, 217–218
   abdominal, 49
Complement system, 44
Compliance, 65
Condylomata acuminata, 194
Congenital adrenal hyperplasia, 83
Congenital cystic adenoid malformation, 220
Congenital heart disease
   anomalous pulmonary venous return, 113
   atrial septal defect, 112
   coarctation of aorta, 113
   hypoplastic left heart, 113
   patent ductus arteriosus, 113
   tetralogy of Fallot, 112
   transposition of great vessels, 112
   truncus arteriosus, 112
   univentricular heart, 113
   vascular rings, 113
   ventricular septal defect, 112
Congenital incontinence, 205
Congenital lobar overinflation, 220
Congenital vascular malformation, 226
Conn's syndrome, 83–84
Contamination, blood products, 9
Contrast dyes, renal toxicity, 67
Controlled trial, 229
Cooper's ligaments, 97
COPD (chronic obstructive pulmonary disease), 65
CO_2 pneumoperitoneum, 200–201
Copper deficiency, 33t
Cori cycle, 3, 33
Coronary artery bypass grafting, 114

Coronary artery disease, 113
Coumadin, 6
Cranial nerves, 77, 214t
   injury in carotid endarterectomy, 118
Craniopharyngioma, 82
Critical care, 62–67
Critical illness polyneuropathy, 67
Crohn's disease, 177–178, 189t
Cronkite-Canada syndrome, 189
Cruciate ligaments, injury, 217
Cryoprecipitate, 5
Cryptococcus, 15
Cryptorchidism, 202
Crypts of Lieberkühn, 184
CT scan, in trauma, 49
Cullen's sign, 167
Curling's ulcer, burn injury, 71
Cushing's disease, 84
Cushing's striae, 72
Cushing's syndrome, 84
Cysteine stones, 202
Cystic artery, 159
Cystic disease of lung, congenital, 220
Cystic duplication, 227
Cystic hygroma, 222
Cystic medial necrosis syndromes, 129
Cystosarcoma phyllodes, 104
Cysts, 76
   brachial cleft, 222
   bronchogenic, 109
   choledochal, 163
   mediastinal, 108
   ovarian, 208
   pilonidal, 194–195
   solitary, hepatic, 157
   splenic, 173
   thyroglossal duct, 89
Cysts choledochal, 221
Cytokines, 41
Cytomegalovirus, anorectum, 195
Cytomegalovirus colitis, 15

Dacron, 201
D cells, 143
Dead space, 65
DeBakey classification, aortic dissection, 119, 119f
Deep venous thrombosis, 7, 131
Delta bilirubin, 164
Demerol, 23
Denonvillier's fascia, 185
Dentate line, 184
DeQuervain's thyroiditis, 90
Dermis, 72
Dermoid cyst, 76
Desmoid tumor, 76, 200
Desmosomes, 1
Dextran, 8
Diabetes insipidus, 211
Diabetes mellitus
   foot infections, 16
   foot ulcer, 47
   wound healing, 47–48
Diabetic neuropathy, 123
Dialysis, indications, 66

Diaphragm, injury, 53–54
Diaphragmatic hernia, pediatric population, 222
Diarrhea, postvagotomy, 150
Dieulafoy's ulcer, 143
Digoxin, 21
Dilutional thrombocytopenia, 9
Dipyridamole, platelet disorders, 6
Disinfectants, 17
Disseminated intravascular coagulation, 6
Diversion colitis, 180
Diverticulitis, 191–192
Diverticulosis, bleeding, 192
Diverticulum(a)
    colonic, 191
    duodenum, 177
    esophageal, 137–138
DKA (diabetic ketoacidosis), 67
DNA transcription, 2f
Dobutamine, 64
Dopamine, 64
Doxorubicin, 35
Drug(s)
    anesthetics, 22–24
    antibiotics, 17–19
    bioavailability, 20
    cardiovascular, 64–65
    kinetics, 20
    nonpolar, 20
    platelet disorders from, 6
    polar, 20
    renal toxicity, 67
    in transplantation, 37–38
Drug metabolism, 20
Ductal carcinoma in situ, breast, 99
Duct of Santorini, 166
Duct of Wirsung, 166
Ducts of Luschka, 159
Dumping syndrome, 149
Duodenum
    anatomy and physiology, 175–176
    arterial blood supply, 175f
    atresia, 225
    carcinoma, 179
    diverticula, 177
    injury, 55–56
    ulcers, 145–146
Dupuytren's contracture, 216
Dysphagia, cervical esophagus, 137
Dysplasia, 34

Ear disorders, 79
Echinococcal abscess, 157
Echocardiography, cardiac tamponade, 115
Ectopia, burn injury, 71
Ectopic pregnancy, 206
Edema, in wound healing, 47
Edrophonium, 23
Efferent-loop obstruction, 150
Ehlers-Danlos syndrome, 47, 129
Eicosanoid production, 44f
Electrical burns, 69
Electrolytes. *See* Fluids and electrolytes; *specific electrolyte*
Elemental formula, 30

Elliptocytosis, 173
Embolism(i), 63–64
    arterial, lower extremity, 124–125
    superior mesenteric artery, 127
Emphysematous gallbladder disease, 161
Empyema, 109
Endocarditis, 115
Endometrial cancer, 208
Endometriosis, 206
Endoplasmic reticulum, 3
End-tidal CO_2 ($ETCO_2$), intraoperative, 25
Enflurane, 22
Enterococcus, antibiotics for, 19
Enterocolitis, neutropenic typhlitis, 193
Eosinophils, 42
Epidermal growth factor, 41
Epidermal inclusion cyst, 76
Epidermis, 72
Epidermoid carcinoma, cervical node, 81
Epidural hematoma, 50
Epiglottitis, 81
Epinephrine, 64
Epiphrenic diverticulum, 138
Epistaxis, 6, 79
    maxillofacial trauma, 52
Epithelial integrity, in wound healing, 46
Epithelialization factors, 42
ERCP (endoscopic retrograde cholangiopancreatography), 161
Erythromycin, 18
Escharotomy, 68
Esophagectomy, 140
Esophagus, 135–141
    achalasia, 138
    anatomy and physiology, 135–137
    arterial blood supply, 135f
    Barrett's, 139
    cancer, 140
    caustic injury, 140–141
    diverticula, 137–138
    endoscopic measurements, 137f
    foreign body, 81
    GERD, 138–139
    hiatal hernia, 139
    injury, 53
    leiomyoma, 140
    lower esophageal sphincter pressure, 136
    perforation, 141
    pharyngoesophageal disorders, 137
    polyps, 140
    Schatzki's ring, 139
    scleroderma, 138
    spasm, 138
    swallowing, 136
    upper esophageal sphincter pressure, 136
    varices, 155
        hemorrhage, 145f
    venous drainage, 136f
Essential fatty acid deficiency, 33t
Estrogen therapy, contraindications, 209
Ethambutol, 19
Etomidate, 22
Eventration, 222

Expiratory reserve volume (ERV), 65
Extracellular fluid compartment, electrolyte concentrations, 1t
Extremity, lower
  acute arterial emboli, 124–125
  arterial circulation, 122f
  collateral circulation, 123
  compartments, 122, 217
  compartment syndrome, 124, 217–218
  leg ulcers, 47
  nerves, 215
  orthopaedic disorders, 217
Extremity, upper
  occlusive disease, 125
  orthopaedic disorders, 216–217
  vascular disorders, 125–127

Facial nerve (CN VII), 77
  injury, 51
Factor VII deficiency, 6
Factor VIII deficiency, 6
Factor X deficiency, 6
Falciform ligament, 151
Familial adenomatous polyposis, 188
Familial hypercalcemic hypocalciuria, 95
Fasciotomy, 58
  forearm, 217
FAST (focused abdominal sonography for trauma) scan, 49
Fat digestion, 31–32
Fat emboli, 63
Fat necrosis, breast, 104
Fatty acids, 32
Febrile nonhemolytic transfusion reaction, 9
Fecal incontinence, 195
Fecalith, 180
Felon, 217
Felty's syndrome, 173
Femoral artery
  aneurysm, 128
  pseudoaneurysm, 128
Femoral fractures, 217
Femoral hernia, 199
Femoropopliteal graft, 123
Femur fracture, 59
Fentanyl, 24
Ferritin, 28
FFP, 5
Fibrin, 4
Fibrinolysis, 5
Fibroadenoma, breast, 98
Fibroblast growth factor, 42
Fibrocystic disease, 98
Fibroids, uterine, 209
Fibromatosis, breast, 104
Fibromuscular dysplasia, 129
Fibrosis, retroperitoneal, 200
Fine-needle aspiration, 88
Fistula
  colovesical, 192
  pancreatic, 167
  rectovaginal, 195
  small bowel, nonhealing, 176–177

Fistula-in-ano, 195
FK-506, 37
Flail chest, 54
Fluids and electrolytes, 26–28
  acid–base balance, 28t
  acute renal failure, 28
  calcium, 27
  chronic renal failure, 28
  extracellular fluid compartment, 1t
  GI electrolyte losses, 26–27
  GI fluid secretion, 26
  intracellular fluid compartment, 1t
  magnesium, 27
  metabolic acidosis, 27
  metabolic alkalosis, 27
  potassium, 27
  sodium, 27
  total body water, 26
  tumor lysis syndrome, 28
  vitamin D, 28
  volume overload, 26
  volume replacement, 26
Fluid therapy, maintenance IV fluids, 220
Flumazenil, 24
5-Fluorouracil, 35
Focal nodular hyperplasia, 157
Folate deficiency, 33t
Follicular thyroid carcinoma, 91
Foot, fractures, 217
Footdrop, 217
Foot infection, diabetic, 16
Foot ulcers, diabetic, 47
Forced vital capacity (FVC), 65
Foregut, 220
Foreign body
  esophageal, 81
  laryngeal, 81
Fournier's gangrene, 14
Fox's sign, 167
Fractures, 59, 215
  laryngeal, 53
  lower extremity, 217
  maxillary, 80
  maxillofacial, 51–52
  open, 219
  orbital, 52
  pathologic, 218
  pelvic, 54–55
  Salter-Harris, 215
  skull, 51
  spinal, 51
  upper extremity, 216
Frey's syndrome, 77
FRIENDS, 176
Functional residual capacity (FRC), 65
Fungal infection, 14–15
Furuncle, 16
Galactocele, 97
Galactorrhea, 97
Gallbladder, 159
  adenocarcinoma, 162–163
  polyps, 164
  porcelain, 163
Gallstone ileus, 161–162, 177
Gallstones, 160

Ganciclovir, 19
Ganglion cyst, 76
Ganglioneuroma, 86
Gangrene, 124
Gap junctions, 1
Gardner's syndrome, 76, 188
Gastrectomy, complications, 149–150
Gastric atony, chronic, 149
Gastric bypass, 149
Gastric cancer, 147–148
Gastric emptying, 143
Gastric inhibitory peptide, 133
Gastric remnant, small, 149
Gastric ulcers, 147
Gastric volvulus, 144
Gastrin, 133
Gastrinoma, 170
Gastritis, 147
    alkaline reflux, 149
Gastroduodenal artery, 159
Gastroenteritis, 180
Gastroepiploic artery, 172f
Gastroesophageal reflux disease (GERD), 138–139
Gastrointestinal hemorrhage
    lower tract, 191, 192f
    upper tract, 144–145
Gastrointestinal hormones, 133–134
Gastrointestinal tract
    electrolyte losses, 26
    fluid secretion, 26
    microflora, 13
Gastroschisis, 226
Gaucher's disease, 173
G cells, 143
Genetics
    cancer, 35–36
    colorectal cancer, 186
    soft tissue tumors, 76
Genital trauma, 60
Genitofemoral nerve injury, 199
Gentamicin, appropriate levels, 17
Germ cell tumors, mediastinal, 108
Giant cell tumor, bone, 218
GIST tumor, 148
Glanzmann's thrombocytopenia, 6
Glasgow Coma Scale, 50
Glioma, 213
Glisson's capsule, 151
Glomus cell tumor, 76
Glossitis, median rhomboid glossitis, 81
Glossopharyngeal nerve (CN IX), 77
    injury in carotid endarterectomy, 118
Glucagon, 133
Glucagonoma, 171
Gluconeogenesis, 3
Gluconeogenesis precursors, in starvation, 30
Glucose, in sepsis, 13
Glucose-6-phosphate dehydrogenase (G6PD) deficiency, 174
Glutamine, 29
Glycogen stores, in starvation, 30
Glycolysis, 3
Goiter, 88
    toxic diffuse, 89
    toxic multinodular, 89–09
Golgi apparatus, 3
Goodsall's rule, 195
Gortex, 201
Gout, 20
G proteins, 1
Grafts
    access, 130
    peripheral vascular disease, 123
Granular cell myoblastoma, 162
Granular cell tumor, breast, 104
Granulocyte colony-stimulating factor (GCSF), 35
Grave's disease, 89
Grey Turner sign, 167
Griffith's point, 193
Growth factors, 41–42
Grynfelt's hernia, 199
Guaiac test, 186
Gynecology, 206–209
Gynecomastia, 97

Hairy cell leukemia, 174
Haldol (haloperidol), 21
Halothane, 22
Hamartoma, pulmonary, 107
Hangman's fracture, 51
Harmonic scalpel, 201
Hartmann's pouch, 180
Hartmann's sign, 141
Hashimoto's thyroiditis, 90
Headache, spinal, 24
Head and neck, 77–81
    abscesses, 80
    anatomy and physiology, 77
    asymptomatic mass lesions, 80–81
    ear, 79
    head injury, 50–51
    laryngeal cancer, 78
    maxillofacial injury, 51–52
    neck and jaw, 80
    neck trauma, 52–53
    nose, 79
    oral cavity cancer, 77–78
    pharyngeal cancer, 78
    salivary gland cancer, 79
    soft tissue sarcoma, 75
Head injury, 50–51
Heart disease
    congenital, 111–112
    coronary artery disease, 113–114
    endocarditis, 115
    tumors, 115
    valve disease, 114–115
Heart transplantation, 40
Helicobacter pylori, gastric ulcers, 147
Hemangioma
    head and neck, 81
    hepatic, 157
    pediatric, 223
    splenic, 173
Hematology, 4–8
    bleeding disorders, 5–7
    coagulation, 4–5

hematologic drugs, 8
Hematoma
    duodenal trauma, 55–56
    epidural, 50, 211, 212f
    intracerebral, 212
    paraduodenal, 55
    pelvic, 55
    rectus sheath, 199
    septal, 79
    subdural, 50, 211
    traumatic, 61t
Hematopoiesis, 172
Hemianopia, bitemporal, 82
Hemobilia, 162
Hemolysis, 9
Hemolytic anemia, 173
Hemophilia A, 6
Hemophilia B, 6
Hemoptysis, massive, 109
Hemorrhage
    cerebral, 211–212
    esophageal varices, 145f
    intraventricular, 213
        traumatic, 50
    lower GI tract, 191, 192f
    mediastinal, 115
    subarachnoid, 212
    upper GI tract, 144–145
Hemorrhagic shock, 63
Hemorrhoids, 194
Hemothorax, 110
Henderson-Hesselbach equation, 28
Heparin, 8
    thrombocytopenia and, 6
Hepatic artery, variants, 151
Hepatic duct, strictures, 162
Hepatic encephalopathy, 154
Hepatic veins, 153
Hepatitis A, 154
Hepatitis B, 154
Hepatitis C, 15, 154
Hepatitis D, 154
Hepatitis E, 154
Hepatoblastoma, pediatric, 224
Hepatocellular carcinoma, 158
Hepatoduodenal ligament, 152, 152f
Hernia
    diaphragmatic, 222
    femoral, 199
    inguinal, 198–199
        pediatric, 227
    umbilical, 227
Herpes simplex virus
    anorectum, 195
    burn wound infection, 71
Hesselbach's triangle, 198
Hetastarch, 9
Heterotopic pancreas, 166
Hiatal hernia, 139
Hiccoughs, 137
HIDA scan, 161
Hidradenitis, 76
Hindgut, 220
Hip dislocation, 217
    congenital, 218

Hirschsprung's disease, 193
    pediatric, 227
Hirudin, 8
Histamine, 42
Histoplasmosis, 15
HIV/AIDS, 15
    anorectal disorders, 195
    Kaposi's sarcoma, 75
    malignancies, 36
HMG-CoA reductase inhibitors, 20
Hodgkin's disease, 174
Hormone-sensitive lipase, 32
Horseshoe kidney, 205
Howship-Romberg sign, 199
Humeral fractures, 216
Humoral immunity, 10
Hürthle cell carcinoma, 92
Hutchinson's freckle, 76
Hydatid cyst, 157
Hydatidiform mole, 209
Hydrocele, 227
Hydrofluoric acid burn, 69
11-Hydroxylase deficiency, 83
17-Hydroxylase deficiency, 83
21-Hydroxylase deficiency, 83
Hyperaldosteronism, 83–84
Hypercalcemia, 27
    causes, 96
Hypercalcemic crisis, 96
Hypercoagulability, 7
Hypercortisolism, 84
Hyperglycemia, pseudohyponatremia, 27
Hyperhidrosis, 76
Hyperkalemia, 27
    succinylcholine and, 23
Hypermagnesemia, 27
Hypernatremia, 27
Hypernephroma, 203
Hyperparathyroidism, 93–95
    primary, 93–94
    secondary, 94–95
    tertiary, 95
Hyperplasia, 34
    adrenal, 83–84, 85
    parathyroid, 94
Hypersensitivity angiitis, 129
Hypersensitivity reactions, 12t
    type I, 42
Hypersplenism, 173
Hyperthyroidism
    causes, 89–90
    treatment, 89
Hypocalcemia, 27
    transfusion-related, 9
Hypocortisolism, 84
Hypoglossal nerve (CN XII), 77
    injury in carotid endarterectomy, 118
Hypokalemia, 27
Hypomagnesemia, 27
Hyponatremia, 27
Hypopharyngeal carcinoma, 78
Hypoplastic left heart, 113
Hyposplenism, 174
Hypotension, 66
Hypothalamus, 82

ICU psychosis, 67
Idiopathic adolescent scoliosis, 218
Idiopathic hypertrophic subaortic stenosis, 115
Idiopathic thrombotic purpura (ITP), 172
Ileostomy, 180
Ileum, anatomy and physiology, 175–176
Ileus, 180
    gallstone, 161–162, 177
Iliac artery, aneurysm, 128
Ilioinguinal nerve injury, 198
Imipenem, 18
Immune arteritis, 129
Immunoglobulins, 12
Immunology, 10–12
    activation sequence, 11
    antibodies, 12
    B cells, 10
    hypersensitivity reactions, 12
    MHC classes, 11
    natural killer cells, 12
    T cells, 10
    transplantation, 37
Imperforate anus, 226
Incidence, 229
Incisional hernia, 199
Incontinence
    anal, 195
    urinary, 205
Indomethacin, 21
Infectious disease, 13–16
    abscesses, 13, 156–157
    aortic graft infection, 121
    bacterial peritonitis, 15, 155
    bacterial thyroiditis, 90
    burn wound infection, 70–71
    Clostridium difficile colitis, 13
    endocarditis, 115
    fungal infection, 14–15
    gastrointestinal microflora, 13
    gram-negative sepsis, 13
    hepatitis C, 15
    HIV, 15
    line infections, 14
    mastitis, 97
    mycotic abdominal aortic aneurysm, 121
    necrotizing soft tissue infections, 14
    transfusion risk, 9t
    viral hepatitis, 154
    wound infection, 13–14
Inflammation, 41–45
    catecholamines, 45
    cell adhesion molecules, 43
    complement system, 44
    cytokines, 42–43
    growth and activating factors, 41–42
    hepatic acute phase response proteins, 43
    interferons, 43
    leukotrienes, 45
    neuroendocrine response, 45
    neutrophil recruitment and activation, 43f
    nitric oxide, 42
    oxidants generated, 45t
    phases, 41
    prostaglandins, 44
    type I hypersensitivity reactions, 42
Inflammatory aneurysm, abdominal aorta, 121
Inflammatory bowel disease, 189–190
Inflammatory cancer, breast, 102
Inguinal hernia, 198–199
    pediatric, 207
Inhalational anesthetics, 22
Injury. *See also* Trauma
    neuroendocrine response, 45
Inspiratory capacity, 65
Insulin, 133
Insulinoma, 170
Interferons, 43
Interleukin(s)
    IL-1, 43
    IL-2, 12
    IL-6, 43
Internal mammary artery, CABG, 113
Intestinal atresia, pediatric, 225
Intra-aortic balloon pump (IABP), 64
Intracellular fluid compartment, electrolyte concentrations, 1t
Intracranial pressure, elevated, 50–51, 212
Intraventricular hemorrhage, 213
Intrinsic factor, 142
Intubation
    chest tube, 53
    prolonged, 81
Intussusception, 224–225
    small bowel, 179
Iodine-131, 89, 92
Ischemia
    cerebral, 117
    mesenteric, 127–128
Ischemic colitis, 193
Isoflurane, 22
Isoniazid, 19
Isoproterenol, 64

Jaundice, 153–154
    workup, 168
Jefferson fracture, 51
Jejunoileal bypass, 149
Jejunum, anatomy and physiology, 175–176
Juvenile polyposis, 188

Kaplan-Meyer, 229
Kaposi's sarcoma, 75
    anorectal, 195
    oropharyngeal, 81
Kawasaki's disease, 129
Keloids, 48, 76
Keratinocytes, 72
Keratoacanthoma, 76
Keratosis, 76
Ketamine, 22
Kidney
    renal cell carcinoma, 203
    trauma, 59–60
Kidney stones, 202

Index 245

Kidney transplantation, 38–39
Klatskin tumor, 163
Kleihauer-Betke test, 61
Knee trauma, 217
Krebs cycle, 3
Krukenberg tumor, 147, 207
Kupffer cells, 152
Kwashiorkor, 31

Laceration
  lip, 76, 81
  pinna, 79
  Stensen's duct, 80
Lactated Ringer's solution, 26
Lactic acid, 3
Langerhans cells, 72
Laparoscopic cholecystectomy, 162
  shock, 164
Laparotomy, in trauma, 49
Laryngeal cancer, 78
Laryngeal fracture, 53
Laryngeal papillomatosis, 228
Laryngomalacia, 228
Larynx, foreign body, 81
Lecithin, 153
LeFort classification, maxillofacial
  fractures, 52f, 52t
Leg. *See* Extremity, lower
Legg-Calvé-Perthes disease, 218
Leiden factor, 7
Leiomyoma
  esophagus, 140
  gastric, 148
  small bowel, 179
  uterine, 209
Leiomyosarcoma
  gastric, 148
  small bowel, 179
Lentigo maligna melanoma, 73
Leriche syndrome, 123
Leukotrienes, 45
Leuprolide, 21
Levamisole, 35
Lichtenstein repair, 198
LiFraumeni syndrome, 36, 76
Ligament of Berry, 87f, 88
Ligamentum teres, 151
Lightning injury, 69
Line infections, 14
Lingual thyroid, 89
Linitis plastica, 148
Lip
  cleft, 81
  laceration, 76, 81
  numbness, 80
Lipoma, 76
Lipoprotein lipase, 32
Littre's hernia, 199
Liver, 151–157
  abscesses, 156–157
  acute phase response proteins, 43
  adenoma, 157
  anatomy and physiology, 151–153
  colorectal metastasis, 36
  focal nodular hyperplasia, 157
  hemangioma, 157
  nitrogen balance, 31
  solitary cyst, 157
  trauma, 57
  tumors
    benign, 157
    malignant, 158
Liver failure, 154
Liver transplantation, 39
Lobular carcinoma in situ, breast, 99
Ludwig's angina, 80
Lumbar disc herniation, 215
Lumbar stenosis, 219
Lung
  abscess, 108
  congenital cystic disease, 220
  functional measurements, 65
  solitary nodule, 110
Lung cancer, 105–107
  mesothelioma, 106
  non-small cell carcinoma, 106
  paraneoplastic syndromes, 106
  small cell carcinoma, 106
Lung injury
  burns, 69
  transfusion-related acute lung injury, 9
Lung transplantation, 40
Lupus anticoagulant, 7
Lymphadenopathy, pediatric population,
  222
Lymphangiectasia, 132
Lymphangiosarcoma, 132
Lymphatic system
  anal canal, 197f
  breast, 97
  disorders, 132
  rectum, 196f
Lymphedema, 132
Lymph nodes
  axillary, anatomic classification, 100
  in cancer, 36
  melanoma, 74
Lymphocele, postoperative, 132
Lymphogranuloma venereum, 191
Lymphoid organs, 12
Lymphoma
  anorectum, 195
  gastric, 148
  in HIV, 15
  mediastinal, 108
  non-Hodgkin's, 173, 174
  small bowel, 179
  splenic, 173
Lynch syndromes, 188
Mafenide sodium, in burns, 70
Magnesium, normal value, 27
Major histocompatibility complex (MHC)
  classes, 11
Malignant hyperthermia, 22–23
Mallory-Weiss tear, 144
Malperforans ulcer, 124
Malrotation, pediatric, 225
Mammary duct ectasia, 97
Mammography, 100
Mandibular injury, 52

Mannitol, for elevated ICP, 51
Marfan's disease, 129
Marfan's syndrome, 47
Marjolin's ulcer, burn injury, 71
Mast cells, 12, 42
Mastectomy
  complications, 103
  preoperative studies, 102
  prophylactic, 101
  surgical options, 103
Mastitis, 97
Mastodynia, 98
Mastoiditis, 81
Maxillary fracture, 80
Maxillofacial fractures, 51–52
M cells, 176
McVay repair, 198
Meckel's diverticulum, 177
  pediatric, 224
Meconium ileus, 226
Median arcuate ligament syndrome, 128
Median nerve, 215
Median rhomboid glossitis, 81
Median sternotomy, 54
Mediastinal masses, in children, 221
Mediastinal tumors, 107–108
Mediastinitis, risk factors, 115
Mediastinoscopy, 106
Mediastinum, thyroid tissue, 88
Medullary thyroid carcinoma, 91–92
Megacolon, 193
Meige's syndrome, 207
Meissner's plexus, 184
Melanocytes, 72
Melanoma, 73–74
  anal, 195
Melena, 191
Menetrier's disease, 143
Meniscus tears, 217
Menorrhagia, bleeding disorders, 6
Merkel cell carcinoma, 76
Mesenteric ischemia, 127–128
Mesenteric tumors, 200
Mesenteric vein thrombosis, 127
Mesothelioma, 106
Meta-analysis, 229
Metabolic acidosis, 27
Metabolic alkalosis, 27
Metaplasia, 34
Metaplastic adenocarcinoma, breast, 102
Metastases, 36
  to adrenal glands, 83
  anal cancer, 196
  colorectal cancer, 186
  esophageal cancer, 140
  hepatic, 158
  melanoma, 74
  pancreatic adenocarcinoma, 169
  pulmonary, 107
Metastatic flare, breast, 104
Methadone, 24
Methemoglobinemia, 67
Methimazole, 89
Methotrexate, 35
Metoclopramide, 21

Metronidazole, 19
Metyrapone, 21
Micelles, 31–32
Microbiology
  gastrointestinal microflora, 13
  surgical wound infection, 13
Microsomal drug metabolism, 20
Midgut, 220
Migrating motor complexes, 176
Milrinone, 64
Minimum alveolar concentration (MAC), 22
Minute ventilation, 65
Mivacurium, 23
Mirizzi syndrome, 164
Misoprostol, 21
Mithramycin, 96
Mitochondria, 2
Mitosis, 1
Mitral regurgitation, 114
Mitral stenosis, 114
Mittelschmerz, 207
Mondor's disease, 98, 131
Monoamine oxidase, 95
Monteggia fracture, 216
Morbid obesity, 148
Morgagni's hernia, 222
Morphine, 23
Motilin, 133
Mucocele, 180
Mucoepidermoid carcinoma
  colorectal, 186
  salivary gland, 79
Mucosa-associated lymphoproliferative
  tissue (MALT), 148
Multiple endocrine neoplasia (MEN)
  syndromes, 95–96
Multiple myeloma, 218
Murphy's sign, 160
Muscle relaxants, 22–23
Musculocutaneous nerve, 215
Myasthenia gravis, 108
Mycotic aneurysm, abdominal aorta, 121
Myelomeningocele, 213
Myocardial contusion, 54
Myocardial infarction
  carotid endarterectomy, 118
  complications, 113
  postoperative, 24
Myofibroblasts, in wound healing, 46
Myoglobin, renal toxicity, 67
Myosin, 3

Narcotics, 23–24
Nasal disorders, 79
Nasogastric suction, 27
Nasopharyngeal angiofibroma, 78
Nasopharyngeal carcinoma, 78
Natural killer cells, 12
ND:YAG laser, 201
Neck. *See* Head and neck
Neck dissection
  modified radical, 77
  radical, 77
Necrotizing enterocolitis, 226
Necrotizing fasciitis, 14

Negative predictive value, 230
Nelson's syndrome, 82
Neostigmine, 23
Nephroblastoma, 223
Nerve injury, 210
    in orthopaedic injury, 59t
Neuroblastoma, 223
Neurofibromatosis, 76
Neurogenic bladder, 204
Neurogenic obstructive uropathy, 204
Neurogenic shock, 63
Neurogenic tumors, mediastinal, 107, 108
Neurohypophysis, 82
Neurologic disorders, liver failure, 154
Neuroma, 76
Neuropathic incontinence, 205
Neurapraxia, 210
Neurosurgery, 210–214
Neurotmesis, 210
Neutropenic typhlitis, 193
Neutrophil(s), in inflammation, 43f
Niacin, 20
Niacin deficiency, 33t
Nipple discharge, 98
Nipride, 64
Nitric oxide, 42
Nitrogen balance, 31
Nitroglycerin, 65
Nitrous oxide (NO_2), 22
Nocardia, 15
Nodular melanoma, 73
Nonparametric statistics, 229
Norepinephrine, 64
Nosebleed. See Epistaxis
Nosocomial pneumonia, 14
NSAIDs, renal toxicity, 67
Nucleolus, 1
Nucleus, 1
Null hypothesis, 229
Nutrition, 29–33
    caloric needs, 29
    carbohydrate digestion, 33
    Cori cycle, 33
    deficiencies, 33t
    fat digestion, 31–32
    nitrogen balance, 31
    preoperative assessment, 29–30
    protein digestion, 33
    starvation/major stress, 30–31

Obesity, morbid, 148
Obstruction
    colonic, 190–191
    neurogenic obstructive uropathy, 204
    small bowel, 177
Obturator hernia, 199
Occlusive disease, upper extremity, 125
Odontoid fracture, 51
Ogilvie's syndrome, 191
OKT3, 38
Oliguria, 67
Omental tumors, 200
Omeprazole, 21
Omphalocele, 226–227
Oncocytoma, renal, 203
Oncogenesis, 34
Oncology, 34–36
Ondansetron, 21
Opioids, 23–24
Opportunistic infections, 15
Oral cavity cancer, 77–78
Orbital fractures, 52
Oriental cholangiohepatitis, 164
Oropharyngeal carcinoma, 78
Orthopaedics, 215–220
    trauma, 59
Osgood-Schlatter disease, 218
Osteitis fibrosa cystica, 94
Osteoblasts, 215
Osteoclasts, 215
Osteogenesis imperfecta, wound healing, 47
Osteogenic sarcoma, 218
Osteomyelitis, 218
Osteosarcoma, 75
    pediatric, 228
Ovarian cancer, 36, 207
Ovarian cysts, 208
Ovarian mass, 209
Ovarian torsion, 209
Overflow incontinence, 205
Oxidants, inflammation and, 45t
Oxygen consumption, 62
Oxygen delivery, in wound healing, 47

Paget's disease
    anal, 196
    breast, 104
Paired tests, 229
Palate, cleft, 81
Palliative surgery, 36
Pancoast tumor, 107
Pancreas, 165–171
    anatomy and physiology, 165–166
    annular, 166
    arterial blood supply, 165f
    endocrine tumors, 170–171
    fistulas, 167
    heterotopic, 166
    injury, 58
    pseudocysts, 167
Pancreas divisum, 166
Pancreas transplantation, 40
Pancreatic adenocarcinoma, 168–169
Pancreatic insufficiency, 168
Pancreatitis
    acute, 166–167
    chronic, 167–168
    spleen in, 174
Pancreatic polypeptide, 133
Pancuronium, 23
Panel reactive antibody, 37
Papillary thyroid carcinoma, 91
Papilloma, intraductal, 98
Papillomatosis
    diffuse, breast, 99
    laryngeal, 228
Parafollicular C cells, 88
Paraganglionoma, 213
Paraneoplastic syndromes, lung cancer, 106

Parapharyngeal abscess, 80
Parathyroid cancer, 95
Parathyroid glands, 93–96
   anatomy and physiology, 93
   disorders, 93–96
Parathyroid hormone (PTH), 93
Parenteral nutrition, 29
Parietal cells, 142
   acid secretion, 143f
Parkland formula, 68
Paronychia, 217
Parotid glands, 77
Parotitis, suppurative, 80
Patellar fracture, 217
Patent ductus arteriosus, 113
Pectus carinatum, 222
Pectus excavatum, 222
Pediatric population
   biliary atresia, 228
   brachial cleft cyst, 222
   brain tumors, 213
   burn injury, 69
   choanal atresia, 228
   choledochal cyst, 221
   congenital cystic disease of lung, 220
   congenital heart disease, 111
   congenital vascular malformation, 226
   cystic duplication, 227
   diaphragmatic hernia, 222
   duodenal atresia, 225
   gastroschisis, 226
   hemangioma, 223
   hepatoblastoma, 224
   Hirschsprung's disease, 227
   hydrocele, 227
   imperforate anus, 226
   inguinal hernia, 227
   intestinal atresia, 225
   intussusception, 224–225
   laryngeal papillomatosis, 228
   laryngomalacia, 228
   lymphadenopathy, 222
   malrotation, 225
   Meckel's diverticulum, 177, 224
   meconium ileus, 226
   mediastinal masses, 221
   necrotizing enterocolitis, 226
   nephroblastoma, 223
   neuroblastoma, 223
   neurosurgery, 213
   omphalocele, 226–227
   orthopaedic disorders, 218
   osteosarcoma, 228
   portal hypertension, 156
   postsplenectomy sepsis syndrome, 173
   pyloric stenosis, 224
   rhabdomyosarcoma, 75
   teratoma, 228
   thyroglossal duct cyst, 223
   tracheoesophageal fistula, 225
   trauma, 60–61
   umbilical hernia, 199, 227
   undescended testicles, 228
   vital signs by age, 61t
   Wilms tumor, 223, 224t
Pediatric surgery, 220–228
   caloric needs, 220
   maintenance IV fluids, 220
Pelvic fractures, 54–55, 55f
Pelvic inflammatory disease, 207
Penicillins, 17–18
Pentoxifylline, platelet disorders, 6
Peptide YY, 134
Percutaneous transluminal angioplasty, 124
Perforation
   duodenal ulcer, 146
   esophagus, 141
Peripheral neuropathy, burn injury, 71
Peripheral vascular disease, 122–125
Peristomal hernia, 199
Peritoneal dialysis, catheter infection, 16
Peritoneal lavage, diagnostic, 49
Peritoneal membrane, 200
Peritoneovenous shunt, 154
Peritonitis, bacterial, 15, 155
Peritonsillar abscess, 80
Petit's hernia, 199
Peutz-Jeghers syndrome, 179, 188
Peyer's patches, 176
Phagosome, 3
Pharmacology, 20–21
Pharyngeal cancer, 78
Pharyngoesophageal disorders, 137
Phenylephrine, 64
Pheochromocytoma, 85–86
Phlegmasia alba dolens, 131
Phlegmasia cerulea dolens, 131
Phrenic nerve, 77
Phytobezoars, 143
Pilonidal cysts, 76, 194–195
Piperacillin, 17–18
Pituitary gland, 82
   adenoma, 84, 213
Placental abruption, traumatic, 61
Plantaris muscle rupture, 217
Plasma cell mastitis, 97
Plasma osmolarity, 26
Plasmin, 5
Platelet(s), in wound healing, 46
Platelet-activating factor, 42
Platelet count, perioperative, 6
Platelet-derived growth factor, 41
Platelet disorders, 6
   idiopathic thrombotic purpura, 172
   thrombotic thrombocytopenic purpura, 173
Pleomorphic adenoma, salivary gland, 79
Pleural effusion, 110
Pleural fluid, 105
Plummer-Vinson syndrome, 78
Pneumatic antishock garment, 49
Pneumatosis intestinalis, 191
Pneumaturia, 205
Pneumocytes, 105
Pneumonia, nosocomial, 14
Pneumoperitoneum, CO_2, 200–201
Pneumothorax, 110
   spontaneous, 109
   tension, 54, 110

Index

PNMT, 85
Poland's syndrome, 98
Polyarteritis nodosa, 129
Polycythemia vera, 7
Polyps
    cancer-containing, 185f
    colonic, 185–186
    esophagus, 140
    familial adenomatous polyposis, 188
    gallbladder, 164
    gastric, 147
Polythelia, 98
Popliteal artery, aneurysm, 128
Popliteal entrapment syndrome, 124
Porcelain gallbladder, 163
Pores of Kahn, 105
Portal hypertension, 155–156
    venous collaterals, 155f
Portal vein, 153
    anatomy, 151f
    injury, 57
Positive predictive value, 230
Posterior cruciate ligament injury, 217
Postpericardiotomy syndrome, 115
Postsplenectomy sepsis syndrome, 173
Posttransplant lymphoproliferative
    disorder, 37
Postvagotomy diarrhea, 150
Potassium, normal value, 27
Pouchitis, 185
Powder burns, 69
Power of test, 229
Pre-albumin, half-life, 29
Predictive value, 230
Pregnancy, 206
    appendicitis during, 180
    breast mass in, 104
    trauma during, 61
Pressure sores, 72–73
Prevalence, 229
Priapism, 205
Primary biliary cirrhosis, 164
Primary sclerosing cholangitis, 163–164
Pringle maneuver, 57f, 153
Procainamide, 21
Procoagulant agents, 8
Prolactinoma, 82
Promethazine, 20
Properdin, 172
Propofol, 22
Propylthiouracil, 89
Prostacyclin, 5
Prostaglandins, 44
Prostate cancer, 203
Prostate gland, benign prostatic
    hypertrophy, 204
Prostate surgery, bleeding disorders, 6
Protein, normal level, 29
Protein C, 5
    activated, 21
Protein C deficiency, 7
Protein digestion, 33
Protein kinase A, 3
Protein kinase C, 3
Protein needs, burn patient, 69

Protein S, 5
Protein S deficiency, 7
Protein synthesis, 2f
Prothrombin complex, 4
Prothrombin time (PT), 5
Proto-oncogenes, 34, 35
Prune belly syndrome, 228
Pseudoaneurysm
    carotid endarterectomy, 118
    femoral, 128
Pseudocysts, pancreatic, 167
Pseudohyperparathyroidism, 95
Pseudohyponatremia, 27
Pseudomembranous colitis, 193
Pseudomonas, antibiotics for, 19
P-450 system, 20
Pulmonary artery, 62t
Pulmonary capillary wedge pressure, 62t
Pulmonary compliance, 65
Pulmonary embolism, 7, 63, 131–132
Pulmonary function parameters, 65
Pulmonary function tests, 105
Pulmonary sequestration, 220
Pyloric stenosis, 224
Pyogenic abscess, 157
Pyrazinamide, 19
Pyruvate kinase deficiency, 173–174

Qualitative variables, 229
Quantitative variables, 229
Quinolones, 18

Raccoon eyes, 51
Radial nerve, 127, 215
Radiation arteritis, 129
Radiation therapy, 34–35
    breast cancer, 103
    colorectal cancer, 187
    thyroid cancer, 92
Radicular cyst, 80
Radiculopathy, cervical, 216
Radioiodine (^{131}I), 89, 92
Ranson's criteria, 166
Raynaud's disease, 129
Receptors, 64
    breast cancer, 102
Rectal trauma, 56
Rectovaginal fistula, 195
Rectum. *See also* Anorectum
    cancer. *See* Colorectal cancer
    carcinoid, 190
    lymphatic drainage, 196f
    prolapse, 194
Rectus sheath, 199
Recurrent laryngeal nerve, 77, 87, 87f
    injury, 53
Red blood cells, 45
Refeeding syndrome, 31
Regional ileitis, 180
Rejection, in transplantation, 38
Renal artery, aneurysm, 128
Renal cell carcinoma, 203
Renal failure
    acute, 28
    chronic, 28

250 The ABSITE Review

Renal osteodystrophy, 95
Renal system, 66–67
Renin, 66
Renovascular hypertension, 125
Reperfusion injury, 45
Residual volume (RV), 65
Resin T_3 uptake, 88
Respiratory quotient (RQ), 30
Respiratory system, 65–66
Resuscitation, burn injury, 68
Retinoblastoma, 76
Retroperitoneal fibrosis, 200
Retroperitoneal sarcoma, 75, 200
Retroperitoneal tumors, 200
Retropharyngeal abscess, 80
Reynolds' pentad, 164
Rhabdomyosarcoma, 75
    ear, 79
Rhinorrhea, cerebrospinal fluid, 79
Richter's hernia, 199
Riedel's struma, 90
Rifampin, 19
Rocuronium, 23
Rokitansky-Aschoff sinuses, 159
Rotator cuff tears, 216
Rotter's nodes, 100
Roux-en-Y gastric bypass, 149
Roux stasis, 149

Sacrococcygeal teratoma, pediatric, 228
Saline, 0.9% normal, 26
Salivary glands, 77
    cancer, 79
Salter-Harris fractures, 215
Saphenous vein, 129, 130f
    CABG, 113
Sarcoidosis, 110
    spleen, 173
Sarcoma, 74–75
    hepatic, 158
    lymphangiosarcoma, 132
    osteogenic, 218
    retroperitoneal, 200
Scaphoid fracture, 216
Scapula fracture, 216
Scars/scarring, 47
    burn injury, 71
    hypertrophic, 76
Schatzki's ring, 139
Schilling test, 176
Schistosomiasis, 157
Sciatic hernia, 199
Scleroderma, esophageal, 138
Sclerosing adenosis, breast, 98
Scoliosis, idiopathic adolescent, 218
Screening
    breast cancer, 100
    colonic polyps, 186
Seat belt injury, 49
Seborrheic keratosis, 76
Secretin, 133
Seizures, burn injury, 71
Selectins, 43
Selenium deficiency, 33t
Seminoma, 202–203
    mediastinal, 108
Sengstaken-Blakemore tube, 155
Sensitivity, 230
Sensory nerves, skin, 72
Sentinel lymph node biopsy (SNLB), 36, 103
Sepsis, 63
    burn wound, 71
    Gram-negative, 13
Septal hematoma, 79
Septic arthritis, 16
Sequential compression devices, 131
Sequestration, 109
Sestamibi-^{131}I scan, 94
Sevoflurane, 22
Sheehan's syndrome, 82
Shock, 63
    laparoscopic cholecystectomy, 164
    spinal, 212
Short-gut syndrome, 176
Shotgun injury, neck, 53
Shoulder dislocation, 216
SIADH (syndrome of inappropriate secretion of antidiuretic hormone), 211
Sickle cell anemia, 174
Sigmoidoscopy, 186
Silvadene, in burns, 70
Silver nitrate, in burns, 70
Silver sulfadiazine, in burns, 70
Sinusitis, 16
SIRS, 65
Skin, anatomy, 72
Skin cancer
    basal cell carcinoma, 74
    melanoma, 73–74
    squamous cell carcinoma, 74
Skin grafts, 72
    burn wound, 69–70
Skin necrosis, warfarin-induced, 7
Skull fractures, 51
Sleep apnea, 81
Slipped capital femoral epiphysis, 218
Small bowel, 175–181. *See also specific segment*
    anatomy and physiology, 175–176
    carcinoid, 178–179
    Crohn's disease, 177–178
    diverticula, 177
    injury, 56
    Meckel's diverticulum, 177
    nonhealing fistula, 176–177
    obstruction, 177
    short-gut syndrome, 176
    stomas, 180
    tumors
        benign, 179
        malignant, 179
Small cell carcinoma, lung, 106
Sodium, normal value, 27
Sodium thiopental, 22
Soft tissue infections, necrotizing, 14
Soft tissue sarcoma, 74–75
Soft tissue tumors, 76
Somatostatin, 133

Somatostatinoma, 170
Spasm, diffuse esophageal spasm, 138
Specificity, 230
Spherocytosis, 173
Spider bite, Brown recluse, 16
Spigelian hernia, 199
Spinal artery, anterior spinal artery syndrome, 213
Spinal cord
  Brown-Sequard syndrome, 213
  central cord syndrome, 213
  injury, 212–213
Spinal headache, 24
Spinal shock, 212
Spine
  cervical radiculopathy, 216
  lumbar disc herniation, 215
  stenosis, 219
  trauma, 51
  tumors, 213
Spleen, 172–174
  anatomy and physiology, 172
  disorders, 172–174
  injury, 58
  rupture, spontaneous, 174
Splenic artery, 172f
  aneurysm, 128
  aneurysms, 174
Splenic vein, thrombosis, 156, 168
Splenorenal shunt, 156
Splenosis, 174
Spondylolisthesis, 218–219
Spontaneous bacterial peritonitis, 155
Squamous cell carcinoma
  anal, 195, 196
  ear, 79
  hypopharyngeal, 78
  laryngeal, 78
  nasopharyngeal, 78
  oropharyngeal, 78
  skin, 74
Staging
  breast cancer, 101
  lung cancer, 106
  melanoma, 73t
Stanford classification, aortic dissection, 119, 119f
Staphylococcus spp., surgical wound infection, 13
Starvation, 30
  metabolic responses, 30, 31t
Statins, 20
Statistics, 229–230
Steatorrhea, 176
Stenosis
  aortic, 114–115, 193
  biliary, 168
  spinal, 219
Stensen's duct, laceration, 80
Stercobilin, 159
Steroids, 1, 37
  wound healing, 48
Stevens-Johnson syndrome, 71
Stewart-Treves syndrome, 104
Stomach, 142–150
  anatomy and physiology, 142–143
  arterial blood supply, 142f
  cancer, 147–148
  leiomyoma, 148
  leiomyosarcoma, 148
  lymphoma, 148
  Mallory-Weiss tear, 144
  morbid obesity, 148
  mucosa-associated lymphoproliferative tissue, 148
  ulcers, 147
Streptokinase, 8
Stress, 30
Stress gastritis, 147
Stress incontinence, 205
Strictures
  common bile duct, 162, 168
  hepatic duct, 162
Stroke, 117
Struvite stones, 202
Student's t test, 229
Subarachnoid hemorrhage, 212
Subclavian artery, 127
Subclavian steal syndrome, 125
Subclavian vein, 127
Subdural hematoma, 50
Sublingual glands, 77
Submandibular glands, 77
Succinylcholine, 22–23
Sudeck's point, 193
Sulfamylon, in burns, 70
Superior laryngeal nerve, 77, 87
Superior mesenteric artery
  embolism, 127
  thrombosis, 127
Superior vena cava syndrome, 115
Suppurative cholecystitis, 160
Suppurative parotitis, 80
Suppurative tenosynovitis, 216
Surgical margins, melanoma, 73t
Surgical technology, 201
SvO_2, 62, 62t
Swallowing, 136
Swan-Ganz catheter, 62
Sweat glands, 72
Symblepharon, burn injury, 71
Syphilis, 207
Systemic vascular resistance, 62t
Takayasu's arteritis, 129
Tamoxifen, 35, 104
Tar burns, 69
T cells, 10
  in HIV, 15
Temporal arteritis, 129
Temporomandibular joint (TMJ) dislocation, 80
Tenosynovitis, suppurative, 216
Tensile strength, in wound healing, 46
Tension pneumothorax, 54, 110
Teratoma
  mediastinal, 108
  pediatric, 228
Testicular atrophy, 198
Testicular cancer, 202–203

Testicular torsion, 204
Tetanus immune globulin, 12
Tetanus toxoid, 12
Tetracycline, 19
Tetralogy of Fallot, 112
Thalassemia, beta, 174
Thallium-tech scan, 94
Thiamine deficiency, 33t
Thoracic aortic disease, 118–120
Thoracic cavity, 105–110
    anatomy and physiology, 105
Thoracic duct, 135
Thoracic outlet, anatomy, 126f
Thoracic outlet syndrome, 125–126
Thoracolumbar spine, 51
Thoracotomy
    ER, 49
    traumatic injury, 53
Thrombin, 4
Thrombocytopenia, 6
Thromboembolic disease, 7
Thrombolytic agents, 8
Thrombophlebitis, 131
Thrombosis
    acute arterial, 125
    mesenteric vein, 127
    ovarian vein, 209
    splenic vein, 156, 168
    superior mesenteric artery, 127
Thrombotic thrombocytopenic purpura, 173
Thromboxane, 5
Thymoglobulin, 37
Thymoma, 107–108
Thyrocervical trunk, 77
Thyroglobulin, 88
Thyroglossal duct cyst, 89, 223
Thyroid carcinoma, 90–92
    follicular, 91
    medullary, 36, 91–92
    papillary, 91
Thyroidectomy, 89
Thyroid gland, 87–92
    anatomy and physiology, 87–88
    descent abnormalities, 89
    disorders, 88–92
    injury, 53
    nodules, 88
Thyroid hormone, 1
Thyroiditis, 90
Thyroid-stimulating hormone, 87
Thyroid storm, 88
Thyrotropin-releasing factor, 87
Tibia fracture, 217
Ticarcillin, 17–18
Ticlopidine, platelet disorders, 6
Tidal volume (TV), 65
Tight junctions, 1
Timentin, 18
Tinsel's test, 126
TIPS, 156
Tissue factor pathway inhibitor, 4
Tissue plasminogen activator, 5, 8
Tissue valves, 114
TNM staging

breast cancer, 101
colorectal cancer, 187
lung cancer, 106
Tonsillar carcinoma, 78
Tonsillectomy, bleeding disorders, 6
Tooth extraction, bleeding disorders, 6
Torus fracture, 219
Torus mandibular, 77
Torus palatini, 77
Total lung capacity (TLC), 65
Toxic epidermal necrolysis, 71
Toxic megacolon, 190
Toxic multinodular goiter, 89–90
Toxic shock syndrome, 209
Trachea, 77
    disorders, 108
Tracheal injury, 53
Tracheobronchial injury, 53
Tracheoesophageal fistula, 108
    pediatric, 225
Tracheo-innominate fistula, 8, 108
Tracheostomy, 81
Traction diverticulum, esophagus, 138
TRAM flaps, 72
Transcription, 1
Transferrin, 28
    half-life, 29
Transforming growth factor-beta, 41
Transfusion reactions, 9
Transitional carcinoma, bladder, 204
Translation, 2
Transplantation, 37–40
    drugs in, 37–38
    heart, 40
    immunology, 37
    kidney, 38–39
    liver, 39
    lung, 40
    pancreas, 40
    rejection, 38
Transposition of great vessels, 112
Trapezius flap, 77
Trapezoid of doom, 199
Trauma, 49–61
    assessment, 49
    bladder, 60
    burns, 68–71
    carotid artery injury, 117
    chest, 53–54
    colon, 56
    duodenal, 55–56
    genital, 60
    head injury, 50–51
    liver, 57–58
    maxillofacial, 51–52
    metabolic responses, 31t
    neck, 52–53
    orthopaedic, 59
    pancreatic, 58
    pediatric, 60–61
    pelvic, 54–55
    penetrating
        chest, 54
        neck, 52
        pelvic injury, 55

pregnant patient, 61
rectal, 56
renal, 59–60
small bowel, 56
spinal, 51
spleen, 58
thoracic aortic transection, 118
ureteral, 60, 204
urethral, 60
vascular, 58–59
Trendelenburg test, 131
Trichilemmal cyst, 76
Trichobezoars, 143
Trigeminal nerve (CN V), 77
Trigger finger, 216
Truncus arteriosus, 112
Trypanosoma cruzi, 193
Tubercles of Zuckerkandl, 88
Tuberculosis, 110
Tuberous sclerosis, 76
Tubular adenoma, 185
Tuftsin, 172
Tumor lysis syndrome, 28
Tumor markers, 34
    CA 19-9, 168
Tumor necrosis factor alpha, 42
Tumors
    bone, 75, 218
    brain, 213
    cardiac, 115
    desmoid, 200
    endocrine, pancreas, 170–171
    hepatic, 157–158
    mesenteric, 200
    omental, 200
    preauricular, 80
    retroperitoneal, 200
    spinal, 213
Tumor suppressor genes, 35
Turcot's syndrome, 188
Typhlitis, neutropenic, 193
Typhoid enteritis, 181
Tyrosine kinase receptors, 1

Ulcerative colitis, 189–190
Ulcers/ulceration
    burn injury, 71
    Curling's, 71
    duodenal, 145–146
    gastric, 147
    lower extremity, 48
    malperforans, 124
    Marjolin's, 71
    pressure sores, 72–73
    venous, 131
Ulnar nerve, 127, 215
Ultrasonography, 201
    colorectal cancer, 186
    FAST scan, 49
Ultraviolet radiation, 73
Umbilical hernia, 199, 227
Unasyn, 17
Undescended testicles, pediatric, 228
Univentricular heart, 113
Urachus, 205

Uremia, 6
Ureteral trauma, 60, 204
Urethral trauma, 60
Urge incontinence, 205
Uric acid stones, 202
Urinary incontinence, 205
Urinary tract infection, 1
Urobilin, 159
Urobilinogen, 153
Urokinase, 8
Urology, 202–205
    benign prostatic hypertrophy, 204
    bladder disorders, 204
    diseases, 205
    incontinence, 205
    kidney stones, 202
    prostate cancer, 203
    renal cell carcinoma, 203
    testicular cancer, 202–203
    testicular torsion, 204
Urticaria, transfusion-related, 9
Uterine bleeding, abnormal, 209
Uterus, rupture, traumatic, 61

Vaginal cancer, 207
Vagotomy, 144
    complications, 149–150
Vagus nerve (CN X), 77, 135
    injury in carotid endarterectomy, 118
Vancomycin, 18
    appropriate levels, 17
Varices, esophageal, 155
    hemorrhage, 145f
Varicocele, 205
Varicose veins, 131
Vascular disorders, 116–132
    abdominal aortic disease, 120–122
    aneurysms. *See* Aneurysms
    atherosclerosis, 116
    cerebrovascular disease, 117–118
    fibromuscular dysplasia, 129
    immune arteritis, 129
    mesenteric ischemia, 127–128
    peripheral vascular disease, 122–125
    renal vascular disease, 125
    thoracic aortic disease, 118–120
    trauma, 58–59
    upper extremity, 125–127
    venous disease, 129–131
Vascular injury, 58–59
    in orthopaedic injury, 59t
    response to, 4
Vascular rings, 113
Vasoactive intestinal peptide, 133
Vasopressin, 21, 64
Venous insufficiency, 131
Venous thrombosis, 7
    central line, 132
Venous ulcers, 131
Ventilation, assisted, 65
Ventricular septal defect, 112
Verner-Morrison syndrome, 171
Verrucae, 76
Vertebral artery, injury, 53
Villous adenoma, 185

VIPoma, 171
Virchow's nodes, 147
Virchow's triad, 131
Virus infection
    hepatitis, 154
    immunology, 11
Visceral sarcoma, 75
Vital signs, pediatric population, 61t
Vitamin D, 28
Vitamin deficiencies, 33t
Vocal cords, 77
Volkmann's contracture, 216
Volume overload, 26
Volume replacement, 26
Volvulus
    cecal, 189
    gastric, 144
    sigmoid volvulus, 189
Von Hippel–Lindau syndrome, 203
Von Willebrand's disease, 5–6
Vulvar cancer, 207
Waldeyer's fascia, 185
Warfarin, 8
    skin necrosis, 7
Warthin's tumor, 79
Warts, 76
Waterhouse-Friderichsen's syndrome, 82
Wernicke's area, 213
Whipple procedure, complications, 169

Whipple's triad, 170
Wilms tumor, 223, 224t
Wolff-Chaikoff effect, 88
Wound healing, 46–48
    abnormal, 48
    collagen in, 47
    epithelial integrity, 47
    essentials, 47
    impediments, 47
    matrix formation, 41f
    myofibroblasts in, 46
    phases, 46
    platelets in, 46
    tensile strength, 47
Wound infection, 13–14
    burn wounds, 70–71
Wound matrix, 41f

Xanthine oxidase, 67
Xanthoma, 76

Yersinia colitis, 193

Zenapax, 38
Zenker's diverticulum, 137
Zinc deficiency, 33t
Zollinger-Ellison syndrome, 146, 170
Zosyn, 18